Supine Percutaneous Nephrolithotomy and ECIRS

Cesare Marco Scoffone • András Hoznek
Cecilia Maria Cracco
Editors

Supine Percutaneous Nephrolithotomy and ECIRS

The New Way of Interpreting PNL

Springer

Editors
Cesare Marco Scoffone
Department of Urology
Cottolengo Hospital
Torino
Italy

Cecilia Maria Cracco
Department of Urology
Cottolengo Hospital
Torino
Italy

András Hoznek
Department of Urology
CHU Henri Mondor
Créteil Cedex
France

ISBN 978-2-8178-0547-4 ISBN 978-2-8178-0459-0 (eBook)
DOI 10.1007/978-2-8178-0459-0
Springer Heidelberg Dordrecht London New York

Printed on acid-free paper

Springer is part of Springer Science+Business Media (www.springer.com)

Preface

Supine percutaneous nephrolithotomy: a new way of interpreting PNL is the culmination of 10 years' intensive work in the field of renal stone surgery. Our strongest desire was to share our extensive experience with ECIRS (Endoscopic Combined Intra Renal Surgery) in the Galdakao-modified supine Valdivia position, a revolutionary approach to percutaneous stone surgery, which we undertook with passion and interest, trying to exploit its advantages and new aspects. In order to do this extensively, we involved renowned surgical urologists, anesthesiologists, radiologists, anatomists, and scrub nurses. Thanks to their essential contribution, the present book finally provides, for the first time as far as we know, a comprehensive and multidisciplinary overview of all the issues relative to percutaneous surgery performed in the emerging supine and supine-modified positions.

The crucial concepts in ECIRS and its synergy and versatility in order to provide the best possible treatment for individual patients affected by large and/or complex urolithiasis are reflected throughout the book. Both synergy and versatility are needed in the preoperative holistic evaluation of the patient. A tailored surgical therapy can be proposed and discussed only after a thorough study of the stone features, the anatomy of the collecting system, and the patient's history, characteristics, and comorbidities. Intraoperatively, synergy is needed both among staff (urologists, anesthesiologists, nurses, radiology technicians) and technical equipment (lithotripsy energies, instruments for antegrade and retrograde access, accessories, imaging assistance); further, all the actors should be as versatile as possible, adapting the procedure to the needs of the patient. Postoperatively, thorough prevention of complications, mainly infectious, and follow-up represent another form of multi-disciplinary synergy.

All the chapters have extensive photographs taken in the operating room, drawings, radiograms, and summarizing tables, with the specific aim to be maximally didactic and to share all our experience in the field, including practical tips and tricks. We hope that this book will be a valuable resource in the field of stone surgery for those currently in training as well as for those already expert in prone percutaneous surgery. It takes into account new ways of performing this technical approach, which has been undergoing continuous improvement since the 1970s and is still riding high.

Our whole-hearted gratitude goes first of all to Professor Roberto Mario Scarpa, who has been the enlightened Chief of the Orbassano University Hospital, allowing us to discover and appreciate this surgical approach and to develop all the subsequent pertinent work. In Créteil, the merit goes to Professor Abbou, one of the pioneers of PNL in France in the early 1980s, who from an early stage acted as a visionary regarding the future role of ECIRS. He prompted his team to follow the Spanish and Italian example and encouraged us to popularize supine PNL in France.

We are also particularly grateful to Dr. Valdivia and Dr. Ibarluzea, the "fathers" of the Galdakao-modified supine Valdivia position, who generously shared their experience with us and supported us in the development of the combined percutaneous approach. Finally, thanks to all the urologists, anesthesiologists, and nurses in the Departments of Urology at the San Luigi Hospital, Orbassano, the Cottolengo Hospital, Torino, and the Henri Mondor Hospital, Créteil, for their valuable cooperation and fundamental support in the development of all the different stages of ECIRS.

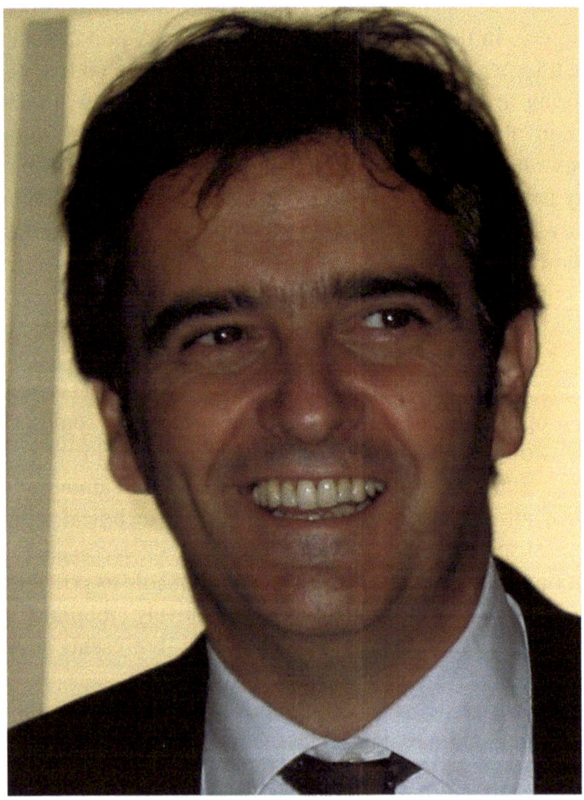

Torino, Italy Cesare Marco Scoffone

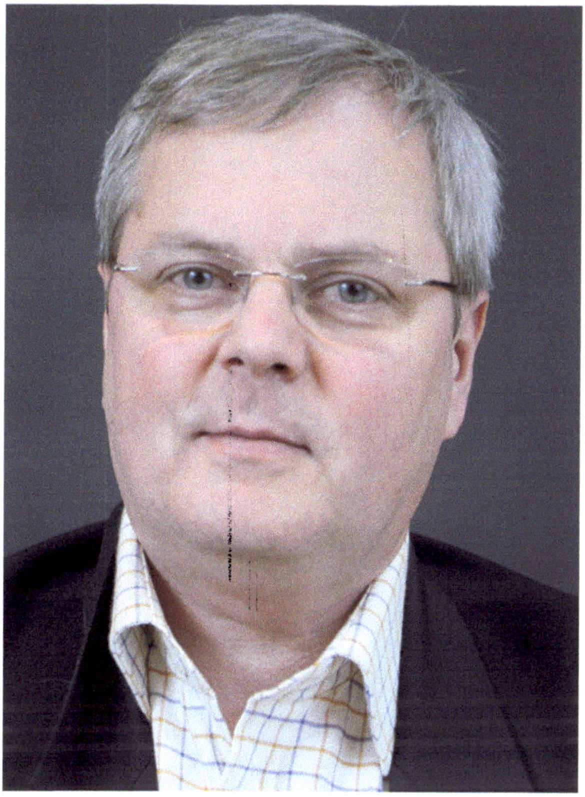

Créteil Cedex, France András Hoznek

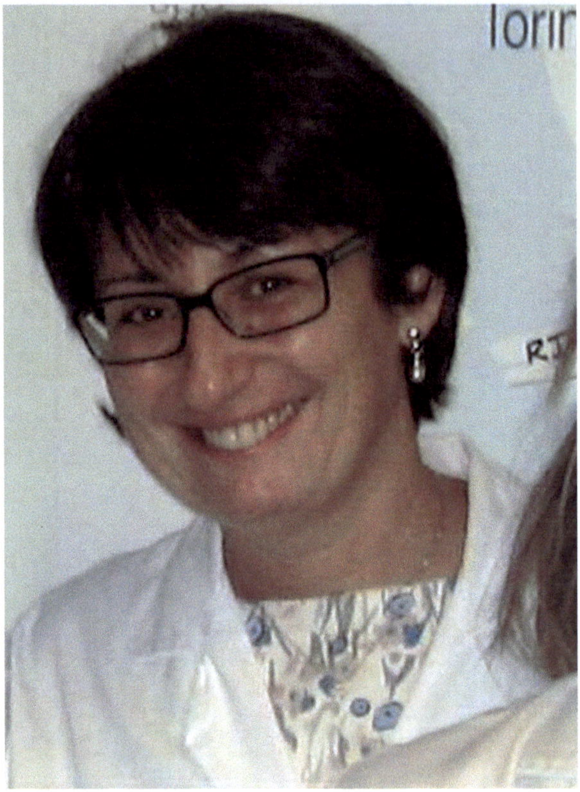

Torino, Italy

Cecilia Maria Cracco

Contents

1 **Introduction** 1
José Gabriel Valdivia Uría

2 **The Early History of Percutaneous Nephrolithotomy (PNL)** 5
Peter Alken

3 **The Evolution from Prone to Supine PNL and from Supine PNL to ECIRS: The Basque History of Endourology** 15
J. Gaspar Ibarluzea, Mikel G. Gamarra, Asier Leibar, and José G. Pereira

4 **PNL: Indications and Guidelines: Urolithiasis** 25
Arvind P. Ganpule and Mahesh R. Desai

5 **PNL: Indications and Guidelines: Stenosis and Tumours** 33
Marianne Brehmer

6 **Anatomy for PNL** 41
Cecilia Maria Cracco and Alessandro Eugenio Vercelli

7 **Imaging in Percutaneous Nephrolithotomy** 57
Susanne Sloth Osther and Palle Jørn Sloth Osther

8 **Anaesthesia for Supine and Modified Supine PNL** 79
Adebanji A.B. Adeyoju and Neil Sutcliffe

9 **Prone PNL: Is It Still the Gold Standard? Review and Results** 89
Thomas Knoll

10 **Endoscopic Combined IntraRenal Surgery (ECIRS): Rationale** 99
Cesare Marco Scoffone, Cecilia Maria Cracco, and Roberto Mario Scarpa

11 **ECIRS: Patient Positioning and Organization of the Operating Room** ... 109
András Hoznek, Francisco Pedro Juan Daels, Michael N'Tege Kimuli, Cecilia Maria Cracco, and Cesare Marco Scoffone

12 **Instruments and Accessories for ECIRS** ... 127
Cesare Marco Scoffone, András Hoznek, and Julie Rode

13 **ECIRS: Access Creation** ... 161
Cesare Marco Scoffone, András Hoznek, and Cecilia Maria Cracco

14 **Stone Fragmentation and Extraction** ... 189
András Hoznek, Michael N'Tege Kimuli, and Cesare Marco Scoffone

15 **Kidney Drainage and Percutaneous Tract Closure** ... 199
Cesare Marco Scoffone, András Hoznek, and Cecilia Maria Cracco

16 **Supine and Supine Modified PNL in Special Situations** ... 209
Cecilia Maria Cracco, Cesare Marco Scoffone, Arvind P. Ganpule, Amit Doshi, and Mahesh R. Desai

17 **PNL in Paediatric Patients** ... 223
Antonio Frattini, Cesare Marco Scoffone, and Stefania Ferretti

18 **Technical Aspects of Percutaneous Management of Ureteral Stenosis and Upper Urinary Tract Transitional Cell Carcinomas (UUT-TCC)** ... 233
Marianne Brehmer

19 **The Scrub Nurse's Point of View on ECIRS (Endoscopic Combined IntraRenal Surgery)** ... 249
Cristian Demelas, Gianni De Masi, Debora Crepaldi, Elena Bertinaria, Michele Trimboli, Angela Palamuso, Tiziana Girodo, and Debora Coda Zabetta

20 **Intraoperative Complications: How to Avoid Them?** ... 265
Francisco Pedro Juan Daels and Mariano Sebastian Gonzalez

21 **Antibiotic Prophylaxis and Infectious Complications in PNL** ... 279
Oscar R. Negrete-Pulido and Jorge Gutiérrez-Aceves

22 **Prone Versus Supine PNL: Results and Published Series** ... 293
András Hoznek, Julie Rode, Cecilia Maria Cracco, and Cesare Marco Scoffone

23 **Micro-ECIRS: A Revolutionary New Tool in the Current Endourologic Armamentarium** ... 303
Cesare Marco Scoffone and Cecilia Maria Cracco

24 **Conclusions and Future Perspectives of PNL** ... 311
András Hoznek, Cecilia Maria Cracco, and Cesare Marco Scoffone

Contributors

Adebanji A.B. Adeyoju, MB, BS, FRCS (Urol) Consultant Urological Surgeon, Department of Urology, Stepping Hill NHS Foundation Trust, Stockport, UK

Peter Alken, MD Department of Urology, University Clinic Mannheim, Mannheim, Germany

Elena Bertinaria Cottolengo Hospital, Torino, Italy

Marianne Brehmer Department of Urology, Institution of Oncology and Pathology, Karolinska Institutet, Aarhus University Hospital, Denmark

Debora Coda Zabetta Cottolengo Hospital, Torino, Italy

Cecilia Maria Cracco, MD, PhD Department of Urology, Cottolengo Hospital, Torino, Italy

Debora Crepaldi Cottolengo Hospital, Torino, Italy

Francisco Pedro Juan Daels, MD Department of Urology, Instituto Universitario del Hospital Italiano de Buenos Aires, Buenos Aires, Argentina

Gianni De Masi Department of Urology, San Luigi Hospital, University of Torino, Orbassano, Torino, Italy

Cristian Demelas Department of Urology, San Luigi Hospital, University of Torino, Orbassano, Torino, Italy

Mahesh R. Desai Department of Urology, Muljibhai Patel Urological Hospital, Nadiad, Gujarat, India

Amit Doshi Department of Urology, Muljibhai Patel Urological Hospital, Nadiad, Gujarat, India

Stefania Ferretti, MD Department of Surgery, Urology Unit, University Hospital of Parma, Parma, Italy

Antonio Frattini, MD Department of Urology, Guastalla Hospital, Guastalla, RE, Italy

Mikel G. Gamarra, MD Department of Urology, Galdakao-Usansolo Hospital, Bizkaia, Basque Country, Spain

Uro-Oncology Section, Urologia Clínica Bilbao, IMQ Zorrotzaurre Clinic, Bilbao, Basque Country, Spain

Arvind P. Ganpule Department of Urology, Muljibhai Patel Urological Hospital, Nadiad, Gujarat, India

Tiziana Girodo Cottolengo Hospital, Torino, Italy

Mariano Sebastian Gonzalez, MD Department of Urology, Instituto Universitario del Hospital Italiano de Buenos Aires, Buenos Aires, Argentina

Jorge Gutiérrez-Aceves, MD Department of Urology, Wake Forest School of Medicine, Winston-Salem, NC, USA

András Hoznek, MD Department of Urology, CHU Henri Mondor, Créteil Cedex, France

J. Gaspar Ibarluzea, MD Endouroloy and ESWL Section, Urología Clínica Bilbao, IMQ Zorrotzaurre Clinic, Bilbao, Basque Country, Spain

Michael N'Tege Kimuli Pyrah Department of Urology, St James's University Hospital, Leeds, UK

Thomas Knoll Department of Urology, Klinikum Sindelfingen-Boeblingen, Sindelfingen, Germany

Asier Leibar, MD Urología Clínica Bilbao, IMQ Zorrotzaurre Clinic, Bilbao, Basque Country, Spain

Department of Urology, Galdakao-Usansolo Hospital, Bizkaia, Basque Country, Spain

Cossu Marco, MD Department of Urology, San Luigi Hospital, University of Torino, Orbassano Torino, Italy

Oscar R. Negrete-Pulido Department of Urology, Lithiasis and Endourology Clinic, Hospital Ángeles LEÓN, Hospital Regional de Alta Especialidad del Bajío, León, Guanajuato, Mexico

Palle Jørn Sloth Osther, MD, PhD Department of Urology, Fredericia Hospital – A part of Hospital Littlebelt, University of Southern Denmark, Fredericia, Denmark

Susanne Sloth Osther, MD Department of Urology, Fredericia Hospital – A part of Hospital Littlebelt, University of Southern Denmark, Fredericia, Denmark

Angela Palamuso Cottolengo Hospital, Torino, Italy

José G. Pereira, MD Robotic Surgery Section, Urología Clínica Bilbao, IMQ Zorrotzaurre Clinic, Bilbao, Basque Country, Spain

Department of Urology, Galdakao-Usansolo Hospital, Bizkaia, Basque Country, Spain

Massimiliano Poggio, MD Department of Urology, San Luigi Hospital, University of Torino, Orbassano, Torino, Italy

Julie Rode Department of Urology, CHU Henri Mondor, Créteil Cedex, France

Roberto Mario Scarpa Department of Urology, San Luigi Hospital, University of Torino, Orbassano, Torino, Italy

Cesare Marco Scoffone, MD Department of Urology, Cottolengo Hospital, Torino, Italy

Neil Sutcliffe, BSc, MBChB, FRCA, FFICM Consultant Urological Surgeon, Department of Urology, Stepping Hill NHS Foundation Trust, Stockport, UK

Michele Trimboli Cottolengo Hospital, Torino, Italy

José Gabriel Valdivia Uría Jefe de Servicio de Urología del Hospital Clínico Universitario "Lozano Blesa" Zaragoza, Cuarte de Huerva, Zaragoza, Spain

Alessandro Eugenio Vercelli, MD, PhD Neuroscience Institute of the Cavalieri Ottolenghi Foundation, Orbassano, Torino, Italy

Department of Neuroscience, University of Torino, Torino, Italy

Chapter 1
Introduction

José Gabriel Valdivia Uría

Abstract In this introduction J.G. Valdivia Uría, the father of the supine position for percutaneous surgery, briefly describes the history of patient positioning for percutaneous renal access, the initial cooperation between urologists and radiologists, and the subsequent birth of percutaneous nephrolithotomy in all its steps, thoroughly developed by various urologists during the years. He underlines the advantages of the supine position and presents the contents of the present book, highlighting its exhaustive approach to all related issues and its practical value.

The percutaneous access to the kidney began to develop in 1954, when radiologists first dared to puncture a hydronephrotic renal pelvis in order to obtain antegrade pyelographies [1, 2].

After these initial experiences, radiologists and urologists began to perform techniques of increasing complexity such as percutaneous nephrostomy [3], extraction of kidney stones through mature tracts of previous percutaneous nephrostomies [4], and finally percutaneous nephrolithotomy (PNL), a technique that afterwards in the urologists' hands got better and better over the years [5–8].

After defining a good technique to puncture the kidney, subsequent improvements were essentially directed at simplifying the procedure of nephrostomy tract dilatation and designing efficient instruments such as nephroscopes, stone extractors, and lithotripsy devices.

At this point it is worth remembering that initially the radiologists aimed at the direct puncture of the renal pelvis without passing through the renal parenchyma, and for that reason they placed the patient in prone position. Although it did not take long to prove the advantages and safety of puncturing the kidney via the calyceal

J.G. Valdivia Uría
Jefe de Servicio de Urología del Hospital Clínico Universitario "Lozano Blesa" Zaragoza, Urbanización Santa Fe, calle 4, n 13, 50410 Cuarte de Huerva, Zaragoza, Spain
e-mail: valdivia@unizar.es

C.M. Scoffone et al. (eds.), *Supine Percutaneous Nephrolithotomy and ECIRS*,
DOI 10.1007/978-2-8178-0459-0_1, © Springer-Verlag France 2014

papilla, all the same it was not considered necessary to modify the patient's position.

The pioneering urologists in these percutaneous techniques described several anatomic references in the lumbar area (points, lines, and angles) in the attempt to simplify the procedure of the renal puncture and make it accessible to all urologists. The radiological C arm was from the very beginning a necessary prerequisite, thanks to its ability to show the path of the puncture needle from different angles.

Some urologists, facing the complexity of this step, refused to perform the initial percutaneous approach themselves, leaving it instead to the radiologists, so that they were used to performing only the endoscopic part of the PNL.

Another fact that dissuaded many urologists from starting with these percutaneous techniques was the laborious way of changing the position of the patient from the initial lithotomic position to the prone decubitus for the main surgery, considering that the patient already had an endotracheal tube, a ureteral catheter, a bladder catheter, and an intravenous access. During the years the anesthetists often reported that prone position was not always well tolerated by all patients and not exempted from possible iatrogenic risks.

The truth is that thousands of percutaneous kidney approaches with patients in the prone position have been performed worldwide, and it is a matter of fact that this procedure is perfectly standardized and made as steady as possible.

Nevertheless, very few urologists would disagree with the fact that percutaneous renal surgery with the patient in the supine position is a well-known and relevant step in the development of the endourological surgery. With the supine technique, there are reduced iatrogenic risks, morbidity, and surgical time. It made the calyceal puncture and the stone fragments extraction easier, and in particular it opened new endourological frontiers allowing the combination of various approaches to the kidney, namely, transurethral, percutaneous, and laparoscopic [9–12].

The idea of the editors of focusing the content of this book on the percutaneous kidney approach with the patient in the supine position is superb, and the publication of this work will be a milestone in the evolution of endourological surgery.

Until now many urologists justified their skepticism in performing PNL in supine position saying that efficacy and safety of this procedure were still to be demonstrated. Many publications tried to compare prone and supine PNL, without fully considering the solid experience of the endourological groups that perform PNL in supine position, nor comparing an equal number of procedures of either technique. I am sure that reading of this book will remove all doubts and will help to encourage those who are still doubtful about supine PNL.

In this book, the reader will find detailed information about the history of PNL and also reviews and results about prone PNL. He will have access to a complete list of indications and guidelines to PNL, as well as to valuable anatomical and radiological details concerning this technique. Additionally, there are also useful practical considerations from the anesthetic point of view, directly related to PNL surgery.

The main body of this work is dedicated to the supine PNL technique, and in their chapters the editors, together with other endourologists with a large and recognized background of experience, make an exhaustive analysis of each one of the practical details that contribute to give brilliance to this technique.

In order to complete the contents of this book, they added consistent practical information on PNL in special situations (including PNL in pediatric patients), Endoscopic Combined IntraRenal Surgery (ECIRS), other indications than urolithiasis for the percutaneous renal surgery (ureteral stenosis, upper urinary tract transitional cell carcinoma), and description and management of the related complications. Finally, the authors make a critical analysis of the results of PNL based on published series and give their own conclusions.

Summarizing, the book that you have in your hands, entitled "Supine Percutaneous Nephrolithotomy and ECIRS: The New Way of Interpreting PNL," is a work of great practical value, not only for those who want to start practicing this technique but also for those that already perform it comfortably.

It is for me a great honor that the editors asked me to write the introduction to this magnificent work, which without doubt will be from now an important landmark for percutaneous renal surgery.

References

1. Ween HS, Florence TJ (1954) The diagnosis of hydronephrosis by percutaneous renal punctures. J Urol 72:589–595
2. Wickbom I (1954) Antegrade pyelography. Acta Radiol 41:505–512
3. Goodwin WE, Casey WC, Woolf W (1955) Percutaneous trocar (needle) nephrostomy in hydronephrosis. JAMA 157:891–894
4. Ferstrom I, Johansson B (1976) Percutaneous pyelolithotomy. A new extraction technique. Scand J Urol Nephrol 10:257–259
5. Karamchetti A, O'Donell WG (1977) Percutaneous nephrolithotomy. An innovative extraction technique. J Urol 118:671–672
6. Smith AD, Reinke DB, Miller RP, Lange PH (1979) Percutaneous nephrostomy in the management of ureteral and renal calculi. Radiology 133:49–54
7. Alken P, Hutschenreiter G, Gunther R, Marberger M (1981) Percutaneous stone manipulation. J Urol 125:463–466
8. Wickham JEA, Kellet MJ (1981) Percutaneous nephrolithotomy. Br Med J 283:1571–1572
9. Valdivia Uría JG, Lanchares E, Villarroya S et al (1987) Nefrolitectomía percutánea: técnica simplificada. (nota previa). Arch Esp Urol 40:177–180
10. Valdivia Uría JG, Valle J, Villarroya S et al (1990) Why is percutaneous nephroscopy still performed with the patient prone? J Endourol 4:269–272
11. Valdivia Uría JG, Valle Gerhold JA, López López JA et al (1998) Technique and complications of percutaneous nephroscopy: experience with 557 patients in the supine position. J Urol 160:1975–1978
12. Valdivia Uría JG (2009) Complete supine percutaneous nephrolithotripsy comparison with the prone standard technique: the time for change from prone to supine position has come! UIJ 2(2). doi:10.3834/uij.1944-5784.2009.04.09

Chapter 2
The Early History of Percutaneous Nephrolithotomy (PNL)

Peter Alken

Abstract The present chapter provides a detailed look into the early history of percutaneous nephrolithotomy (PNL), showing that many have contributed to the development of this procedure including the author, who has taken active part in it. PNL has become an integral part of urology since more than 30 years, quickly expanding during the 1980s, but was not widely accepted until the 1970s. Many other urologists have contributed to this technique, reinventing it many times, and of course, the beneficial effects of the introduction of new instruments, accessories, technologies, and devices are evident.

A look into the early history of percutaneous nephrolithotomy (PNL) shows that many have contributed to the development of this procedure, which has become an integral part of urology since more than 30 years.

2.1 The Beginning

2.1.1 Percutaneous Nephrostomy

Percutaneous nephrostomy was not widely accepted until the 1970s [1]. There are many hints on early percutaneous procedures in the old urological literature of different countries. Simple puncture of the kidney from the flank was performed, e.g., by Hillier in 1865 [2], and described as a frequently performed procedure for instance by Küster [3]. J. Israel and W. Israel mentioned percutaneous nephrostomy

P. Alken, MD
Department of Urology, University Clinic Mannheim, Theodor Kutzer Ufer 1-3, D-68167 Mannheim, Germany
e-mail: peter.alken@umm.de

C.M. Scoffone et al. (eds.), *Supine Percutaneous Nephrolithotomy and ECIRS*,
DOI 10.1007/978-2-8178-0459-0_2, © Springer-Verlag France 2014

drainage in 1925 in their German textbook "Chirurgie der Niere und des Harnleiters." They used the technique of trocar puncture of hydronephrotic kidneys from the flank and introduction of a tube for drainage in the second half of the nineteenth century [4]. They quote Schede to have performed this procedure around 1880 [5].

The technique of percutaneous nephrostomy was described again 150 years later by the American urologist Goodwin in 1955 [6], although remaining relatively disregarded and in the hands of the radiologists. Percutaneous nephrostomy under ultrasound control was performed in 1974 by Pedersen [7]. In the author's experience, the introduction of ultrasound into clinical routine in the early 1980s had an important impact on percutaneous procedures in Europe. In many countries where urologists had direct access to ultrasound, they took the puncture away from the radiologists' hands, and the whole procedure was then performed by the urologist alone. Since 1980 the author established all his percutaneous accesses under combined ultrasound and fluoroscopic control himself and has taught his coworkers accordingly [8]. Especially in North America, urologists have only very limited experience in establishing an autonomous percutaneous access [9, 10] and sometimes invent complicated or not well-accepted endourological techniques to bypass the problem that radiologist governs this step of PNL [11–13].

2.1.2 Percutaneous Stone Removal

The credit for the first stone extraction through a previously established nephrostomy tract is given to Rupel and Brown in 1941 [14], but Chester Allen described this procedure already in 1935 [15], and the early literature in various countries will probably show further descriptions of this procedure.

An operatively established access was used to remove larger stones by disintegration with an electrohydraulic lithotrite in 1970 by Sachse [16], and the same results were achieved with an ultrasound lithotrite that was originally designed for the disintegration of bladder stones by Rathert in Aachen, Germany [17], and by Kurth in Mainz, Germany [18].

An essential publication by Fernström (radiologist) and Johansson (urologist) reported on three successful cases of primary percutaneous nephrostomy, subsequent tract dilatation for several days, and stone extraction under fluoroscopic control [19]. Their first case was done in 1974, and they concluded that the technique was suitable for stones up to 15 mm in diameter. But they did not realize the full potential of percutaneous stone removal: in a later publication in 1982 [20] with 33 patients treated in that manner they still stated: "*… the canal is ready for instrumentation after 8 days and the stone is removed after 10–12 days. The patient can be discharged 17 days after the performance of the percutaneous nephrostomy.*" and "*Calculi greater than 20 mm are not suitable for percutaneous nephrolithotomy because of the excessive degree of dilatation which would be required.*" At that time one session stone removal with ultrasound or electrohydraulic disintegration had already become routine for several urologists. Nowadays it is especially the stone above 20 mm in diameter which is regarded as the standard indication for percutaneous nephrolithotomy. This was only possible by putting all the pieces of the puzzle together in the right way (Fig. 2.1).

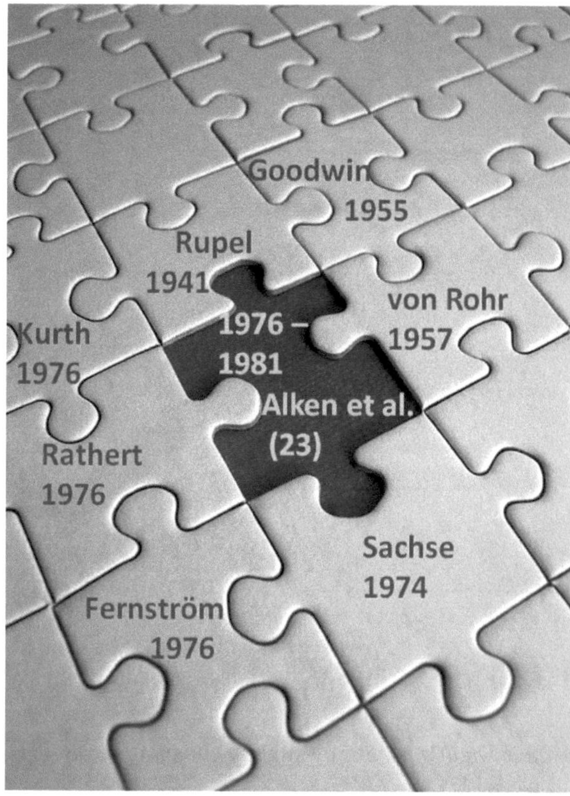

Fig. 2.1 The puzzle of PNL history [6, 14, 16, 17, 18, 19, 23, 42]

Between 1976 and 1979 the author, the radiologist Rolf Günther and the urologist Gerd Hutschenreiter contributed to the further development of the PNL technique. Initially the radiologist did the puncture, but when ultrasound became available, the whole procedure became urologic. Our first report of a case treated by percutaneous ultrasound lithotripsy [21] was followed by presentations with increasing patient numbers and refinement of the technique at the 1979 annual meeting of the European Intrarenal Surgery Society in Bern and the meeting of the German Urological Society in the same year [22]. Our 1980 presentation at the 75th American Urological Association (AUA) annual meeting in San Francisco was the basis for the manuscript on PNL that was submitted to the Journal of Urology at that AUA meeting. It was accepted with minor modifications. Dr. Scott, who was at that time the editor of the Journal, disliked some concluding remarks in the last three paragraphs of the discussion: "*With a set of instruments currently being developed, we expect to reduce the time for the whole procedure to two ambulant sessions for dilation and a one-week hospital stay for stone removal... Percutaneous stone manipulation as a deliberate alternative to open surgery has to compete with the techniques for operative stone removal established over the past 100 years. Its specific place among the various techniques of stone therapy will be defined on the basis of further experience.*" We respected his comment "*The Journal of Urology is not a*

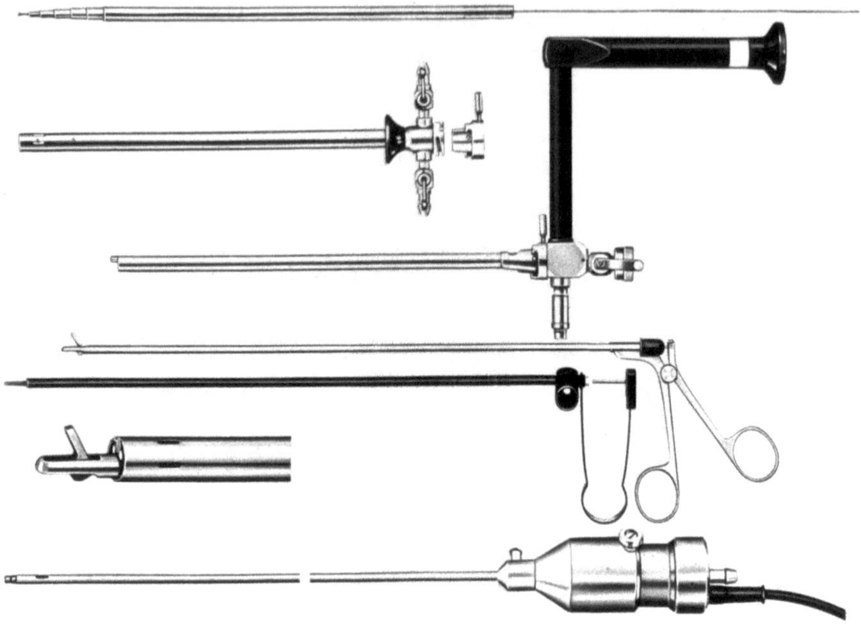

Fig. 2.2 The PNL instruments

medicine man's paper" by slightly changing these statements, but without changing our ideas [23].

At the time of the presentation at the AUA meeting in May 1980, the telescope dilators designed by the author and produced by Karl Storz were already in use [24]. These dilators were the first instruments purposely built for percutaneous stone removal. They were developed as a consequence of the problems met with serial plastic or metallic dilators initially used and developed as part of a set of instruments (Fig. 2.2) to establish a large, straight nephrostomy tract with minimal bleeding in one session and to allow a complete one session procedure. Percutaneous stone removal in one session is of course desirable for the patient, but it was not easy to achieve. Clayman et al. in their report on 100 cases in 1984 succeeded in only 31 % of their patients [25]. In the authors' initial series published in 1983, the one-session stone-free rate was also only 60 % [26].

Fragmentation of large stones was obtained with an electrohydraulic system [25] or preferably with an ultrasound lithotrite, as the latter caused no harm to tissue [27].

2.1.3 *Prone or Supine?*

The prone position was the classic position described for percutaneous nephrostomy. For many years the author did not use cystoscopy with retrograde ureteral catheterization before the nephrostomy puncture [24]. Thus it was not necessary to turn the patient from the supine-cystoscopy-position to the prone-nephrostomy-position. Bolsters underneath the abdomen were not used because we felt that they pushed the kidney cephalad instead of exposing it. Thus breathing of the patient was unimpeded, and the anesthetists had no problems with control of the patient as they used epidural anesthesia and could communicate with the patient during the whole procedure.

Experience with a supine percutaneous access was gained with patients that required emergency drainage of a kidney that got obstructed after open surgery. It was easy to do but did not change our PNL procedure.

2.2 The Progress

Many others have contributed to the development of percutaneous nephrolithotomy: Clayman and coworkers were the first to describe the use of angioplasty balloon dilatation catheters for tract dilatation as another alternative to the sequential dilatation with plastic dilators in 1983 [28]. This group published an experience with 100 cases in 1984 [25].

The term endourology was coined by Smith et al. in 1979 [29] when they described the possible future application of percutaneous nephrostomy. Nowadays stone therapy is only a minor aspect of this continuously developing field.

The use of PNL quickly expanded. After personal experience with PNL since 1980, Marberger and collaborators designed a purposely built nephroscope and ultrasound lithotrite for percutaneous use together with the Richard Wolf GmbH, Knittlingen, Germany [30], and Korth with Olympus Winter und Ibe, Hamburg, Germany [31]. Clayman and Castaneda-Zuniga were the first to publish a book on almost every aspect of percutaneous renal surgery [32]. Wickham, who had learned about the technique of PNL during his visits to the Department of Urology at the University of Mainz and the author's presentation at the meeting of the European Intrarenal Surgery Society in Bern in 1979, was probably the first person to reintroduce a pelvic stone into the kidney to demonstrate the ease of the procedure to the patient and the first to try not to insert a nephrostomy after a percutaneous procedure, as no bleeding from the tract was observed (Wickham, personal communication). But he was also the one who realized the potential of PNL and organized the first world meeting on this topic [33]. One-session PNL was initiated by the design of telescopic dilators [24] which are still very popular after 30 years [34]. Also the Amplatz dilators and sheath became widespread access instruments [35]. Segura and coworkers were the first to publish a series of 1,000 procedures [36]. Many other urologists have contributed to this technique and they, like Clayman and collaborators in 1984 [25], reported in the early 1980s that PNL had replaced 90 % or more of their surgical procedures for renal stone removal. But at that time, minimally invasive PNL was being continuously replaced by a noninvasive technique, namely, extracorporeal shock wave lithotripsy (ESWL) [37, 38]. The worldwide

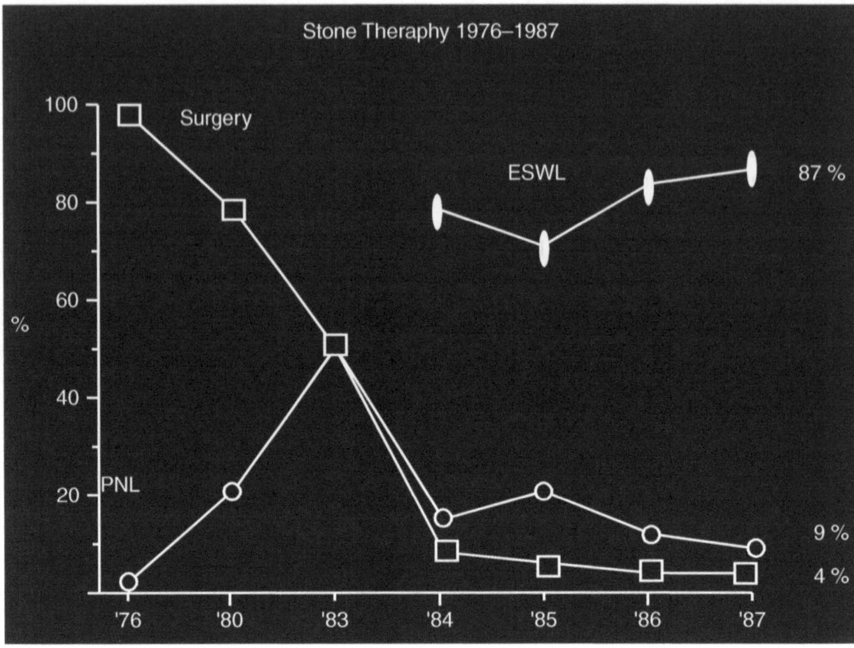

Fig. 2.3 Frequency of stone therapy from 1976 to 1987 in the Department of Urology, University Clinic, Mainz, Germany

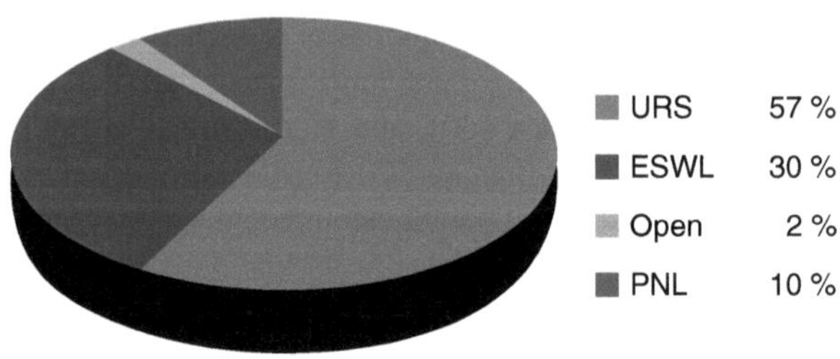

Fig. 2.4 Frequency of stone therapy from 2007 to 2008 in the Department of Urology, University Clinic, Mannheim, Germany

fourth extracorporeal lithotripter was installed in 1983 at the Department of Urology at Mainz University Clinic in Germany, where the author worked until 1987. ESWL immediately reduced the frequency of PNL to approximately 10 % (Fig. 2.3), because all the small stones that could have been removed by percutaneous extraction were now shocked. Today PNL ranges in this 10 % level in most of the affluent countries, as data from the authors department in Mannheim show (Fig. 2.4). The situation is different in countries where there are still a lot of big stones as in India, as shown by the statistics from Muljibhai Patel Urological Hospital, India (Fig. 2.5). With the enormously high PNL working load in his country and several thousands of cases having been treated in his department, Dr. Desai has somehow reinvented PNL [39, 40] and has of course already a positive experience with the supine position [41].

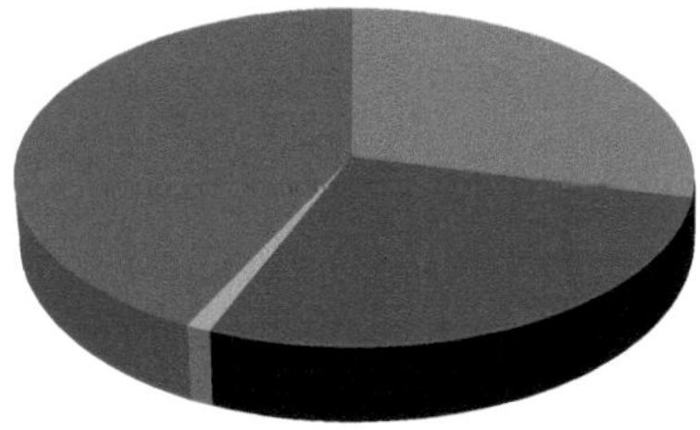

Fig. 2.5 Frequency of stone therapy from 2007 to 2008 in the Muljibhai Patel Urological Hospital, Nadiad Gujarat, India (courtesy of Dr. Mahesh Desai)

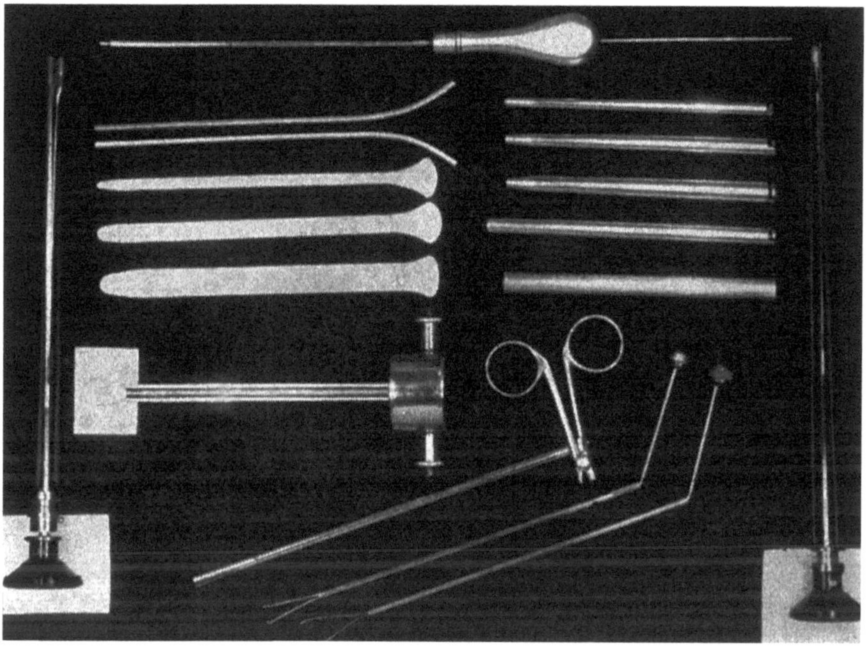

Fig. 2.6 Instruments designed for percutaneous pyeloscopy by H. von Rohr (Illustration 19. Preliminary pyeloscopic instruments. Above: Hemispherical polished puncture probe with a sort of withdrawn guiding stylet. Below on the left: Two half-sheathed guides. Below: Flat guides with increasing width to spread the half-sheathed guides. Below: Loop fixation to be inserted into the outer shaft with a tightening device, bearing the optic shaft or for the drilling shaft and space for a lamp-holder. On the right: Conical "third-pin" from I to III, below: cylindrical "third-pin" IV. Below: Outer tube with a lumen of 8 millimeters. Below: stone-crusher and grasping forceps. Left and right to the side: straight view telescope with a lamp holder and side view optics)

2.3 Conclusions

This brief look into the past of PNL might have missed some aspects, but like the future is difficult to predict, the past is difficult to "*re*-dict" In 1994 the author learned that the German urologist Heinrich von Rohr (1911–1978) had developed instruments (Fig. 2.6) for percutaneous endoscopic procedures and had designed an

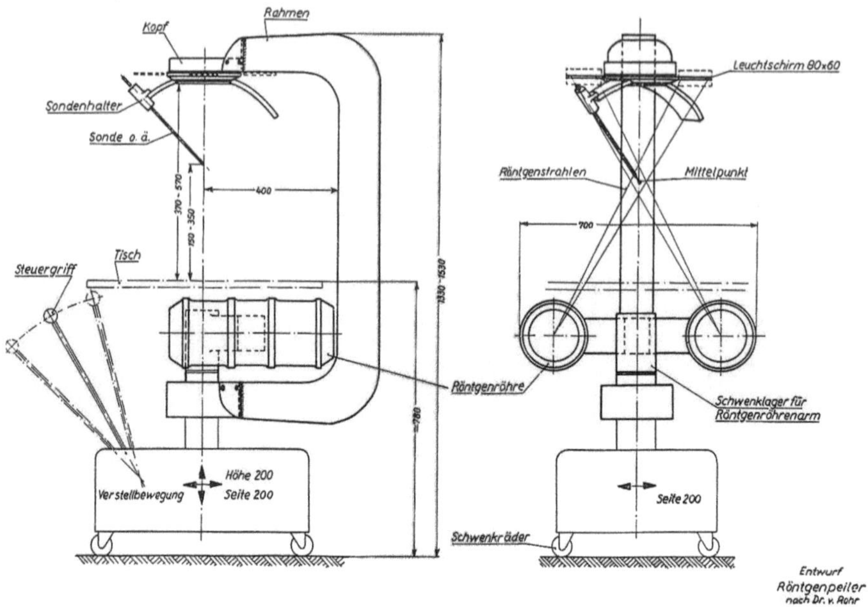

Fig. 2.7 X-ray localization and needle guide apparatus for percutaneous puncture of the renal collecting system designed by H. von Rohr (Illustration number 17, general construction drawing of the X-ray detector, Spring 1954, by Mr. Engineer Kretschmer of the German Federal Office for Material testing in Berlin-Dahlem)

X-ray apparatus (Fig. 2.7) to guide a puncture needle to the right place in the kidney. He had published studies on cadavers and animals in the East German Zeitschrift für Urologie und Nephrologie in 1958 [42]. At that time this periodical was probably only read in East Germany. We do not know why von Rohr never proceeded to clinical studies. But sometimes the right thoughts need the right time to become reality.

References

1. Günther RW, Alken P (1982) Percutaneous nephropyelostomy: applications, technique and critical evaluation. In: Wilkins RA, Viamonte M (eds) Interventional radiology. Blackwell, Oxford, pp 333–356
2. Bloom DA, Morgan JR, Scardino PL (1989) Thomas Hillier and percutaneous nephrostomy. Urology 33:346–350
3. Küster EGF (1896–1902) Die Chirurgie der Nieren. Verlag von Ferdinand Enke, Stuttgart
4. Israel J, Israel W (1925) Chirurgie der Niere und des Harnleiters. Thieme, Leipzig, p 222
5. Israel J, Israel W (1925) Chirurgie der Niere und des Harnleiters. Thieme, Leipzig, p 501
6. Goodwin WE, Casey WC, Woolf W (1955) Percutaneous trocar (needle) nephrostomy in hydronephrosis. J Am Med Assoc 157:891–894

7. Pedersen JF (1974) Percutaneous nephrostomy guided by ultrasound. J Urol 112:157–159
8. Osman M, Wendt-Nordahl G, Heger K et al (2005) Percutaneous nephrolithotomy with ultrasonography-guided renal access: experience from over 300 cases. BJU Int 96:875–878
9. Bird VG, Fallon B, Winfield HN (2003) Practice patterns in the treatment of large renal stones. J Endourol 17:355–363
10. Preston MA, Blew BD, Breau RH et al (2010) Survey of senior resident training in urologic laparoscopy, robotics and endourology surgery in Canada. Can Urol Assoc J 4:42–46
11. Hunter PT, Hawkins IF, Finlayson B et al (1983) Hawkins-Hunter retrograde transcutaneous nephrostomy: a new technique. Urology 22:583–587
12. Leal JJ (1988) Percutaneous removal of renal and ureteral stones with and without concomitant transurethral manipulation by a urologist using antegrade and retrograde techniques without a radiologist's assistance. J Urol 139:1184–1187
13. Khan F, Borin JF, Pearle MS et al (2006) Endoscopically guided percutaneous renal access: "seeing is believing". J Endourol 20:451–455
14. Rupel E, Brown R (1941) Nephroscopy with removal of stone following nephrostomy for obstructive calculus anuria. J Urol 46:177–182
15. Allen CD (1935) Notes on nephrostomy drainage. Urol Cut Rev 39:389–393
16. Sachse H (1970) Erfahrungen mit der Elektrolithotripsie. Verh Deutsche Ges Urologie 23:171–173, Springer, Berlin
17. Kurth KH, Hohenfellner R, Altwein J (1977) Ultrasound litholapaxy of a staghorn calculus. J Urol 117:242–243
18. Rathert P, Stumpf U, Pohlman R, Lutzeyer W (1976) Ultraschall-Lithotripsie von Ureter- und Nierensteinen: experimentelle und erst klinische Untersuchungen. Verh Deutsche Ges Urologie 28:365–367, Springer, Berlin
19. Fernström I, Johannson B (1976) Percutaneous pyelolithotomy: a new extraction technique. Scand J Urol Nephrol 10:257–259
20. Fernström I, Johansson B (1982) Percutaneous extraction of renal calculi. Front Eur Radiol 1:1–24
21. Alken P, Kurth KH, Günter R (1977) Die perkutane Instrumentation bei Nierensteinen. In: Gasser G, Vahlensieck W (eds) Fortschritte der Urologie und Nephrologie. Steinkopf Verlag, Darmstadt, pp 393–397
22. Alken P, Altwein J (1979) Die perkutane Nephrolitholapaxie. Verh Deutsche Ges Urol 31:109–112, Springer, Berlin
23. Alken P, Hutschenreiter G, Günter R, Marberger M (1981) Percutaneous stone manipulation. J Urol 125:463–466
24. Alken P (1985) The telescope dilators. World J Urol 3:7–10
25. Clayman RV, Surya V, Miller RP et al (1984) Percutaneous nephrolithotomy: extraction of renal and ureteral calculi from 100 patients. J Urol 131:868–871
26. Alken P, Günther R, Thüroff J (1983) Percutaneous nephrolithotomy – a routine procedure? Br J Urol Suppl:1–5 ISSN No: 0007–1331
27. Alken P (1982) Percutaneous ultrasonic destruction of renal calculi. Urol Clin North Am 9:145–151
28. Clayman RV, Castaneda-Zuniga WR, Hunter DW et al (1983) Rapid balloon dilatation of the nephrostomy tract for nephrostolithotomy. Radiology 147:884–885
29. Smith AD, Lange PH, Fraley EE (1979) Applications of percutaneous nephrostomy. New challenges and opportunities in endo-urology. J Urol 121(3):382
30. Marberger M, Stackl W, Hruby W (1982) Percutaneous litholapaxy of renal calculi with ultrasound. Eur Urol 8:236–242
31. Korth K (1983) A new percutaneous pyeloscope with permanent irrigation. Br J Urol Suppl: 31–33 ISSN No: 0007–1331
32. Clayman RV, Castaneda-Zuniga WR (1984) Techniques in endourology: a guide to the percutaneous removal of renal and ureteral calculi. Heritage, Dallas
33. Wickham JEA, Miller R (1983) Percutaneous renal surgery. Br J Urol Special Suppl ISSN: 0007–1331

34. Yamaguchi A, Skolarikos A, Buchholz NP et al (2011) Operating times and bleeding complications in percutaneous nephrolithotomy: a comparison of tract dilation methods in 5537 patients in the Clinical Research Office of the Endourological Society Percutaneous Nephrolithotomy Global Study. J Endourol 25:933–939
35. Rusnak B, Castaneda-Zuniga W, Kotula F et al (1982) An improved dilator system for percutaneous nephrostomies. Radiology 144:174
36. Segura W, Patterson OE, Le Roy AJ et al (1985) Percutaneous removal of kidney stones: review of 1000 cases. J Urol I134:1077–1081
37. Chaussy C, Eisenberger F, Wanner K et al (1976) The use of shock waves for the destruction of renal calculi without direct contact. Urol Res 4:175
38. Chaussy C, Brendel W, Schmiedt E (1980) Extracorporeally induced destruction of kidney stones by shock waves. Lancet 316:1265–1268
39. Desai M, Ganpule A, Manohar T (2008) "Multiperc" for complete staghorn calculus. J Endourol 22:1831–1833
40. Desai M, Jain P, Ganpule A et al (2009) Developments in technique and technology: the effect on the results of percutaneous nephrolithotomy for staghorn calculi. BJU Int 104:542–548
41. Manohar T, Jain P, Desai M (2007) Supine percutaneous nephrolithotomy: effective approach to high-risk and morbidly obese patients. J Endourol 21:44–49
42. von Rohr H (1958) Die (endoskopische) Pyeloskopie: Neues Verfahren der Nierenheckendiagnostik und Grundlage der vereinfachten Entfernung von Nierenbeckensteinen: Ein Arbeitsbericht. Z Urol Nephrol 12:697–712

Chapter 3
The Evolution from Prone to Supine PNL and from Supine PNL to ECIRS: The Basque History of Endourology

J. Gaspar Ibarluzea, Mikel G. Gamarra, Asier Leibar, and José G. Pereira

Beautiful ships usually sail well (marine saying)

Abstract The Basque history of PNL shows the fundamental role of the reciprocal interactions among urologists, thanks to books, publications, and congresses, in an era without internet or other nowadays obvious technological supports. G. Ibarluzea experienced also as sometimes practical problems or occasional events (like the limitations of a fixed radiologic table or the Steinstrasse complications of ESWL of large stones) can trigger new ideas like the introduction of the Galdakao-modified supine Valdivia position for percutaneous surgery, first born with the intent to simultaneously treat concomitant ureteral calculi.

J.G. Ibarluzea, MD (✉)
Endouroloy and ESWL Section, Urología Clínica Bilbao, IMQ Zorrotzaurre Clinic, Bilbao, Basque Country, Spain
e-mail: gibarluzea@urologiaclinica.biz

M.G. Gamarra, MD
Department of Urology, Galdakao-Usansolo Hospital, Bizkaia, Basque Country, Spain

Uro-Oncology Section, Urología Clínica Bilbao, IMQ Zorrotzaurre Clinic, Bilbao, Basque Country, Spain
e-mail: mgamarra@urologiaclinica.biz

A. Leibar, MD
Department of Urology, Galdakao-Usansolo Hospital, Bizkaia, Basque Country, Spain

Urología Clínica Bilbao, IMQ Zorrotzaurre Clinic, Bilbao, Basque Country, Spain
e-mail: aleibar@urologiaclinica.biz

J.G. Pereira, MD
Department of Urology, Galdakao-Usansolo Hospital, Bizkaia, Basque Country, Spain

Robotic Surgery Section, Urología Clínica Bilbao, IMQ Zorrotzaurre Clinic, Bilbao, Basque Country, Spain
e-mail: jpereira@urologiaclinica.biz

C.M. Scoffone et al. (eds.), *Supine Percutaneous Nephrolithotomy and ECIRS*,
DOI 10.1007/978-2-8178-0459-0_3, © Springer-Verlag France 2014

3.1 At the Beginning (During the 1980s)

Endourology was born in the early 1980s of the last century. Dr. Peter Alken [1] in percutaneous renal surgery and Dr. Enrique Perez Castro [2] in transurethral ureteroscopy were for our group the reference figures.

We started the practice of rigid ureteroscopy at the end of 1984, thanks to our close relationship with Dr. Perez Castro. By the middle of 1985, we started working with percutaneous renal surgery following Dr. Alken's method, and we learned from the very beginning to make the ultrasound-guided puncture as it seemed to us the simplest and safest way to reach the kidney cavities.

In those years there was nobody near to us from whom to learn, and three books, published before 1985, were our sources of inspiration:

- "Percutaneous Renal Surgery" by Wickham JE and Miller RA, 1983 [3];
- "Percutaneous Surgery of Renal Stones. Techniques and tactics" by Korth K, 1984 [4];
- "Techniques in Endourology: A guide to the percutaneous removal of renal and ureteral calculi" by Clayman RV and Castañeda-Zuñiga W, 1984 [5].

We especially considered Dr. Knut Korth book as the PNL Bible in those days. It was sometime before the advent of extracorporeal shock wave lithotripsy (ESWL), and therefore the cases with which to practice the technique were abundant. We were very lucky under this respect, because this situation allowed us to choose the best stones to improve our learning curve.

Late in 1989 a new period started with the opening of our lithotripsy section with a Dornier HM4 lithotriptor. All around us staghorn and complicated stones started arriving at our hospital. The ESWL was considered the panacea in the treatment of urolithiasis, and we soon found ourselves with a lot of impossible cases after many ESWL sessions and enormous Steinstrasse to solve. As we performed percutaneous renal surgery in the classical prone position, the percutaneous nephrolithotomy (PNL) and the transurethral ureteroscopy (URS) had to be carried out separately and with complicated changes in the patient's position.

To make things more complicated in our ESWL unit, we had designed an operating room exclusively for endourology, which was an exact copy of the one that Dr. Korth had in the Loretto-Krankenhaus of Freiburg, with a Philips radiological table specific for urology. This operating room gave us great agility for our urological practice in all procedures where X-rays were needed, but we soon started to find several problems for the percutaneous renal surgery. The radiological table only allowed access from one side. When the case involved a right kidney, after placing the ureteral catheter, we had to turn the patient over to put him in prone position, and this, although time consuming, was fairly simple. But when the kidney was the left one, things were much more complicated. We had to turn the patient around 180° and then turn him over, all this under general anesthesia with a catheter in place and in a relatively small operating room full of anesthesiological equipment and urologic instruments. The radiological table also had another problem, in that it could only accommodate anteroposterior X-ray projections, even though this didn't affect us very much as we always made the initial puncture with ultrasound.

In cases of large lithiasis erroneously treated with ESWL, it happened frequently that we performed a transurethral rigid ureteroscopy first, followed by the placement of a ureteral balloon catheter before changing completely position and surgical field to perform PNL.

The same happened when at the end of a PNL, we realized that there were stone fragments in the ureter and we could not clean them from upwards with our flexible instruments. We had to put the patient in the lithotomic position again to perform a transurethral URS.

This was the situation in which we were in the early 1990s. We were acquainted with the papers of Dr. Gabriel Valdivia Uría of the Hospital Clinico Universitario de Zaragoza [6] on the percutaneous renal surgery in supine position with an air bag under the flank, but given the prevailing view among the great popes of the endourology, we did not pay much attention to this issue.

3.2 Starting the Evolution (During the 1990s)

One day at the end of 1992, in a left kidney case, tired of so many complicated maneuvers, after placing the ureteral catheter, I exploited the idea of putting an air bag under the flank of the patient. Performing ultrasound I was surprised to see how accessible the kidney was, and so I performed my first PNL in the position described by Valdivia in 1987. Anesthesiologists, nurses, and all personnel involved in the operating room were overjoyed about having eliminated all the usual complicated maneuvers.

Unfortunately, when the case was a right kidney, the radiological table mentioned above compelled us to make the same complicated maneuvers if we wanted to use the supine position, and for this reason I decided to keep performing right PNL in prone position.

After 8 years of prone PNL, I continued to operate right kidneys in prone position and left kidneys in supine position, with an air bag under the ipsilateral flank. To say the truth, I did not find any difference between the two positions in the endoscopic procedure or in the ultrasound-guided puncture. Only my inclination to go below in the puncture when working in the supine position was due to the habit of working for so many years in the prone position. However, there was a problem due to the features of the radiological table. As I said, being only the anteroposterior projection possible, the kidney and the urinary tract were superimposed on the spine hampering the vision during dilatation of the percutaneous tract.

The PNL technique in supine followed the same steps as in prone. We first placed the ureteral catheter with the patient in the lithotomic position, and then we placed the patient supine with the air bag under the side, leaving the transurethral tract abandoned with the catheter perfusing a saline solution with contrast and some methylene blue, as we had always done with the prone position (Fig. 3.1).

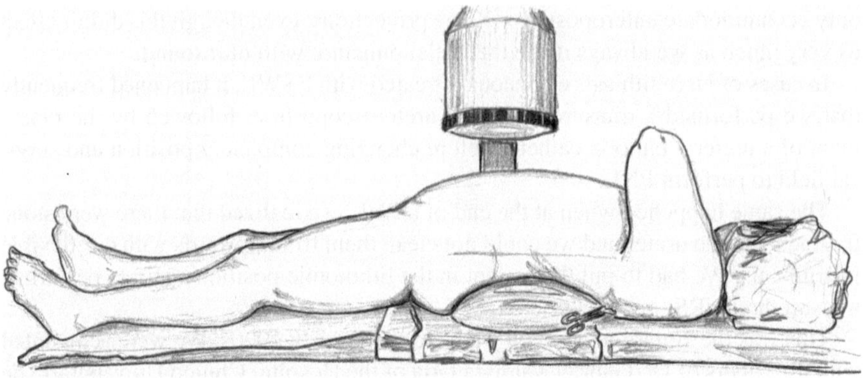

Fig. 3.1 We started the percutaneous renal surgery in supine position with the same protocol we have been using in prone position. Lithotomy position was used to catheterize the ureter, and then we changed the field placing the patient in the Valdivia position and leaving the transurethral way with the perfusion of contrast and dye through the catheter

3.3 Discovering the Endoscopic Combined IntraRenal Surgery (ECIRS)

A short time after starting to operate in the Valdivia position, we found ourselves, at the end of a PNL, with a large number of fragments dislodged in the distal ureter. This particular case was of a woman previously treated with ESWL for a stone of considerable size in the left kidney. After fighting a long time to remove the whole Steinstrasse, my assistant, Dr. Aurelio Jorge, asked for a rigid ureteroscope, dismantled the field, and improvised a transurethral access with the patient in supine position and the knees flexed (Fig. 3.2). We solved the case very quickly and numerous fragments pushed upwards were easily extracted through the Amplatz sheath.

This was, as far as I remember, the first “rendezvous,” opening the way to a new concept in endourology: the simultaneous transurethral and percutaneous access to the whole urinary tract.

3.4 In Search of the Best Position

Since then we began to place the patient in the lithotomic position, placing the ureteral catheter almost simultaneously to the percutaneous puncture. Perfusion through the catheter was no more necessary as the assistant could inject contrast when needed, and if we thought it convenient, we could also perform a transurethral URS.

Although, the classical lithotomic position was uncomfortable, and above all, depending on the type of leg support employed, it could produce pain to the lower limbs during the postoperative period, especially after long procedures. We gradually

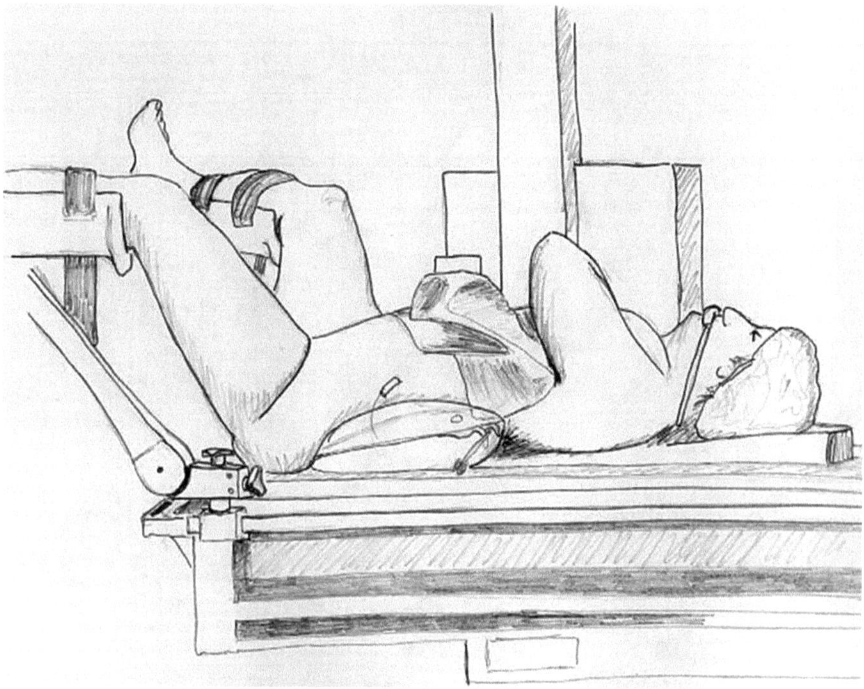

Fig. 3.2 The residual fragments and the Steinstrasse after an incorrect indication to ESWL forced us to perform transurethral URS and PNL. The lithotomic position was uncomfortable for performing both procedures simultaneously, and the stirrups could cause pain to the patient's legs

started changing the position of the ipsilateral leg, looking for more ergonomic leg holders until we found a position comfortable for both surgeon and patient (Fig. 3.3).

We always used a three-liter saline solution bag filled with air clamped with a Kocher forceps, allowing volume control until the best position was found (Fig. 3.4). The bag can be very full with the patient more sideways if we have to enter through a posterior calyx and can contain less air with the patient practically in supine position if we have a very accessible anterior calyx. We have tried to replace the irrigation bag by other devices, but by now we always came back to it.

We have discovered that it was very easy to treat the patient in this position, obtaining a through and through passage of the guidewire from the skin to the urethra which makes much easier to dilate the tract, especially with the Amplatz set, and provides a greater security during the whole procedure, with no fear of losing the tract.

3.5 ECIRS Comes of Age

In the late 1990s, after 10 years of intensive work, our Philips table (Fig. 3.5) broke down and for budgetary reasons, it was decided not to repair it. We did not mind as we discovered that the ideal place to work with our position was a large

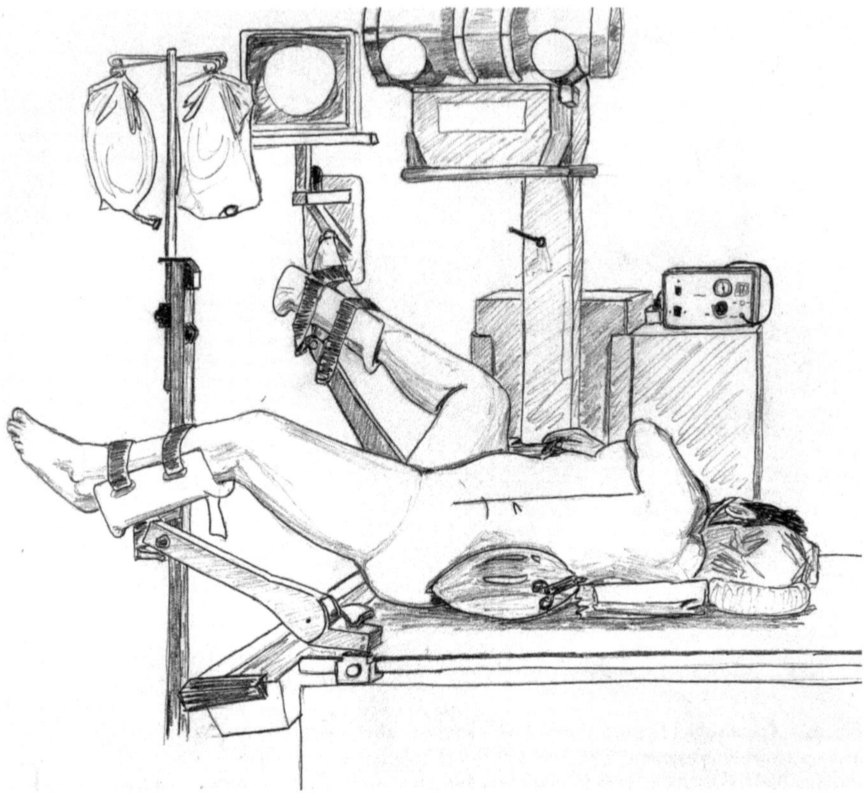

Fig. 3.3 Gradually we developed a more comfortable position for both patient and surgeon, finding more appropriate leg holders. The ipsilateral leg was extended with a small knee flexion, and the contralateral leg was well abducted

conventional operating room with a good radiolucent table and a good fluoroscopic C arm (Fig. 3.6).

Now, at the beginning of the new century, our position is totally consolidated and it is known as the Galdakao-modified supine Valdivia position [7].

I can't remember precisely the date, but from approximately 1988/1989, we never performed renal surgery in prone position anymore, having solved all our endourological problems in a satisfactory way with the supine position.

Two urologists from Orbassano (Torino), Dr. Roberto Mario Scarpa and Dr. Cesare Marco Scoffone [8], enthusiastic about the simultaneous endourological access, were the ones who created the acronym ECIRS (Endoscopic Combined IntraRenal Surgery), which has become the general term to define this technique ever since.

Fig. 3.5 Our early Philips table only allowed anteroposterior radiological projection, so there was conflict between the backbone and the kidney in the supine position with the air bag under the flank

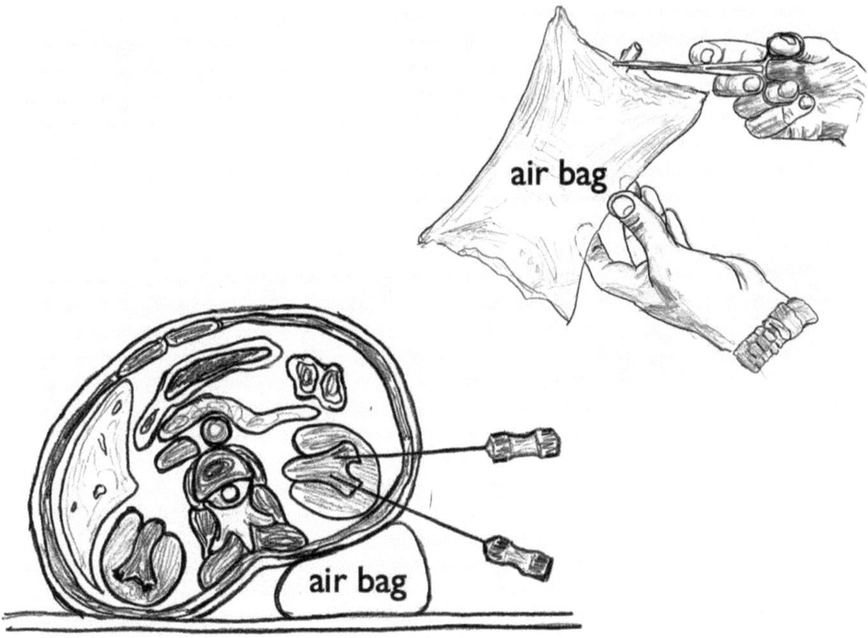

Fig. 3.4 A three-liter saline bag filled with air and clamped with a Kocher forceps permits volume control until the most comfortable position is found. Depending on the need to enter through an anterior or a posterior calyx, there will be more or less need of air

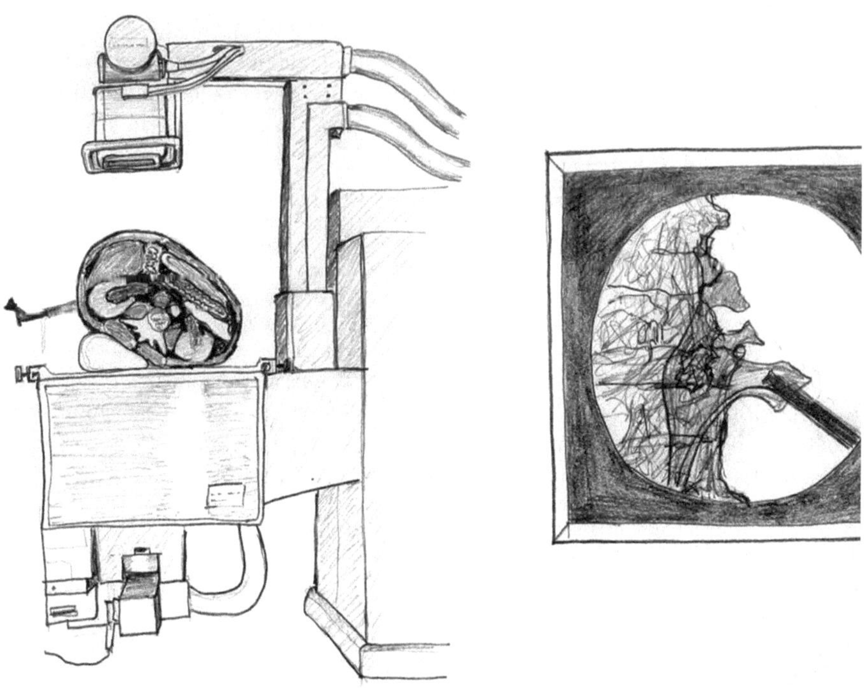

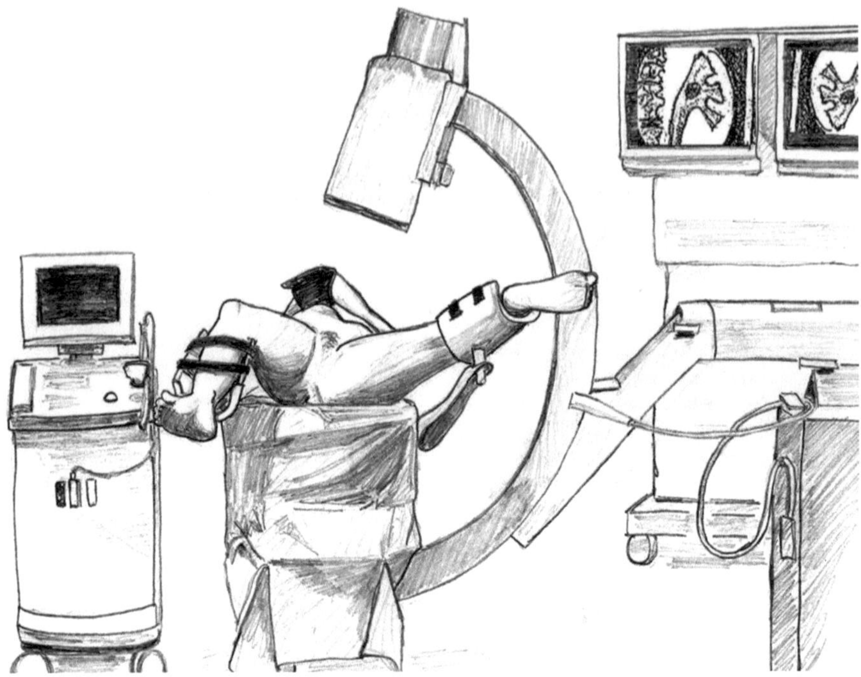

Fig. 3.6 Soon we learned that the best place for this technique was the standard operating room with a good C arm. With a small shift in the orbital axis, 10° or 20°, we got an interference-free X-ray image

In this type of surgery, all details are relevant, including suitable nephroscopes and ergonomically leg holders which do not protrude laterally too much. But what is critically important is the correct positioning of the patient. Don't start the procedure before you feel reasonably comfortable and have explored the possible access with ultrasound and X-ray (Fig. 3.7).

3.6 Conclusions

In different chapters of this book, the new generations of urologists who practice this technique will sort out all the details of it, so that the little tricks and small technical expedients learned from experience will be shared. Our target has been to make things in the easiest and simplest way, having always in mind and first of all the safety of our patients.

It is a beautiful technique, which, together with the current technological advances, will for sure sail well with future generations of endourologists.

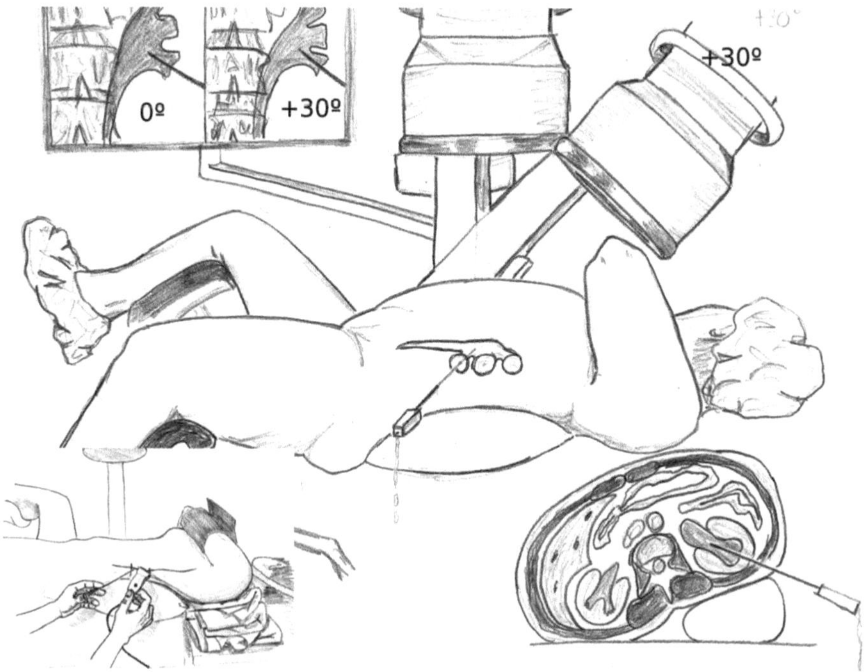

Fig. 3.7 The perfect puncture technique. Ultrasound exploration and puncture, complemented with the fluoroscopic trick, 30° sagittal projection with the C arm, simplify the access, increase feasibility, and minimize radiation exposure

References

1. Alken P, Hutschenreiter G, Günter R, Marberger M (1981) Percutaneous stone manipulation. J Urol 125:463–466
2. Perez Castro E, Martinez Pineiro JA et al (1980) La ureterorenoscopia transuretral. Un actual proceder urologico. Arch Esp Urol 33:445–460
3. Wickham JE (1983) Percutaneous renal surgery. Churchill Livingstone, London
4. Korth K (1984) Percutaneous surgery of renal stones. Techniques and tactics. Springer, Heidelberg
5. Clayman RV, Castaneda-Zuniga WR (1984) Techniques in endourology: a guide to the percutaneous removal of renal and ureteral calculi. Heritage, Dallas
6. Valdivia Uría JG, Valle J, Villarroya S et al (1990) Why is percutaneous nephroscopy still performed with the patient prone? J Endourol 4:269–272
7. Ibarluzea Gonzàlez G, Gamarra Quintanilla M, Gallego Sànchez JA et al (2001) Percutaneous kidney lithotripsy. Clinical course, indications and current methodology in our Lithotripsy unit. Arch Esp Urol 54:951–969
8. Ibarluzea G, Scoffone CM, Cracco CM et al (2007) Supine Valdivia and modified lithotomy position for simultaneous anterograde and retrograde endourological access. BJU Int 100:233–236

Chapter 4
PNL: Indications and Guidelines: Urolithiasis

Arvind P. Ganpule and Mahesh R. Desai

Abstract It is essential to clearly define the indications for PNL according to established guidelines for the treatment of urolithiasis. A thorough preoperative workup should identify stone (size, location, composition and hardness) and patient features (including special situations like urinary malformations, skeletal deformities, paediatric age or pregnancy), in order to define the indication to the percutaneous approach and possibly find out the best candidates for the supine position.

4.1 Introduction

The American Urological Association (AUA) has been the frontrunner in formulating guidelines for urolithiasis since 1991. Since then, a number of editions of guidelines have been published, the 2005 guidelines on staghorn calculi being the latest [1]. The European Association of Urology (EAU) has published similar guidelines since 2000. The latest updates have been published in 2012 [2].

In this chapter, we discuss the indications for percutaneous nephrolithotomy (PNL). Literature with robust level of evidence was reviewed and cited whenever

A.P. Ganpule (✉) • M.R. Desai
Department of Urology, Muljibhai Patel Urological Hospital, Civil Hospital Road, Nadiad 387001, Gujarat, India
e-mail: doctorarvind1@gmail.com; mrdesai@mpuh.org

C.M. Scoffone et al. (eds.), *Supine Percutaneous Nephrolithotomy and ECIRS*,
DOI 10.1007/978-2-8178-0459-0_4, © Springer-Verlag France 2014

necessary. The EAU, AUA and the 2nd International Consultation on Urolithiasis guidelines were taken as reference for discussion [1–3].

4.2 Indications for PNL According to the Guidelines

The factors which determine the indications for PNL include stone factors (stone size, stone composition, stone location), patient factors (body habitus, renal anomalies) and previous failure of other treatment modalities (extracorporeal shock wave lithotripsy, flexible ureteroscopy or other surgery).

The usual indications for PNL are stones larger than 20 mm^2, staghorn stones, partial staghorn calculi and stones in patients with chronic kidney disease. The contraindications for PNL include pregnancy, bleeding disorders and uncontrolled urinary tract infections [2].

4.3 Preoperative Workup

The recommendations and guidelines suggest intravenous urography (IVU) as the gold standard in the preoperative workup for urolithiasis. Non-contrast computerised tomography (NCCT) scan is quick and safe, contrast-free alternative to IVU. Randomised studies have shown that NCCT has similar or superior results to excretory urography in acute flank pain [4]. Contrast media should not be given or should be avoided when there is an elevated creatinine level, pregnancy or lactation [5, 6]. Additional information can be gained by contrast-enhanced CT scan (CTU); however at the moment there is no level 1 evidence to suggest that CTU is superior to IVU in the workup of urolithiasis [7]. Computerised tomography (CT) is a useful tool in planning PNL, particularly in anomalous kidneys [8]. Besides identification of stones, CT provides information regarding selection of appropriate treatment modality. It helps in this regard, by providing information regarding the size, number and attenuation number of the stone, presence and degree of hydronephrosis and skin to stone distance. All these factors help in determining the selection of appropriate treatment modality. X-ray KUB and ultrasound are used by few clinicians as a measure of preoperative investigations; however this cannot be considered as a standard. These investigations help to plan access and predict the possible success rates. Ultrasound is useful as a tool in the preoperative workup if the method of access is ultrasound guided.

Recently the applicability of 3D reconstruction is described for planning percutaneous access. Staghorn stone volume and its distribution ("staghorn morphometry") predict the requirement of tract and stage for PNL monotherapy, also helping to classify staghorn calculi accordingly. The model of staghorn morphometry differentiates staghorn into type 1 (single tract and stage), type 2 (single tract-single/multiple stage or multiple tract-single stage) and type 3 (multiple tract and stage) [8].

The EAU guidelines [2] state that for all patients with infection stones, recent history of urinary tract infection and bacteriuria, antibiotics should be administered before the stone-removing procedure and continued at least for 4 days afterwards. For septic patients with obstructing stones, urgent decompression of the collecting system with either percutaneous drainage or ureteral stenting is indicated. Definitive treatment of the stone should be delayed until sepsis is resolved.

4.4 Stone Factors

4.4.1 Stone Size

PNL monotherapy is the treatment of choice for "large stones". Generally speaking the definition of large stones includes those which measure 2 cm in diameter [9]. PNL attains stone-free rates up to 95 %, as it offers direct removal of stone fragments through the nephrostomy tract. For stones smaller than 2 cm in size, the treatment algorithm becomes more complicated because of the multiple variables involved. AUA guidelines recommend PNL as a treatment of choice for staghorn calculi. A retrospective study with 200 patients has shown that renal deterioration occurs in 28 % of patients with staghorn calculi treated conservatively. This emphasises the fact that staghorn stones should be aggressively and surgically managed [10]. PNL should be the recommended modality for staghorn calculi as clearance rates are greater three times than those reported for ESWL [11].

The following are the treatment options in staghorn calculi [1]:

1. PNL should be the first treatment utilised for most patients (level 2 of evidence).
2. ESWL should not be used as the preferred treatment modality for staghorn stones.
3. Open surgery should be recommended only if the stones are not expected to be removed in a reasonable number of stages.
4. Nephrectomy should be considered in nonfunctioning kidneys.

To summarise, PNL is the first choice for staghorn calculi treatment. Open surgery is desirable in the situation when expertise is not available and the stones cannot be cleared with a reasonable number of stages and tracts. Nephrectomy should be considered for nonfunctioning kidneys.

4.4.2 Location of Stones

Larger stones of the lower pole are best managed by PNL as a first treatment option irrespective to the lower pole anatomy [2, 3]. Treatment of lower polar stones should be guided by the diameter of the stone. Data from meta-analysis suggest that larger lower polar stones have lower clearance rates and higher retreatment rates [11] (level 1 of evidence). A large multicentric prospective randomised trial comparing with ESWL showed PNL to have a significantly higher stone-free rate (91 %) compared to ESWL (21 %); in addition the need for ancillary procedures and retreatment rates was higher for ESWL as compared to PNL (level 1 of evidence) [12, 13]. The calyceal stone burden is the most important factor in predicting the clearance.

Calyceal diverticulum is nonsecretory urothelium-lined compartment in communication with the renal collecting system. Asymptomatic stones in the diverticulum may be left alone; however stones causing pain, haematuria and infection should be treated. PNL offers better stone-free rates. Although there have been no randomised trials comparing laparoscopy with PNL and ureteroscopy, PNL is considered to be a gold standard in management of calyceal diverticular stones. In comparison to ESWL, PNL has higher stone-free rates with similar recurrence rates and complication rates [14]. The stone-free rates for PNL range in between 85 and 93 %; the added advantage of PNL is that it provides excellent access for obliteration of the diverticular sac [15].

4.4.3 Composition and Hardness of Stone

Stone composition and fragility is a "key" factor in determining the modality of treatment to be chosen. The composition of the stone is an important factor for predicting the success rates of renal calculi. Specific stone compositions have different clearance rates because of the varying fragility of stones. Cystine stones are harder to fragment; hence cystine stones larger than 15 mm should not be treated with ESWL. PNL would be a good option in these patients [2]. The measurement of stone density with NCCT helps in predicting success rates of ESWL and the need for PNL. Stones with greater than 1,000 Hounsfield units (HU) show poor results with ESWL [16, 17]. Struvite stones are best dealt with PNL.

The EAU guidelines state that for large ESWL-resistant stones, PNL is the best alternative for efficient removal, thereby avoiding too much shock wave energy to the renal tissue [2].

4.5 PNL in Special Situations

4.5.1 Anomalous Kidneys

This group of patients includes those patients with stones in ectopic, horseshoe or kidneys with fusion anomalies (see also Chap. 16). The approach to managing these stones should be individualised [8]. The factors to be taken into consideration are the stone bulk, the location of the stone, the vascularization and the anatomy of the pelvicalyceal system. Ultrasound helps in gaining access in ectopic kidney apart from being a diagnostic tool. CT is pivotal in deciding the management and choosing the method of treatment in anomalous kidney.

CT will also give the attenuation values and be a deciding factor in deciding ESWL or flexible ureteroscopy. Flexible ureteroscopy will be useful tool in small burden stones in size with the availability of smaller flexible ureteroscopes and access sheaths. However the surgeon should consider complete "on table" clearance in these patients as the drainage is likely to be impaired. Ultrasound-guided approach for ectopic kidneys should be done by surgeons well versed with it. Laparoscopic-assisted PNL has shown good clearance rates with minimal morbidity and less likelihood of ancillary procedures. Although adequate fragmentation can be achieved with ESWL, the drainage of fragments might be impaired due to the anatomical abnormalities. The choice of ESWL and flexible ureteroscopy as a "sandwich" treatment option should be done prudently.

4.5.2 Paediatric Urolithiasis

Although the treatment modalities used are same in children as in adults, specific points should be noted in children (see Chap. 17). The indications for ESWL are similar to those in adults. Stones in children with a diameter of less than 20 mm are ideal cases for ESWL. The success rates decrease as stone burden increases, and larger stones should be treated with PNL [2].

The recommendations are the following:

1. Children have a tendency to pass larger fragments.
2. Ultrasound should be the modality for localisation of stone when ESWL is the modality chosen.
3. Smaller instruments should be used for endourologic manipulations.

4.5.3 Percutaneous Antegrade Ureteroscopy

Percutaneous antegrade removal of ureteral stones is a consideration in selected cases, for treatment of such large (>15 mm diameter) impacted stones in the proximal ureter between the ureteropelvic junction and the lower border of the fourth lumbar vertebra. In these cases the stone-free rates range between 85 and 100 %; percutaneous antegrade removal of ureteral stones is an alternative, when ESWL is not indicated or has failed and/or when the upper urinary tract is not amenable to retrograde ureteroscopy [2].

4.5.4 Urolithiasis in Pregnancy

Urolithiasis in pregnancy remains a diagnostic and therapeutic challenge (see also Chap. 16). Ultrasound is the method of choice for the practical and safe evaluation of a pregnant woman with urolithiasis. The management depends on the degree of obstruction and time of presentation. If conservative methods fail, a temporary diversion is warranted. Due to the established risks of radiation exposure on the growing fetus, ESWL and PNL are contraindicated in pregnancy [2].

4.6 Summary of Recommendations on PNL "Technique" by the 2nd International Consultation on Stone Disease

PNL has been performed traditionally in a prone position; however it can technically also be performed in supine/lateral decubitus. The access to the collecting system can be gained either ultrasound guided or fluoroscopy guided, depending on the availability of instruments and expertise. The access site should be the posterior calyx whenever possible. The tract should be the shortest possible tract from the skin to the desired calyx traversing the papilla. Depending on the stone configuration, the calyx should be selected (supracostal, infracostal or subcostal), so that maximum stone bulk can be cleared with the minimum number of tracts. Renal tract dilation (either with balloon, Amplatz or metallic dilators) is a matter of surgeon preference or availability. Balloon dilator is regarded as the gold standard. In complicated cases or when secondary intervention is required, a nephrostomy tube which serves the dual purpose of tamponade and a conduit for second look is placed. In uncomplicated cases, tubeless PNL with or without application of tissue sealants is a safe alternative [3].

References

1. Preminger GM, Assimos DG, Lingeman JE et al (2005) Nephrolithiasis guideline panel Chapter 1, AUA guidelines on management of staghorn calculi: diagnosis and treatment recommendation. J Urol 173:1991–2000
2. Türk C, Knoll T, Petrik A et al (2012) Guidelines on urolithiasis, European Association of Urology. http://www.uroweb.org/gls/pdf/20_Urolithiasis_LR%20March%2013%202012.pdf
3. Denstedt J, Khoary S (2008) Stone disease. In: 2nd international consultation on stone disease. Health Publications (Editions 21), Paris
4. Worster A, Preyra I, Weaver B et al (2002) The accuracy of non contrast helical computed tomography versus intravenous pyelography in the diagnosis of suspected acute urolithiasis: a meta-analysis. Ann Emerg Med 40:280–286
5. Morcos SK, Thomsen HS, Webb JA (2001) Contrast media safety committee of the European society of urogenital radiology prevention of generalized reactions to contrast media: a consensus report and guidelines. Eur Radiol 11:1720–1728

6. Thomsen HS, Morcos SK (2003) Contrast media and the kidney: European society of urogenital radiology (ESUR) guidelines. Br J Radiol 76:513–518
7. Aga P, Bansal R (2010) Is intravenous urogram no longer an imaging of choice for percutaneous nephrolithotomy? Indian J Urol 26:303–304
8. Mishra S, Sabnis RB, Desai MR (2012) Staghorn morphometry: a new tool for clinical classification and prediction model for percutaneous nephrolithotomy monotherapy. J Endourol 26:6–14
9. Tiselius HG, Ackermann D, Alken P et al (2001) Working party on lithiasis, European Association of Urology. Eur Urol 40:362–371
10. Teichman JM, Long RD, Hulbert JC (1995) Long term renal fate and prognosis after staghorn calculus management. J Urol 153:1403–1407
11. Meretyk S, Gofrit ON, Gafni O et al (1997) Complete staghorn calculi: randomized prospective comparison between extracorporeal shock wave lithotripsy monotherapy and combined with percutaneous nephrolithotomy. J Urol 157:780–786
12. Lingeman JE, Siegel YI, Steele B (2005) Management of lower pole nephrolithiasis. J Urol 173:469–473
13. Albala DM, Assimos DG, Clayman RV et al (2001) A prospective randomized trial of extracorporeal shock wave lithotripsy and percutaneous nephrostolithotomy for lower pole nephrolithiasis: initial results. J Urol 166:2072–2080
14. Turna B, Raza A, Moussa S et al (2007) Management of calyceal diverticular stones with extracorporeal shock wave lithotripsy and percutaneous nephrolithotomy: long term outcome. BJU Int 100:151–156
15. Wen CC, Nakada SY (2007) Treatment selection and outcomes: renal calculi. Urol Clin North Am 34:409–419
16. Shah K, Kurien A, Mishra S et al (2010) Predicting effectiveness of extracorporeal shockwave lithotripsy by stone attenuation value. J Endourol 24:1169–1173
17. El Nahas AR, El Assmy AM, Manour O et al (2007) A prospective multivariate analysis of factors predicting stone disintegration by extracorporeal shock wave lithotripsy: the value of high resolution non contrast computed tomography. Eur Urol 51:1688–1693

Chapter 5
PNL: Indications and Guidelines: Stenosis and Tumours

Marianne Brehmer

Abstract A stenosis in the upper urinary tract (UUT) can be of non-malignant or malignant origin.

In stenosis in the UUT, factors of significance for the choice of the treatment modality and for its results are location and length of the stricture, and renal function. Also the origin of the stricture, malignant or non-malignant, should be taken into consideration. Therefore, these factors should be adequately investigated prior to treatment.

Symptoms and/or findings suspicious for transitional cell carcinoma (TCC) in the UUT are strong indications for endoscopic examination. In case of TCC, for patients with solitary kidney or poor renal function the choice of endoscopic organ-sparing treatment or of radical nephroureterectomy will have important impact on the quality of life.

5.1 Stenosis

A stenosis in the upper urinary tract (UUT) can be of non-malignant or malignant origin. It can be located in the ureteric orifice, in the ureteroenteric anastomosis, in the ureter, in the ureteropelvic junction (UPJ) or within the pyelocalyceal system. Non-malignant strictures may be caused by previous transurethral resection in the bladder, inflammatory reactions (in the ureteric wall or retroperitoneal), previous impacted ureteric stone, previous electrocoagulation or laser ablation of tumours in the upper tract, open surgery of the ureter (including reimplantation), previous pyeloplastic surgery or congenital malformations. Malignant strictures may be caused by tumours in the bladder, ureter or UPJ or by malignant lesions outside the ureter causing extrinsic compression. In this section, mainly non-malignant strictures will be discussed.

M. Brehmer
Department of Urology, Institution of Oncology and Pathology, Karolinska Institutet, Aarhus University Hospital, 8200 Aarhus N, Denmark
e-mail: marianne.brehmer@rm.dk, marianne.brehmer@ki.se, mail@mbrehmer.com

C.M. Scoffone et al. (eds.), *Supine Percutaneous Nephrolithotomy and ECIRS*,
DOI 10.1007/978-2-8178-0459-0_5, © Springer-Verlag France 2014

5.2 Choice of Treatment Modality

Factors of significance for the choice of the treatment modality and for its results are (a) location of the stricture, (b) length of the stricture and (c) renal function. Therefore, these factors should be investigated prior to treatment.

Several studies have shown that retrograde and antegrade endopyelotomy is safe and effective if the patients are properly selected [1–6]. The length of the stricture seems to be the most important factor for a favourable outcome of endoureterotomy [7, 8]; however, some authors have proved good results despite of the stricture being >2 cm [9]. Other factors of relevance for the outcome of endopyelotomy in UPJ strictures are a large renal pelvis, high UPJ and renal function <20 %, which are all associated with a poor outcome [4, 10–12].

The grade of the renal function may determine whether treatment should be carried out or not. If the function of the affected kidney is 5 % or less of the total renal function, that function is presumably not sufficient to avoid haemodialysis if something would happen to the contralateral kidney. Consequently, treatment may be questioned. However, if the impaired function is enough to cause problems such as pain or infections, treatment of the stricture, or nephrectomy, may be indicated.

5.3 Indications for Antegrade Percutaneous Investigation and Approach

The location of the stenosis is essential for the choice of treatment approach. Strictures in the UUT may be managed with retrograde, antegrade or combined approach. A retrograde approach is less invasive than a percutaneous antegrade one; however, in some cases the retrograde approach is not possible, and in other cases a combined retrograde and antegrade approach is necessary. In a tight stricture located in the distal part of the ureter, an antegrade approach is usually more likely to be successful than a retrograde one. Additionally, in patients who have a urinary diversion, the retrograde approach is usually difficult or even impossible. In those cases, antegrade or combined approach is recommendable.

In case of a ureteric obstruction where the patient has been equipped with a nephrostomy tube and if malignancy is suspected, antegrade ureteroscopy can be used for visual investigation and for taking selective cytology and biopsies. The technical aspects of these procedures will be discussed in Chap. 18.

5.4 Tumours

Transitional cell carcinoma (TCC) is relatively common in the urinary bladder whereas is rather rare in the UUT. Only 5–10 % of all TCC tumours occur in the UUT [13–15]. Patients with primary TCC in the renal pelvis or ureter have 30–50 % risk of developing TCC in the urinary bladder [16, 17], whereas patients with primary bladder cancer have only a 2–3 % risk to develop TCC in the UUT [18, 19]. Patients with TCC in the UUT on one side have a risk of 2–6 % of developing a contralateral tumour [15, 20, 21].

TCC in the UUT is more common in the Caucasian population, principally at the age over 60 years. The reasons are unknown; however, smoking is a recognised risk factor. Balkan nephropathy, analgesics including phenacetin, labour in paint or petroleum industries are other possible risk factors. Artificial sweetening, coffee, stone formation and previous radiation therapy have been discussed as possible ethiological factors but have not been proven yet [22].

5.5 Symptoms

The most common symptom of TCC in the UUT is macroscopic haematuria followed by flank pain, due to obstruction. Weight loss, tiredness and anaemia occur at more advanced stages of the disease. However, today most tumours are detected accidentally due to urinary cytology or computerised tomography (CT) used for investigation on wider indications.

5.6 Diagnostic Methods

The diagnosis of TCC in the UUT is sometimes difficult. Studies have revealed that up to 75 % of the TCC tumours in the UUT were not detected by intravenous radiography [23]. CT scan with native, loading and excretion phases enhances the diagnostic sensitivity [24, 25]. However, the sensitivity decreases if lesions are <5 mm (Fig. 5.1). Also relatively flat lesions, especially in the ureter, that cover a large area are difficult to detect by CT scan (Fig. 5.2). Moreover, some suspicious lesions identified by radiography are not malignant [26], for example, prominent papillae (Fig. 5.3). The development of radiographic methods, from intravenous pyelography to CT and magnetic resonance imaging (MRI), has increased the sensitivity, but the radiographic grading of detected lesions is not always corresponding to the pathological grading (Fig. 5.4). Adding cytology may further enhance the diagnostic accuracy, although sensitivity may be variable. For high-grade tumours, the sensitivity is around 80 %, but for low-grade tumours, the sensitivity is low [27, 28]. Consequently, the combined use of radiographic examination and urine cytology presents a significant risk of false positive as well as false negative findings.

5.7 Indications for Ureterorenoscopy

By ureterorenoscopic examination, using semirigid and flexible ureteroscopes, ureter, renal pelvis and calyces can be explored and biopsies and selective cytology can be obtained. Indications for diagnostic ureterorenoscopy are:

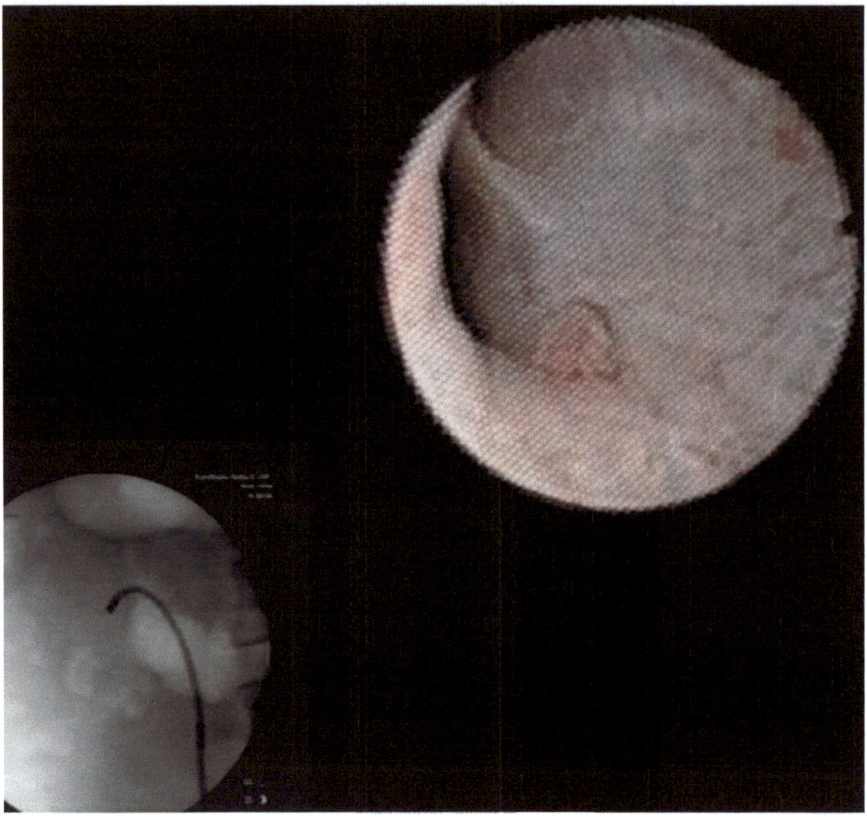

Fig. 5.1 Small renal pelvic tumour, not detected by CT scan

- Suspicious radiographic findings in the UUT with or without malignant cells in bladder cytology.
- Malignant cells in bladder cytology without diagnosed malignancy in the bladder.
- Macroscopic haematuria from the UUT without radiographic findings.

In the latter case, one single episode of macroscopic haematuria with no malignant cells found in urine cytology and no radiographic findings in a low-risk patient does not require diagnostic ureteroscopy. However, if persistant bleeding or in a high-risk patient (heavy smoker, previous bladder cancer, occupational risk), diagnostic ureteropyeloscopy should be performed. The patient should be prepared for simultaneous laser treatment if tumours, suitable for localised treatment, are found.

If possible, a diagnostic and therapeutic ureterorenoscopy should be performed through a retrograde approach. The reason for this is that a percutaneous puncture may imply seeding of tumour cells in the access tract. However, in some cases, an antegrade

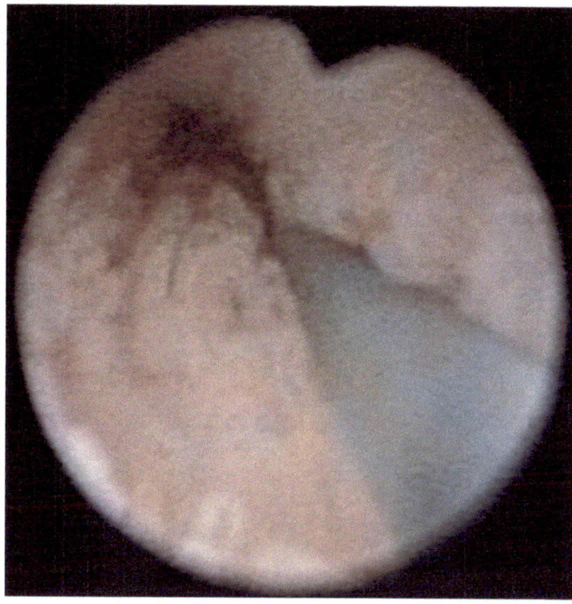

Fig. 5.2 Low papillary growth in the ureter, not detected by CT scan

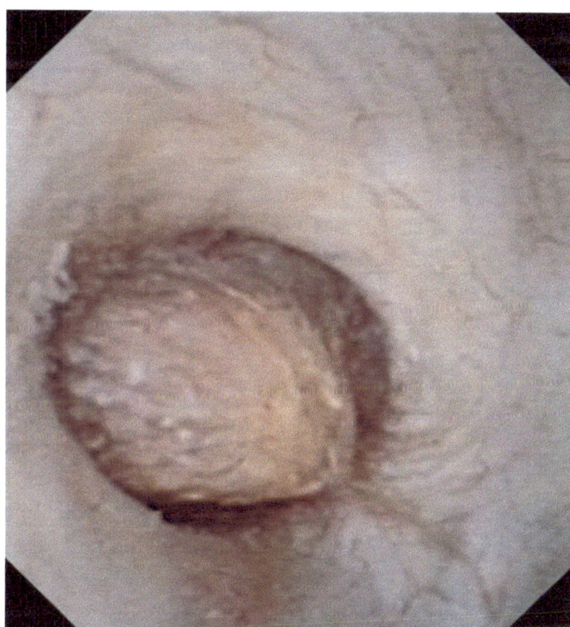

Fig. 5.3 Prominent papilla

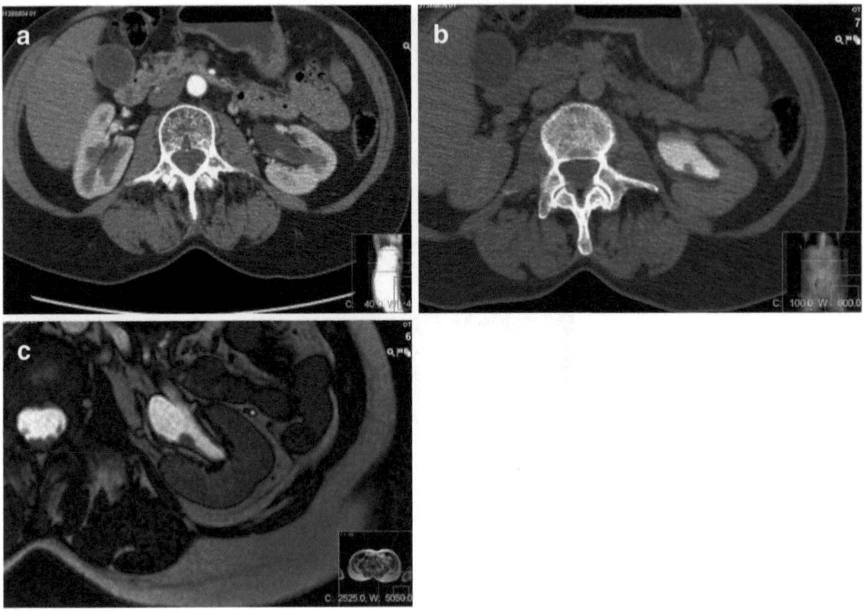

Fig. 5.4 (**a**) Renal pelvic tumour visualised in CT artery phase; (**b**) in the CT scan excretion phase, the tumour appears superficial; (**c**) by MRI it seems even more obvious that the tumour is superficial. However, the patient was operated on by radical nephroureterectomy, and pathology revealed that the tumour was high grade. Six months after the surgery, the patient was dead

or combined approach is needed. Such situations may be when a tumour is located in a lower calyx that cannot be reached via ureteroscopic retrograde approach or when a patient has been operated on with urinary diversion. Reimplanted ureters and ureteric strictures caused by other reasons such as radiation therapy may make it impossible to use a retrograde approach. The technical aspects will be further discussed in Chap. 18.

5.8 Treatment and Indications

The standard therapy for TCC in the UUT is radical nephroureterectomy. The reason is that the recurrence rate is relatively high, the sensitivity of cytology, as previously mentioned, is not very reliable and the radiographic methods not very sensitive for small tumour lesions. However, in patients with a solitary kidney or with severe renal failure, this will inevitably lead to haemodialysis, a condition with severe impact on the quality of life and on the costs for the society.

Consequently, indications for organ-sparing endoscopic treatment of TCC in the UUT are solitary kidney and kidneys with severely impaired function. A total renal function with a clearance <10 ml/min is not sufficient to avoid haemodialysis.

Therefore, these patients should be offered an organ-sparing treatment. The option of radical nephroureterectomy should also be offered to the patient; however, the patient has to be informed that he or she cannot come into consideration for a renal transplant until after 5 years of no tumour recurrence. Moreover, in some countries, patients over the age of 70 are not eligible for renal transplantation. Another absolute indication is the presence of severe comorbidities, considered a contraindication for radical nephroureterectomy. Endoscopic organ-sparing treatment is less burdening for the patient and can usually be carried out in spinal anaesthesia in those cases.

References

1. Stilling NM, Jung H, Nørby B et al (2009) Retrograde ureteroscopic holmium laser endopyelotomy in a selected population of patients with ureteropelvic junction obstruction. Scand J Urol Nephrol 43:68–72
2. Acher PL, Nair R, Abburaju JS et al (2009) Ureteroscopic holmium laser endopyelotomy for ureteropelvic junction stenosis after pyeloplasty. J Endourol 23:899–902
3. Ponsky LE, Streem SB (2006) Retrograde endopyelotomy: a comparative study of hot-wire balloon and ureteroscopic laser. J Endourol 20:823–826
4. El-Nahas AR, Shoma AM, Eraky I et al (2006) Percutaneous endopyelotomy for secondary ureteropelvic junction obstruction: prognostic factors affecting late recurrence. Scand J Urol Nephrol 40:385–390
5. Conlin MJ, Bagley DH (1998) Ureteroscopic endopyelotomy at a single setting. J Urol 159:727–731
6. Minervini A, Davenport K, Keeley FX, Timoney AG (2006) Antegrade versus retrograde endopyelotomy for pelvi-ureteric junction (PUJ) obstruction. Eur Urol 49:536–542, discussion 542–543
7. Braga LH, Lorenzo AJ, Skeldon S et al (2007) Failed pyeloplasty in children: comparative analysis of retrograde endopyelotomy versus redo pyeloplasty. J Urol 178:2571–2575, discussion 2575
8. Lin CM, Tsai TH, Lin TC et al (2009) Holmium: Yttrium-Aluminum-Garnet laser endoureterotomy for benign ureteral strictures: a single-centre experience. Acta Chir Belg 109: 746–750
9. Hatsuse K, Ono Y, Kinukawa T et al (2002) Long-term results of endopyeloureterotomy using the transpelvic extraureteral approach. Urology 60:233–237, discussion 237–238
10. Biyani CS, Cornford PA, Powell CS (2000) Ureteroscopic endopyelotomy with the holmium: YAG laser. Mid-Term results. Eur Urol 38:139–143
11. Renner C, Frede T, Seemann O, Rassweiler J (1998) Laser endopyelotomy: minimally invasive therapy of ureteropelvic junction stenosis. J Endourol 12:537–544
12. Rassweiler JJ, Subotic S, Feist-Schwenk M et al (2007) Minimally invasive treatment of ureteropelvic junction obstruction: long-Term experience with an algorithm for laser endopyelotomy and laparoscopic retroperitoneal pyeloplasty. J Urol 177:1000–1005
13. Babjuk M, Oosterlinck W, Sylvester R et al (2011) EAU guidelines on non-muscle-invasive urothelial carcinoma of the bladder, the 2011 update. Eur Urol 59:997–1008
14. Munoz JJ, Ellison LM (2000) Upper tract urothelial neoplasms: incidence and survival during the last 2 decades. J Urol 164:1523–1525
15. Kirkali Z, Tuzel E (2003) Transitional cell carcinoma of the ureter and renal pelvis. Crit Rev Oncol Hematol 47:155–169
16. Hisataki T, Miyao N, Masumori N et al (2000) Risk factors for the development of bladder cancer after upper tract urothelial cancer. Urology 55:663–667

17. Azémar MD, Comperat E, Richard F et al (2011) Bladder recurrence after surgery for upper urinary tract urothelial cell carcinoma: frequency, risk factors, and surveillance. Urol Oncol 29:130–136
18. Hurle R, Losa A, Manzetti A, Lembo A (1999) Upper urinary tract tumors developing after treatment of superficial bladder cancer: 7-year follow-up of 591 consecutive patients. Urology 53:1144–1148
19. Millán-Rodríguez F, Chéchile-Toniolo G, Salvador-Bayarri J et al (2000) Upper urinary tract tumors after primary superficial bladder tumors: prognostic factors and risk groups. J Urol 164:1183–1187
20. Novara G, De Marco V, Dalpiaz O et al (2009) Independent predictors of contralateral metachronous upper urinary tract transitional cell carcinoma after nephroureterectomy: multi-institutional dataset from three european centers. Int J Urol 16:187–191
21. Holmäng S, Johansson SL (2006) Bilateral metachronous ureteral and renal pelvic carcinomas: incidence, clinical presentation, histopathology, treatment and outcome. J Urol 175:69–72, discussion 72–73
22. Colin P, Koenig P, Ouzzane A et al (2009) Environmental factors involved in carcinogenesis of urothelial cell carcinomas of the upper urinary tract. BJU Int 104:1436–1440
23. Keeley FX, Bibbo M, Bagley DH (1997) Ureteroscopic treatment and surveillance of upper urinary tract transitional cell carcinoma. J Urol 157:1560–1565
24. Browne RF, Meehan CP, Colville J et al (2005) Transitional cell carcinoma of the upper urinary tract: spectrum of imaging findings. Radiographics 25:1609–1627
25. Dillman JR, Caoili EM, Cohan RH et al (2008) Detection of upper tract urothelial neoplasms: sensitivity of axial, coronal reformatted, and curved-planar reformatted image-types utilizing 16-row multi-detector CT urography. Abdom Imaging 33:707–716
26. Wang J, Wang H, Tang G et al (2009) Transitional cell carcinoma of upper urinary tract vs. benign lesions: distinctive MSCT features. Abdom Imaging 34:94–106
27. Williams SK, Denton KJ, Minervini A et al (2008) Correlation of upper-tract cytology, retrograde pyelography, ureteroscopic appearance, and ureteroscopic biopsy with histologic examination of upper-tract transitional cell carcinoma. J Endourol 22:71–76
28. Messer J, Shariat SF, Brien JC et al (2011) Urinary cytology has a poor performance for predicting invasive or high-grade upper-tract urothelial carcinoma. BJU Int 108:701–705

Chapter 6
Anatomy for PNL

Cecilia Maria Cracco and Alessandro Eugenio Vercelli

Abstract A good preoperative knowledge of the anatomy of the kidney of a given patient (including vascularization and collecting system) and of the topographic relationships of the kidney with the surrounding organs is fundamental in order to choose the best therapeutic approach, foresee possible intraoperative technical difficulties, inform the patient about success and complication rates, prepare a proper and complete endourological armamentarium of instruments and accessories, and plan the best renal puncture. Static anatomy data obtained from preoperative studies should then be integrated with dynamic real-time anatomy investigated by preliminary endoscopy.

6.1 Introduction

For the treatment of urolithiasis, many anatomical studies have been performed to improve the results of minimally invasive techniques such as extracorporeal shock wave lithotripsy (ESWL), retrograde intrarenal surgery (RIRS), and percutaneous nephrolithotomy (PNL) [1–4]. A good preoperative knowledge of the anatomy of the kidney of a given patient (including vascularization and collecting system) and of the topographic relationships of the kidney with the surrounding anatomical

C.M. Cracco, MD, PhD (✉)
Department of Urology, Cottolengo Hospital, Via Cottolengo 9, 10152 Torino, Italy
e-mail: cecilia.cracco@libero.it

A.E. Vercelli, MD, PhD
Neuroscience Institute of the Cavalieri Ottolenghi Foundation,
Regione Gonzole 10, 10043 Orbassano (Torino), Italy

Department of Neuroscience, University of Torino,
Corso M. D'Azeglio 52, 10126 Torino, Italy
e-mail: alessandro.vercelli@unito.it

C.M. Scoffone et al. (eds.), *Supine Percutaneous Nephrolithotomy and ECIRS*,
DOI 10.1007/978-2-8178-0459-0_6, © Springer-Verlag France 2014

structures is fundamental in order to choose the best therapeutic approach. In fact it allows to foresee possible intraoperative technical difficulties, to inform the patients about success and complication rates, and to prepare a proper and complete endourological armamentarium of instruments and accessories [5, 6]. In case of PNL the preoperative analysis of all these anatomical details is essential for the planning of the best renal puncture (see also Chap. 13).

6.2 General Anatomy of the Kidney

The kidneys are characteristically bean shaped and have a superior and an inferior pole, an anterior and a posterior aspect, a convex lateral border, and a concave medial border with a depression, consisting of the hilum containing renal vessels and renal pelvis.

The kidneys are located laterally to the spine, at the level of T12–L2 vertebrae (Fig. 6.1a): the right kidney is positioned a half vertebra below the other (Fig. 6.1c),

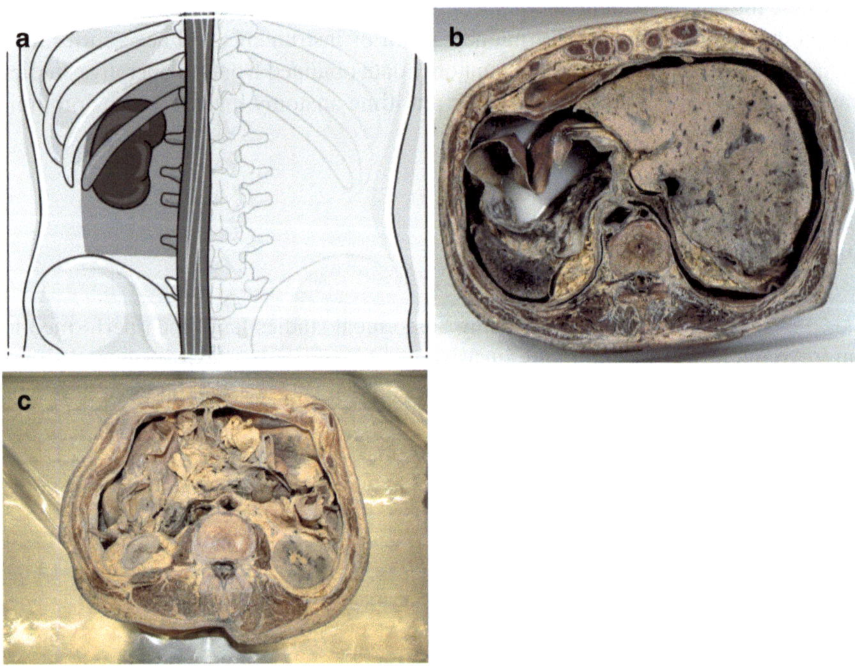

Fig. 6.1 Drawing of the anatomical location of the kidneys in the retroperitoneum (**a**) (© Carole Fumat); coronal macrosection from a formalin-fixed cadaver at the level of the adrenal space (**b**), just above the kidneys, crossing both the liver and spleen, and at the level of L1 (**c**), showing the perirenal and pararenal spaces and that the right kidney is lower than the left one (Courtesy of Prof. Giacomo Giacobini and Dr. Vittorio Monasterolo, Department of Neuroscience, University of Torino, Italy)

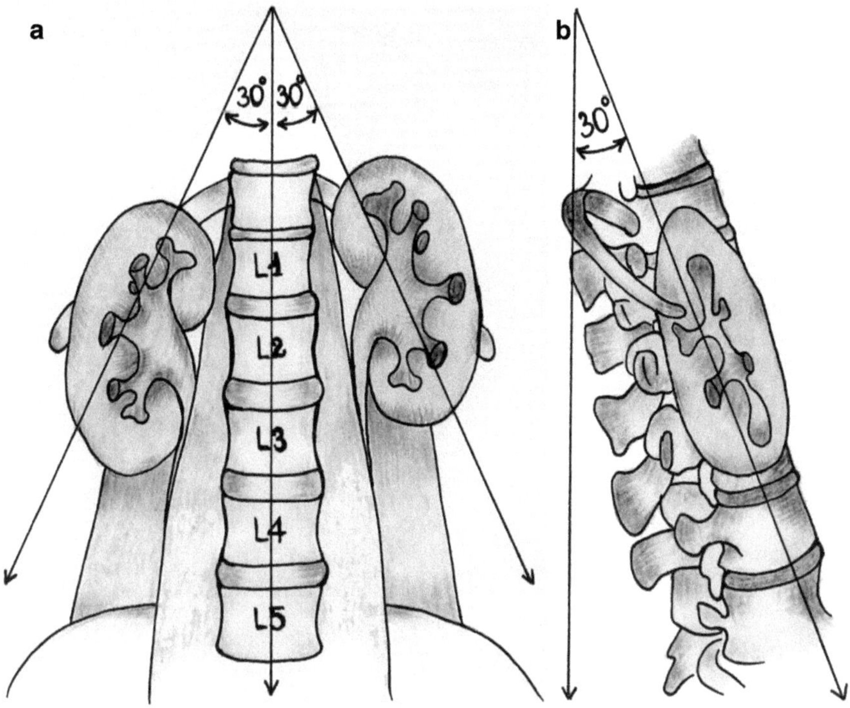

Fig. 6.2 Kidney orientation on the frontal plane (**a**) and on the sagittal plane (**b**) (© Cracco)

for the interposition of the liver on the right side (Fig. 6.1b). In average, the kidneys are 11/12 cm high, 6 cm wide, and 3 cm thick, their length being correlated with the height of the individuals. It has been reported that the superior pole has a greater width than the inferior one and that the left kidney is generally larger, higher, and thicker than the right one.

Their main axis is directed downwards, laterally, and anteriorly parallel to the oblique course of the psoas major muscles, with the superior poles closer to each other, more medial and more posterior than the inferior ones (Fig. 6.2a, b). Kidneys are angled 30°–50° behind the frontal coronal plane and their hilar region is rotated anteriorly with the lateral border rotated posteriorly (Fig. 6.3a, b). The supine or prone positions of the patient have no effect on the orientation of the kidneys [7].

The renal parenchyma basically consists of a cortex and a medulla. The medulla is characterized by 14–20 pyramidal structures, whose base is in contact with the cortex, and apex (also called renal papilla) directed to the renal sinus. It contains the loops of Henle and the collecting ducts, joining to form about 20 papillary ducts, opening at the area cribrosa papillae renalis, draining the urine out of the parenchyma into the renal collecting system. The cortex penetrates between two adjacent pyramids, giving rise to the renal columns (of Bertin). It contains the glomeruli with the proximal and distal convoluted tubules [8, 9].

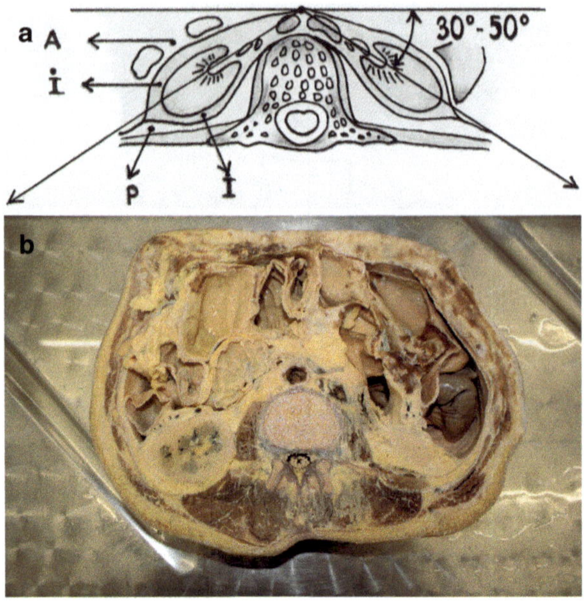

Fig. 6.3 Kidney orientation on the coronal plane, drawing (**a**) (*P* posterior pararenal space, *I* intermediate perirenal space, *A* anterior pararenal space) (© Cracco) and picture from a coronal macrosection from a formalin-fixed cadaver (**b**) (Courtesy of Prof. Giacomo Giacobini and Dr. Vittorio Monasterolo, Department of Neuroscience, University of Torino, Italy)

6.3 Topographic Anatomy of the Kidney

The kidneys are a paired organ located in the retroperitoneum on the posterior abdominal wall, against the psoas major and the quadratus lumborum muscles, in a space surrounded by a connective sheath named Gerota's or renal fascia. This space is closed cranially (where the sheaths are fused above the adrenal glands with the infradiaphragmatic fascia) and laterally (where the sheaths are fused behind the ascending and descending colon), whereas the anterior (prerenal fascia) and posterior (retrorenal fascia) sheaths of the fascia fade caudally in the retroperitoneum, weakly fused around the ureters, allowing renal fluid connections to drain into the sacral fossa. Laterally, Gerota's fascia is continued by the subperitoneal fascia, located between the parietal peritoneum and the fascia transversalis. Medially, the posterior sheaths of the two sides fade in the prevertebral fascia (giving rise to the Zuckerkandl's fascia), whereas the anterior ones join to each other ventrally to the blood vessels (aorta and inferior caval vein) forming the Toldt's fascia immediately below the parietal peritoneum. Therefore it is rare that a hematoma, a urinoma, or an abscess of one side involves the contralateral side.

Between the Gerota's fascia and the capsula fibrosa (renal capsule or true renal capsule) of the kidney, a though capsula which adheres to the organ, there is the perirenal adipose tissue (capsula adiposa), which surrounds the kidney and adrenal gland. The adipose tissue located anteriorly and posteriorly outside the renal fascia is the pararenal fat. Therefore there are three potential compartments created by the anterior and posterior layers of the renal fascia (Fig. 6.3a):

1. The posterior pararenal space, containing only fat.
2. The intermediate perirenal space, containing the adrenal glands, separated from the kidneys by an additional fascial layer, the kidneys, the proximal ureters and the perirenal fat.
3. The anterior pararenal space, extending across the midline and containing the ascending and descending colon, the duodenal loop, and the pancreas.

6.4 Relationships with Neighboring Viscera

6.4.1 Posterior Relationships

The relations of the two kidneys are similar posteriorly:

- The superior poles, to the upper limit of the renal sinus, lay on the diaphragm and, through it, are in contact with the costodiaphragmatic sinuses, the pleura, and the 12th rib (also the 11th rib on the left). Therefore, the diaphragm as well as the pleura is traversed by all intercostal renal punctures and also by some subcostal ones [10]. The lowermost lung edge lies above the 11th rib, at the 10th intercostal space regardless of the degree of respiration. With a supracostal 11th rib approach, the risk is 14 % on the left side and 29 % on the right side in prone position and 16 % on the left and 8 % on the right side in the supine position. A 10th rib supracostal approach is prohibitive, with more than 50 % risk of puncturing the lung [11]. Any intercostal puncture should be made in the lower half of the intercostal space, to avoid injury to the intercostal neurovascular bundles above, and also far from the vertebrae to avoid lung puncture because the lower margin of the lung is more horizontal than the axis of the ribs.
- Medially, they lay on the fascia of the psoas muscle (Fig. 6.4).
- Laterally, they lay on the quadratus lumborum and transversus abdominis muscles (Fig. 6.4).

6.4.2 Anterior Relationships

Anteriorly (Fig. 6.5), the left kidney is in relation with the spleen (laterally), the stomach, the pancreas and the jejunum (medially), and the colon (at the inferior pole); the right kidney with the liver (the bare area), the duodenum (medially), and the colon (at the inferior pole).

In mid- or full inspiration, especially in case of hepatomegaly or splenomegaly, the liver and spleen are displaced caudally, thus increasing the risk of lesion of

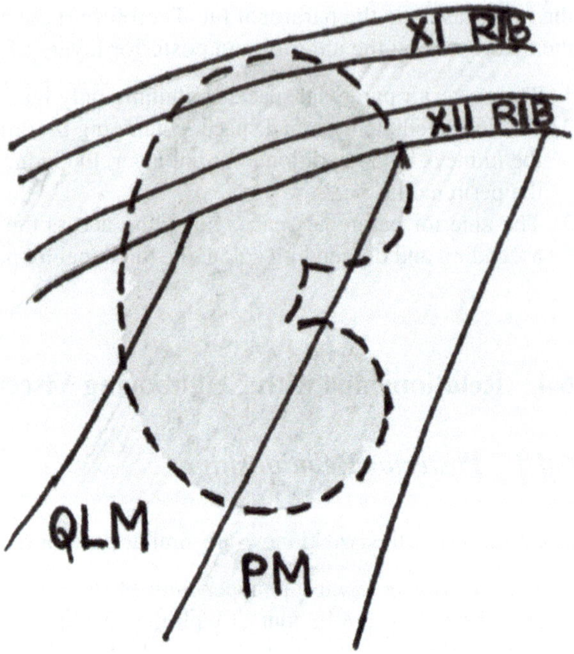

Fig. 6.4 Schematic drawing of the posterior relationships of the kidneys. *PM* psoas muscle, *QLM* quadratus lumborum muscle (© Cracco)

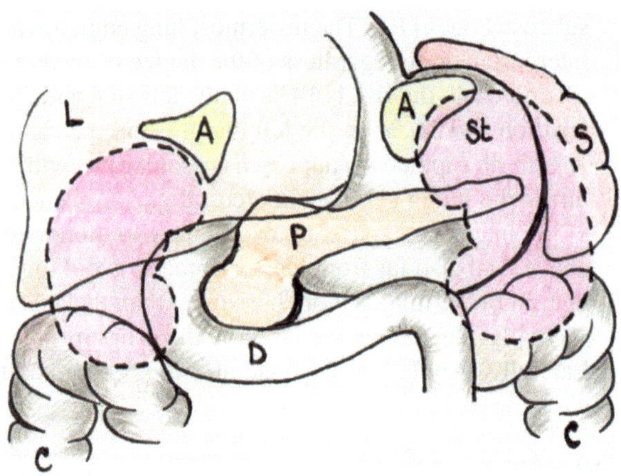

Fig. 6.5 Schematic drawing of the anterior relationships of the kidneys. *A* adrenals, *S* spleen, *L* liver, *St* stomach, *C* colon, *P* pancreas, *D* duodenum (© Cracco)

puncture. The prone position displaces the colon posteriorly, with an increased risk of bowel injury, the supine one with the flank elevated 30° more anteromedially with a longer access tract (although a shortest distance may not necessarily be the best one). This happens because the anterior body wall is more compliant than the posterior one, so that in the prone position the anterior wall pushes the kidney backwards. The position of the retroperitoneal colon (that can be foreseen with the preoperative CT scan) is particularly relevant, being occasionally posterolateral or even posterior to the kidney, thus at risk of being injured in the percutaneous approach, especially to the inferior poles of the kidneys and when the patient is in the prone position (10 % versus 1.9 % in supine) [12–16].

On the superior pole, the adrenal glands are in contact, through the interposition of the interadrenorenal fascia, with the lower lateral side of the kidneys. Medially, the kidneys show a concavity, a deep groove, the renal sinus, which contains the renal hilum, through which the ureter/renal pelvis, renal artery, renal vein, lymphatic vessels, and nerves enter or exit the kidney. The renal hilum relates to the gonadal vessels and the aorta on the left and to the inferior caval vein on the right.

6.5 Renal Vascularization (Fig. 6.6)

6.5.1 Arteries

The distribution of the intrarenal arteries was described a long time ago in man [5, 8, 9] and divides the renal parenchyma into anatomic segments. In human kidney the anterior (ventral) and posterior (dorsal) ones are the most important segments. The pattern of kidney segmentation in humans has been described as formed by 4 or 5 arterial segments.

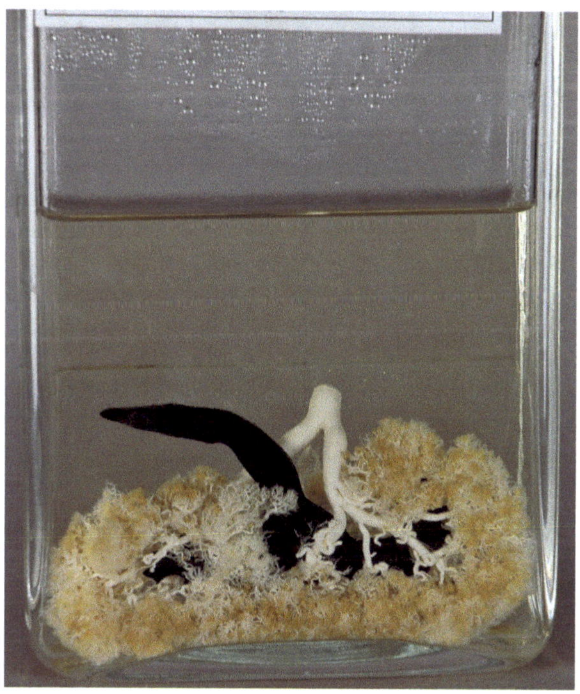

Fig. 6.6 Isolated and fixed vascularization of the kidney. Veins in *black*, arteries in *white* (Courtesy of Prof. Giacomo Giacobini, Museum of Human Anatomy, Torino, Italy)

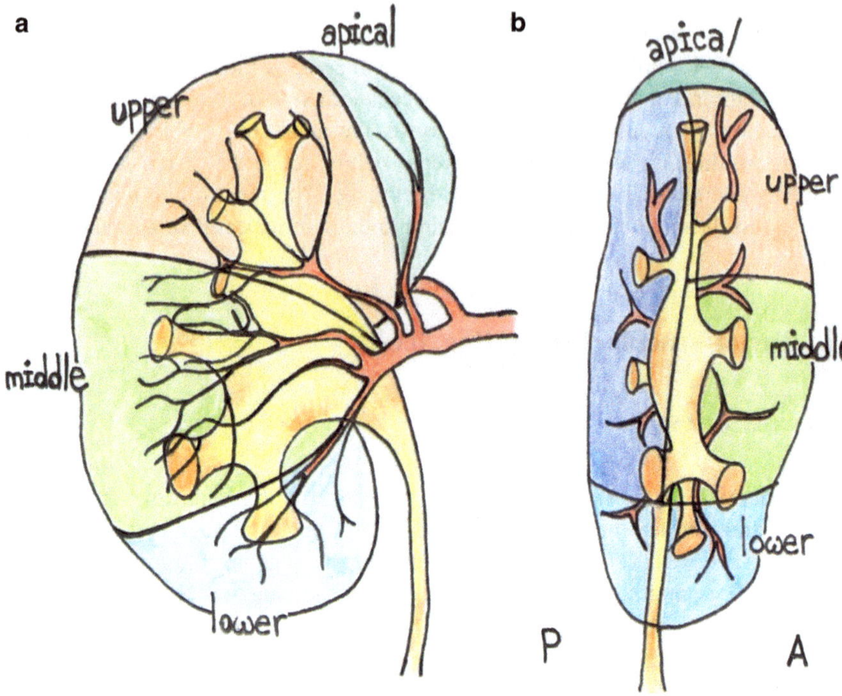

Fig. 6.7 Schematic drawing of the anterior (*A*) and posterior (*P*) segmental distribution of the arterial renal branches, frontal (**a**) and lateral (**b**) views (© Cracco)

The renal artery, located in between the vein (anterior) and the pelvis (posterior), gives off the inferior suprarenal artery, then divides in an anterior and a posterior branch (Fig. 6.7). The posterior branch becomes the posterior segmental artery, to supply the homonymous anatomical segment of the kidney (50 % of the parenchyma). The anterior branch provides 3 or 4 segmental arteries for the superior pole, the anterosuperior segment, the anteroinferior segment, and the inferior pole.

Before entering the parenchyma the segmental arteries give off the interlobar arteries, which enter in the renal columnae between the pyramids. Close to the base of the pyramids, they give off the arcuate arteries, usually by dichotomous division, which change direction turning parallel to the base. From the convex side of the arcuate arteries originates the interlobular arteries, which in turn originate the afferent arterioles of the glomeruli (Fig. 6.8b). In addition, from the efferent arteries of the glomeruli originate the arterioles rectae spuriae, whereas the rectae verae originate from the concavity of the arcuate arteries.

Taking into consideration this arterial distribution, it is easy to understand why the safest access to the renal urinary tract passes through the longer axis of a lower renal calyx papilla, generally a posterior one. This is the least traumatic access, reducing the risk of bleeding, because the needle passes along the Brodel's bloodless line, i.e., the avascular field between anterior and posterior divisions of the main renal artery, avoiding contact with large vessel (Fig. 6.8).

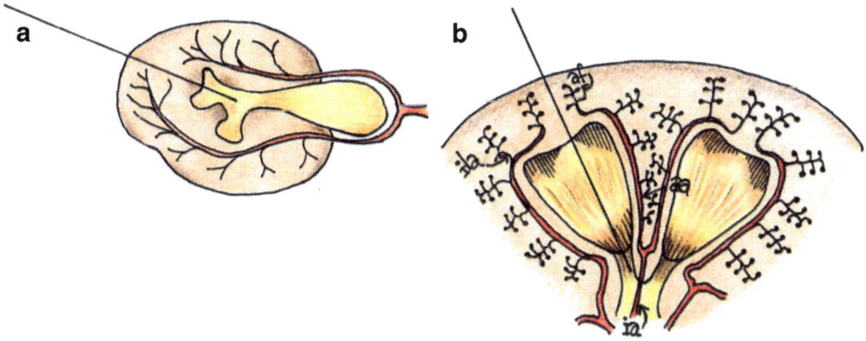

Fig. 6.8 Schematic drawing of the Brodel's bloodless line on a coronal plane (**a**) and of the relatively avascular space between the branches of the interlobular arteries (**b**). *ia* interlobar artery, *aa* arcuate artery, *ila* interlobular artery, *af* afferent arteries (© Cracco)

6.5.2 Veins

Despite the existence of free circulation throughout this venous system, the renal veins are worth of attention because a lesion of a large one may result in important back bleeding during and after PNL.

The venous drainage does not follow the segmental scheme [5, 8, 9, 17, 18]: the veins are diffusely anastomosed to each other, thus preventing parenchymal congestion and ischemia. The cortex is drained by the stellate veins, which drain into the arches of the interlobular veins and some of them into the retroperitoneum.

There are three systems of longitudinal free anastomotic arcades: of first, second, and third order from periphery to center, with anastomoses between the stellate veins (more peripherally in the cortex), the arcuate veins (at the base of the pyramids), and the interlobar, also called infundibular, veins (close to the renal sinus). There are also transverse anastomoses which link the ventral and the dorsal veins at different levels. Around the minor calyces they form a large venous anastomosis, similar to a collar. This is the reason why a percutaneous puncture should always aim for the tip of the papilla and never the fornix/infundibulum.

The interlobar veins converge to produce large venous trunks, which form the renal vein. In humans two trunks (cranial and caudal) are present in 29 % of cases and three (cranial, middle, and caudal) in 54 %. In all cases the venous drainage of the superior and inferior calyces originates only from ventral plexuses, the dorsal drainage emptying into the ventral drainage by transverse anastomoses. In humans the superior calyceal group is involved by a dorsal and a ventral venous plexus in 85 % of cases, and the inferior calyceal group in 50 % of cases, where large veins originate their course parallel to the anterior and posterior surfaces of the calyceal infundibula.

There are large veins in close relationship to the ventral and dorsal surface of the ureteropelvic junction (UPJ) (90 and 3 %, respectively). Therefore, UPJ endoscopic incision to relieve its obstruction must be done posterolaterally to avoid the risk of dividing a large vein.

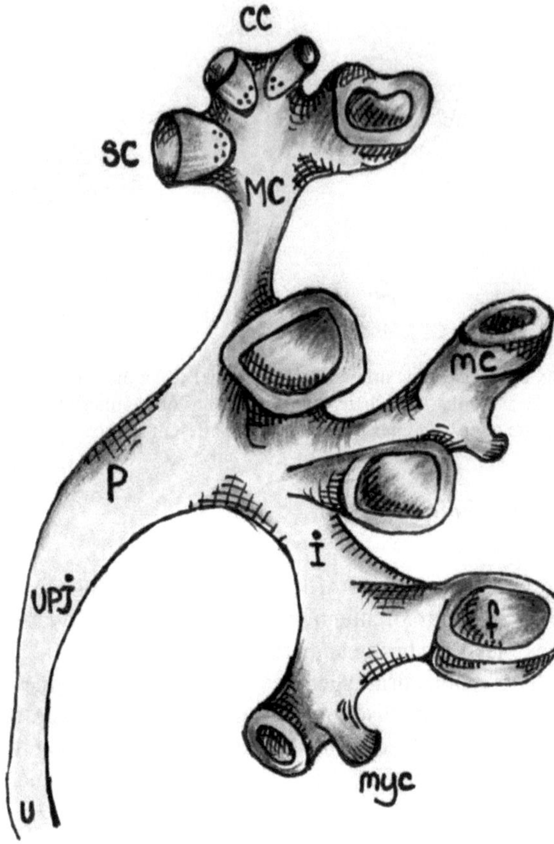

Fig. 6.9 Schematic drawing of the normal anatomy of the collecting system. *U* ureter, *UPJ* ureteropelvic junction, *P* pelvis, *MC* major calyx, *mc* minor calyx, *myc* microcalyx, *SC* single calyx, *CC* compound calyx, *I* infundibulum, *f* fornix (© Cracco)

6.6 Configuration of the Renal Collecting System

6.6.1 Normal Anatomy (Fig. 6.9)

The pelvis renalis or renal pelvis is the expansion from the upper end of the ureter into which the calyces of the kidney open. Ordinarily lodged within the renal sinus (intrarenal pelvis), under certain conditions, as in a long kidney or obstruction of the ureteropelvic junction, a large part of it may be outside the kidney (extrarenal pelvis).

The calices renales or renal calyces are the recesses of the pelvis of the kidney which enclose the pyramids. The calices renales majores or major renal calyces are the two or more larger subdivisions of the renal pelvis, into which the minor calyces open. The calices renales minores or minor renal calyces are a varying number (5–14, 8 in average) of smaller subdivisions of the renal pelvis which enclose the pyramids (sometimes compound, i.e., enclosing 2–3 papillae) and open into the major calyces, directly or into an infundibulum.

The microcalix/microcalyx is a very small renal calyx arising by calyceal branching, usually at the side of a calyx of normal size [5, 6, 8, 9].

6.6.2 *Variability of the Pelvicalyceal System Anatomy*

Pelvicalyceal system (PCS) anatomy is one of the most neglected aspects during endourological stone removal [19, 20]. The Brodel's kidney type (present in 69 % of the right kidneys) has a short and medially directed anterior calyx, whereas the posterior one is longer and laterally directed; the Hodson's kidney type (present in 79 % of left kidneys) has a longer anterior calyx, closer to the lateral border of the kidney, and a shorter and more medial posterior calyx (Fig. 6.10).

The overall morphology of the PCS is quite variable and can be ascribed to two major phenotypes [9] (Fig. 6.11): A and B. In A1 the middle zone is drained by the superior or inferior or both the superior and inferior calyceal groups simultaneously; in A2 the middle zone is drained by crossing calyces simultaneously, one draining into the superior one and one into the inferior one. In B1 the middle zone drains into the major calyx with a connection free from the superior and inferior calyceal groups; in B2 the middle zone drains into minor calyces which open directly into the renal pelvis. All PCS types had similar success rates, although one might expect B2 to be more favorable for introduction and manipulation of the nephroscope. Recently type B1 has been identified as the PCS type requiring an increased number of accesses for achieving stone clearance [21]. The PCS is usually oriented on a frontal plane. Thinking to a percutaneous access, it is important to study preoperatively the anteroposterior position of the collecting system relative to the lateral margin.

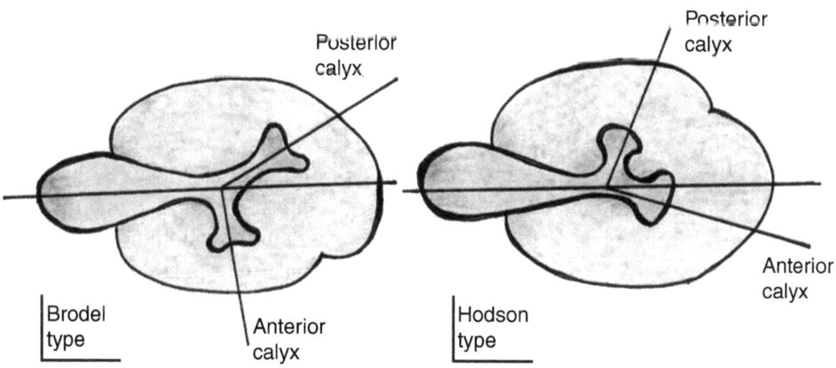

Fig. 6.10 Schematic drawing of the Brodel's and Hodson's kidney types (see text) (© Cracco)

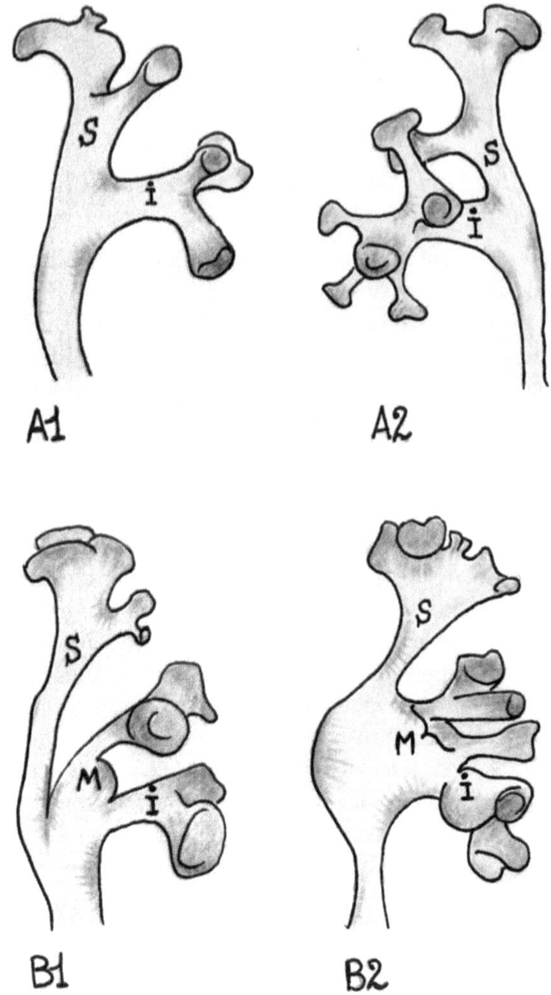

Fig. 6.11 Schematic drawing of the morphology of the pelvicalyceal system, classified according to Sampaio into type A (*A1* and *A2*) and type B (*B1* and *B2*). *S* superior calyceal group, *M* middle calyceal group, *I* inferior calyceal group (see text) (© Cracco)

6.6.3 Pelvicalyceal Parameters Influencing Surgical Choices

The morphology of the PCS plays a role in stone formation, but also definitely influences the indications and the success of various minimally invasive procedures, including ESWL, RIRS, and PNL. Morphometric analysis of the PCS and morphometric values of a number of parameters on imaging studies (including pelvicalyceal biomodeling with 3D computed tomography reconstructions) may be of help in the preoperative evaluation of patients suffering from urolithiasis [22, 23]. However, it has been argued that, as the pelvicalyceal structures are dynamic, the diameter or other measurements of any particular structure within the collecting system might also change during peristalsis [22].

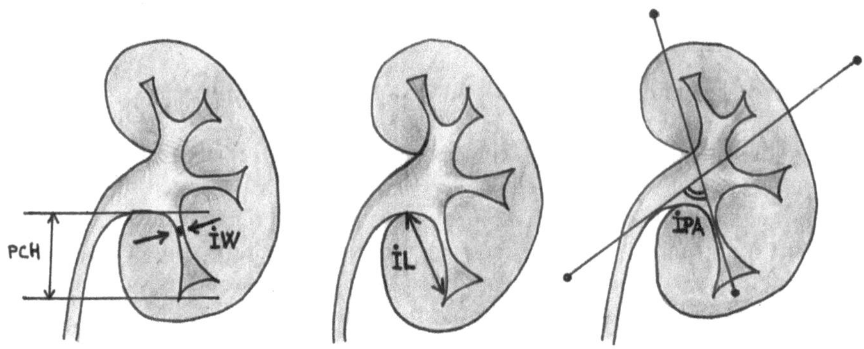

Fig. 6.12 Schematic drawing of the pelvicalyceal morphometric parameters. *IW* infundibular width, *IL* infundibular length, *IPA* lower pole infundibulopelvic angle, *PCH* pelvicalyceal height (© Cracco)

Relevant parameters might be (Fig. 6.12):

- Infundibular width (IW), the narrowest point along the infundibular axis.
- Infundibular length (IL), the distance between the most distal point of the calyx containing the calculus and the pelvic-infundibular junction.
- Lower pole infundibulopelvic angle (IPA), the inner angle formed at the intersection of the ureteropelvic and central axes of the lower pole infundibulum.
- Pelvicalyceal height (PCH), the distance between the lower lip of the renal pelvis and the bottom of the lower calyx.
- Upper-lower calyx angle (ULA), the angle between the central axes of the upper and lower calyx infundibula.

Let's cite some practical examples. The presence of an inferior calyx infundibulum >3 cm in size and the presence of an IPA <30° are predictive factors for failed flexible RIRS and ESWL when performed on patients with lower pole stones [1–3]. A wide IPA (>70°) or short IL (<3 cm) and broad IW (>5 mm) regardless of IPA are significant favorable factors predicting stone clearance [1]. An IPA higher than 45° is related to a high success rate for RIRS [24]. Some authors put in evidence the relevance of a PCH <15 mm [25].

As to PNL, the impression is that sometimes it can be difficult to obtain an optimal access through a narrow and long calyx infundibulum, and stones can be hard to reach or can be lost after fragmentation when the pelvicalyceal system is extremely large. In a study carried out on the PCS of about 500 patients by means of preoperative intravenous urography, no difference was seen in the success rates among the PCS types, although it was higher when the PCS had a surface area smaller than 20.5 cm^2. The mean IPA, upper-lower calyx angle, IL, and IW did not significantly affect the PNL success rate. The surface area of the renal collecting system can be measured using a 1-mm^2 grid from the intravenous urography. Severely dilated and large PCS generally have lower PNL success rates. PCS surface area and degree of hydronephrosis have no direct relationship, although no hydronephrosis will be present in kidneys with large extrarenal pelvis [4].

6.7 Conclusions

Preoperative planning to select the optimal target calyx for renal access is the most critical step for PNL success. The renal access step can be facilitated by thorough preoperative studies with a three-dimensional knowledge of the kidney anatomy and of the stone, as well as by preliminary retrograde flexible ureteroscopy during ECIRS for direct visualization and determination of the relationship of the calyx selected for puncture to the stone location. Incorporation of these clinical technical considerations into the treatment plan could decrease the possible negative effect of some anatomic parameters on PNL success.

References

1. Elbahnasy AM, Shalkhav AL, Hoenig DM et al (1998) Lower caliceal stone clearance after shock wave lithotripsy or ureteroscopy: the impact of lower pole radiographic anatomy. J Urol 159:676–682
2. Gupta NP, Singh DV, Henal AK, Mandal S (2000) Infundibulopelvic anatomy and clearance of inferior caliceal calculi with shock wave lithotripsy. J Urol 163:24–27
3. Geavlete P, Multescu R, Geavlete B et al (2008) Influence of pyelocalyceal anatomy on the success of flexible ureteroscopic approach. J Endourol 22:2235–2239
4. Binbay M, Akman T, Ozgor F et al (2011) Does pelvicaliceal system anatomy affect success of percutaneous nephrolithotomy? Urology 78:733–738
5. Kaye KW (1983) Renal anatomy for endourologic stone removal. J Urol 130:647–648
6. Francisco JBS, Carlos AM (1988) 3-dimensional and radiological pelvicaliceal anatomy for endourology. J Urol 140:1352–1355
7. Das S, Dhanraj P, Shyamkumar N et al (2008) Redefining caliceal anatomy in axial plane: selective overlapping of the appropriate contiguous sections on delayed post-contrast CT. Internet J Urol 5(2). doi:10.5580/fc4
8. Testut L, Latarjet A (1971) Anatomia Umana, V edizione. UTET, Torino
9. Sampaio FJB (1996) Surgical anatomy of the kidney. In: Smith AD, Badlani GH, Bagley DH et al (eds) Smith's textbook of endourology, (part II: percutaneous surgery), chapter 6. Quality Medical Publishing, St. Louis (USA)
10. Munver R, Delvecchio FC, Neuman GG, Preminger GM (2001) Critical analysis of supracostal access for percutaneous renal surgery. J Urol 166:1242–1246
11. Lang E, Thomas R, Davis R et al (2009) Risks, advantages, and complications of intercostal versus subcostal approach for percutaneous nephrolithotripsy. Urology 74:751–755
12. Hopper KD, Sherman JL, Luethke JM et al (1987) The retrorenal colon in the supine and prone patient. Radiology 162:443–446
13. Tuttle DN, Yeh BM, Meng MV et al (2005) Risk of injury to adjacent organs with lower-pole fluoroscopically guided percutaneous nephrostomy: evaluation with prone, supine, and multiplanar reformatted CT. J Vasc Interv Radiol 16:1489–1492
14. Cormio L, Annese P, Corvasce T et al (2007) Percutaneous nephrostomy in supine position. Urology 69:377–380
15. Duty B, Okhunov Z, Smith A, Okeke Z (2011) The debate over percutaneous nephrolithotomy positioning: a comprehensive review. J Urol 186:20–25
16. Azhar RA, Szymanski KM, Lemercier E et al (2011) Visceral organ-to-percutaneous tract distance is shorter when patients are placed in the prone position on bolsters compared with the supine position. J Endourol 25:687–690

17. Pereira-Sampaio M, Favorito LA, Henry R, Sampaio FJB (2007) Proportional analysis of pig kidney arterial segments: differences from the human kidney. J Endourol 21:784–788
18. Bagetti Filho HJS, Pereira-Sampaio MA, Favorito LA, Sampaio FJB (2008) Pig kidney: anatomical relationships between the renal venous arrangement and the kidney collecting system. J Urol 179:1627–1630
19. Filho DB, Favorito LA, Costa WS, Sampaio FJB (2009) Kidney lower pole pelvicaliceal anatomy: comparative analysis between intravenous urogram and three-dimensional helical computed tomography. J Endourol 23:2035–2040
20. Kaye KW, Reinke DB (1984) Detailed caliceal anatomy for endourology. J Urol 132:1085–1087
21. Yazici O, Binbay M, Akman T, Kewer C et al (2013) Is there a difference in percutaneous nephrolithotomy outcomes among various types of pelvicaliceal system? World J Urol 31:1267–1272
22. Sampaio FJB (2001) Renal collecting system anatomy: its possible role in the effectiveness of renal stone treatment. Curr Opin Urol 11:359–366
23. Sampaio FJB, D'Anunciacao AL, Silva ECG (2007) Comparative follow up of patients with acute and obtuse infundibulum-pelvic angle submitted to extracorporeal shockwave lithotripsy for lower caliceal stones: preliminary report and proposed study design. J Endourol 11:157–161
24. Resorlu B, Oguz U, Resorlu EB et al (2012) The impact of pelvicaliceal anatomy on the success of retrograde intrarenal surgery in patients with lower pole renal stones. Urology 79:61–66
25. Madbouly K, Sheir KZ, Elsobky E (2001) Impact of lower pole renal anatomy on stone clearance after shock wave lithotripsy: fact or fiction? J Urol 165:1415–1418

Chapter 7
Imaging in Percutaneous Nephrolithotomy

Susanne Sloth Osther and Palle Jørn Sloth Osther

Abstract With regard to patient selection for PNL, planning of percutaneous access, intraoperative guidance and postoperative evaluation of potential complications and stone-free status, imaging plays a crucial role. In this chapter the role of current imaging modalities is discussed, and focus is made on how appropriate imaging studies may lead to safe and efficacious percutaneous renal surgery. The role of the various preoperative, intraoperative and postoperative imaging tools is discussed. Furthermore, possible future scenarios with regard to imaging in PNL are briefly touched.

7.1 Introduction

Percutaneous nephrolithotomy (PNL) is the preferred treatment of patients with large and/or complex renal calculi and for those in whom other treatment modalities (extracorporeal shock wave lithotripsy, (ESWL), retrograde ureteroscopic procedures, etc.) have failed. With regard to patient selection for PNL, planning of percutaneous access, intraoperative guidance and postoperative evaluation of potential complications and stone-free status, imaging plays a crucial role. In this chapter we will discuss the role of current imaging modalities and focus on how appropriate imaging studies may lead to safe and efficacious percutaneous renal surgery. Furthermore, possible future scenarios with regard to imaging in PNL will be briefly touched.

S.S. Osther, MD • P.J.S. Osther, MD, PhD (✉)
Department of Urology, Fredericia Hospital – A part of Hospital Littlebelt,
University of Southern Denmark, Dronningensgade 97, DK-7000 Fredericia, Denmark
e-mail: susanne.sloth.osther@rsyd.dk; palle.joern.osther@rsyd.dk

C.M. Scoffone et al. (eds.), *Supine Percutaneous Nephrolithotomy and ECIRS*,
DOI 10.1007/978-2-8178-0459-0_7, © Springer-Verlag France 2014

7.2 Preoperative Imaging

Preoperative imaging should enable the surgeon to select the right treatment approach for the right patient, define stone burden, delineate renal anatomy as well as relationship of the kidney to neighbouring organs and estimate renal function [1].

7.2.1 Defining Stone Burden and Renal Anatomy

7.2.1.1 Plain Abdominal Radiography (KUB)

KUB (kidney-ureter-bladder plain radiography) is readily available and inexpensive. With regard to detection of upper urinary tract stones, it has however a rather low sensitivity and specificity both with regard to renal (58 and 62 %, respectively) and ureteral (67 and 69 %, respectively) calculi [1, 2]. It visualizes most calcium stones: calcium oxalate monohydrate (COM) and brushite being the most radiopaque and calcium oxalate dihydrate (COD) and calcium carbonate apatite the least radiopaque. Cystine and struvite stones are weakly radiopaque, whereas uric acid stones are radiolucent (Fig. 7.1). This information is useful, since it gives you an idea whether stones and fragments can be visualized on fluoroscopy during operation. Although KUB in combination with ultrasonography and/or retrograde pyelography may be enough to present the calyceal anatomy for puncture, it is inferior to other imaging modalities with regard to presentation of overall and kidney anatomy, and furthermore it does not give any information on renal function.

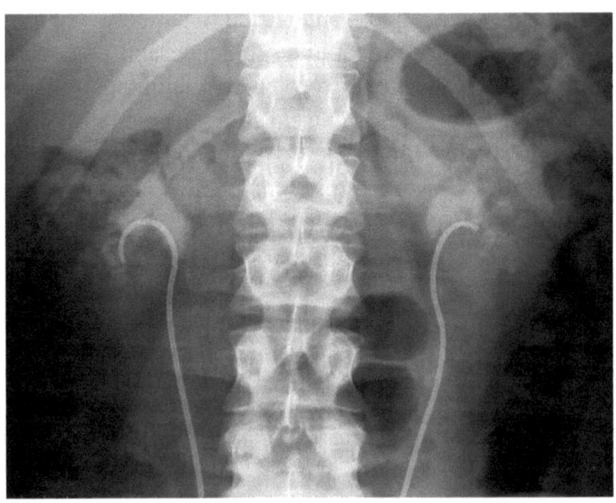

Fig. 7.1 Bilateral weak radiopaque staghorn stones in a patient with cystinuria. The patient was referred with bilateral JJ stents

7.2.1.2 Intravenous Urography (IVU)

Traditionally, IVU was the preferred imaging modality for both diagnosis of the stone disease and planning of treatment including access in PNL. With use of both anterior-posterior (AP) and oblique views, IVU presents the anatomy of the collecting system as well as its relationship to the ribs, thereby predicting the need for a supracostal access [1]. IVU is usually performed in the supine position. If a prone position or a modified supine position is chosen for PNL, this information may be of limited value, since changing the position also modifies the anatomic interrelations. For instance, it has been shown that by changing from the prone to the prone-flexed position, a supra-11th rib access may be converted to a supra-12th rib and a supra-12th to an infracostal access with obvious advantages when it comes to potential complications [3, 4]. Furthermore, in supine positions a supracostal access is rarely needed.

7.2.1.3 Computerized Tomography (CT)

Non-contrast CT (NCCT or CT KUB) unequivocally performs significantly better than IVU (level of evidence 1a) in the evaluation of acute flank pain and the diagnosis of urolithiasis [5, 6], and indeed in many institutions IVU is no longer available [1]. Both sensitivity and specificity of NCCT in the evaluation of renal and ureteral calculi approach 100 % [7].

However, with regard to anatomical information, NCCT is a poor substitute for IVU, and most patients undergoing PNL require additional anatomical imaging after an otherwise diagnostic NCCT [8]. This may be achieved by a retrograde pyelography at the time of surgery, which in many instances may be enough to delineate the collecting system sufficiently for a safe puncture. Standard CT urography, which has been proposed as the 'catch-all' diagnostic procedure for all renal tract anomalies [9], has its own limitations for calculus management, since excretory phase studies (ECT) may mask calculi [8]. Whether three-dimensional (3-D) CT pyelography offers any value over conventional IVU and NCCT has been questioned [1]. We will argue, however, that multidetector CT pyelography with multiplanar reconstruction and 3-D reformatting (3-D CT) is highly valuable in cases with complex anatomy/stone burden in which you anticipate surgical difficulty. A 3-D CT not only presents exact volume, orientation and location of stone(s) in relation to the collecting system, thereby facilitating selection of the optimal calyx for percutaneous access (Fig. 7.2), it also provides excellent perirenal organ mapping in combination with the CT images used for the 3-D reconstruction, thereby presenting the optimal plane of access in order to avoid injury of adjacent organs such as the liver, spleen, colon and pleura, which is of special value in patients with unusual body habitus (Fig. 7.3) and renal anomalies (Fig. 7.4). A 3-D CT demonstrates accurately the presence of parallel calculus-bearing calyces, and it displays calyceal orientation, thickness of narrowed calyces or the neck of a calyceal diverticulum [8, 10]. In special situations this may be highly valuable, when deciding the best

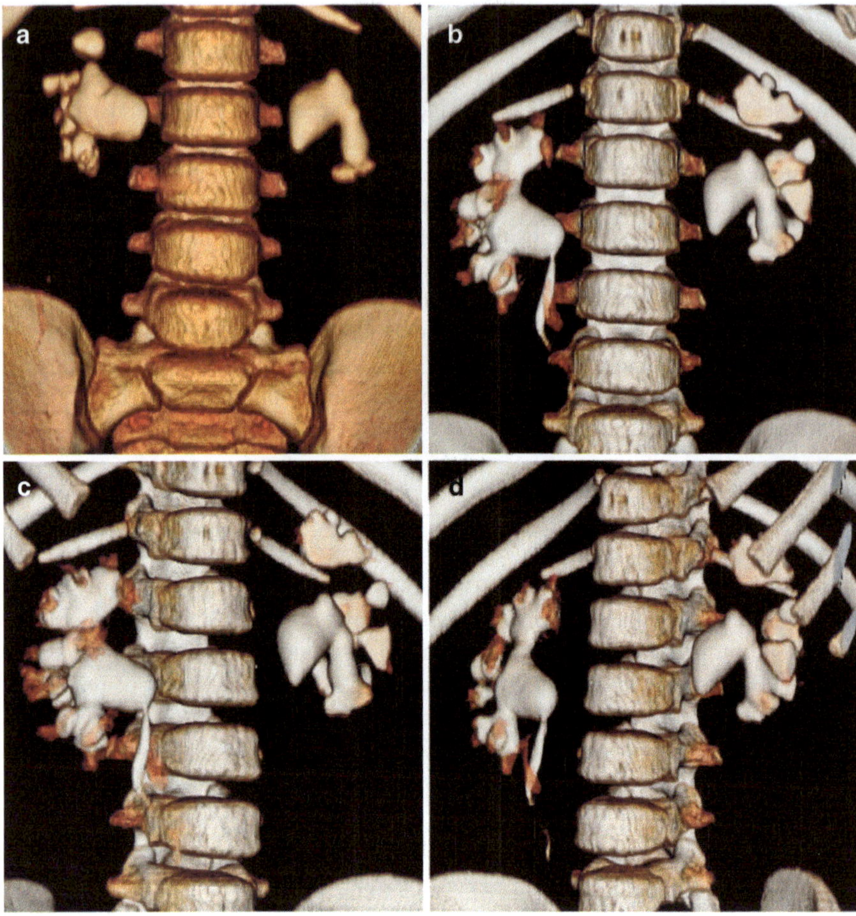

Fig. 7.2 Three-dimensional (3-D) reconstruction of bilateral staghorn stones. (**a**) Non-contrast CT (NCCT); (**b–d**) excretory CT (ECT). The 3-D reconstruction details the stone volume in relation to the collecting system from different angles, thereby guiding the optimal access

route of access and when performing Endoscopic Combined IntraRenal Surgery (ECIRS) in order to be guided around 'from above and below' in very complex systems [11]. Previously, 3-D CT was considered time-consuming and its reconstructions unreliable and therefore unsuitable for routine use [12]. Recent studies using interobserver statistics have, however, confirmed that 3-D CT in routine daily clinical practice is applicable, visualizing clinically significant calculi and accurately reconstructing the upper tract in rich 3-D format [8]. We are currently using this imaging modality in patients with renal anomalies and anticipated access difficulties, such as horseshoe kidneys (Fig. 7.5), malrotated kidneys, pelvic kidneys and calyceal diverticulum stones (Fig. 7.6). In the Clinical Research Office of the Endourological Society (CROES) PCNL Global Study, it was shown that PNL in

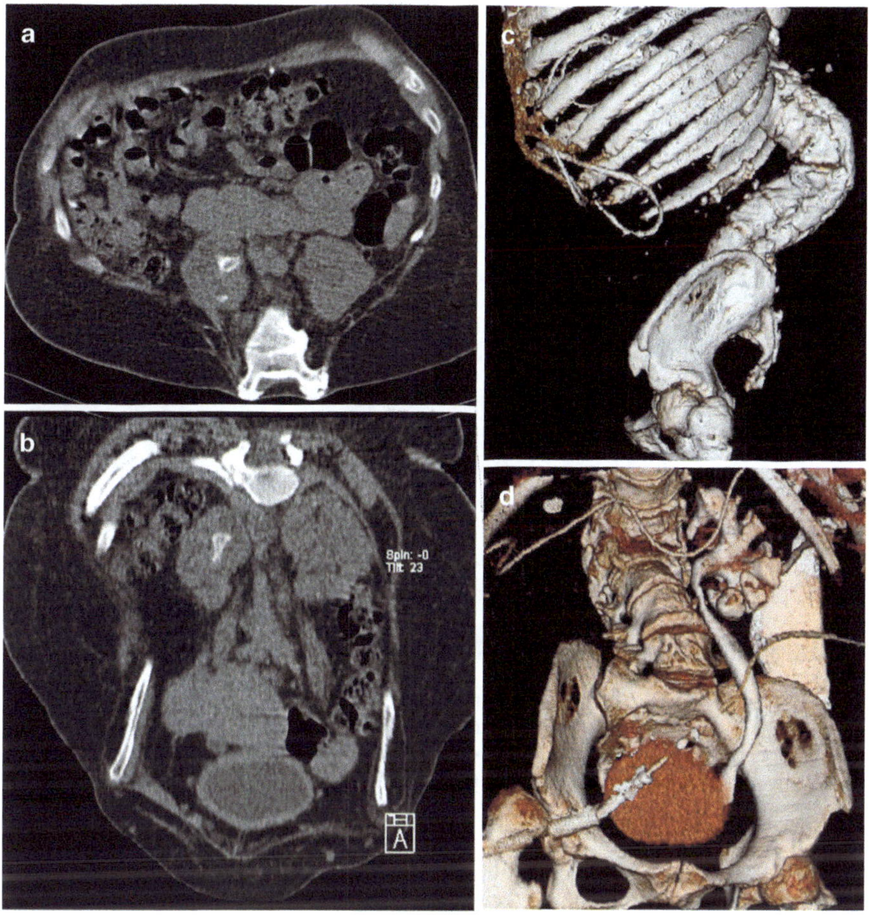

Fig. 7.3 Patient with severely altered body habitus due to myelomeningocele. (**a**) Axial reconstruction showing spina bifida and medially located kidneys with a pelvic and a calyceal stone in the right kidney; (**b**) coronal reconstruction showing the right-sided stone in the renal pelvis, note the malformed columna pointing towards you at top of the image; (**c**) 3-D lateral view showing the relation of the kyphoscoliosis to the ribs; (**d**) 3-D reconstructed excretory phase, note the ventriculoperitoneal shunt catheter

anomalous kidneys was just as successful with regard to stone-free rates as PNL in normal kidneys [13]. Median operative time was significantly longer, however, and access for PNL was unsuccessful in significantly more patients in whom renal anomalies were present. In our experience access difficulties in such cases may be limited and consequently operative time reduced using preoperative 3-D CT. CT has been considered inferior to IVU when evaluating stone-bearing calyceal diverticula [1]. As demonstrated in Figs. 7.6 and 7.7 it is clear, however, that 3-D CT is capable of delineating the collecting system anatomy including diverticulum size, location and stone burden excellently, and we believe that 3-D CT ultimately will replace

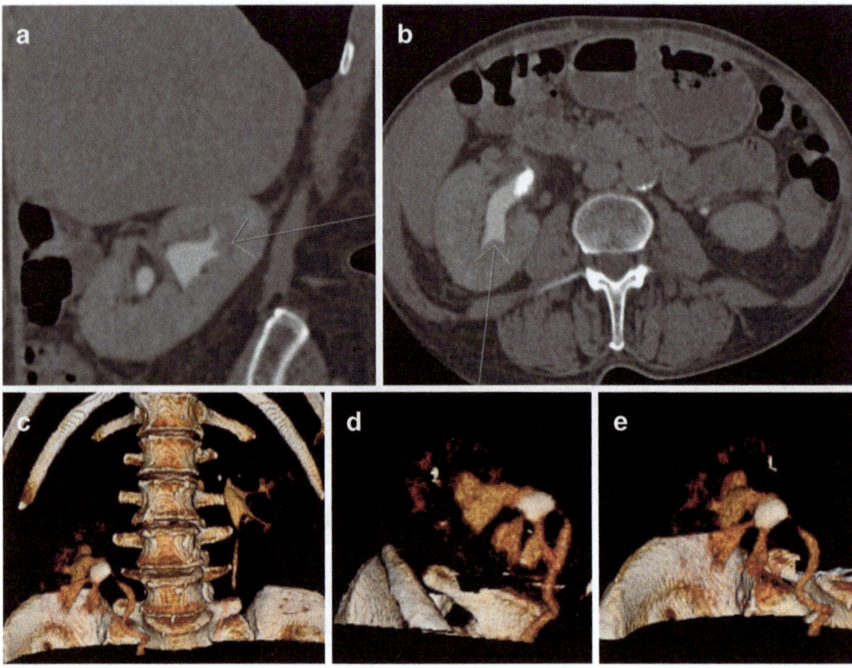

Fig. 7.4 Coronal (**a**) and axial (**b**) views of a kidney located just at the entry of the bony pelvis. *Arrows* show safe puncture line away from the liver and intestines. A 3-D reconstruction (**c, d**) from different angles demonstrating that an upper pole puncture will be most appropriate due to narrowing of the calyceal necks of the lower and middle calyces. Furthermore, the working space away from the bony pelvis makes the upper pole puncture most appealing (**e**)

IVU for preoperative access planning in patients with suspected renal anomalies, also in cases presenting with calyceal diverticula.

In some centres a KUB is added to the initial CT examination to evaluate whether the calculi are radiopaque on fluoroscopy, which is important information, when access is performed and presence of residual fragments are evaluated during and after surgery. This is unnecessary exposure of the patient to ionized radiation; however, since it has been shown that if the calculi are visible on the CT planning image (CTI, scout, topogram, etc.), they are also visible on KUB/fluoroscopy (positive predictive value 100 %) [14].

7.2.1.4 Magnetic Resonance Imaging (MRI)

Although MRI has the ability to detect the secondary effects of obstructive urolithiasis [15], MRI is unreliable in identifying both renal and ureteral calculi, and at present MRI has no role in the preoperative evaluation of patients undergoing PNL. In case of younger patients, pregnancy and patients that have undergone multiple prior CT exams in which you want to avoid ionized radiation, ultrasound seems to be the better alternative.

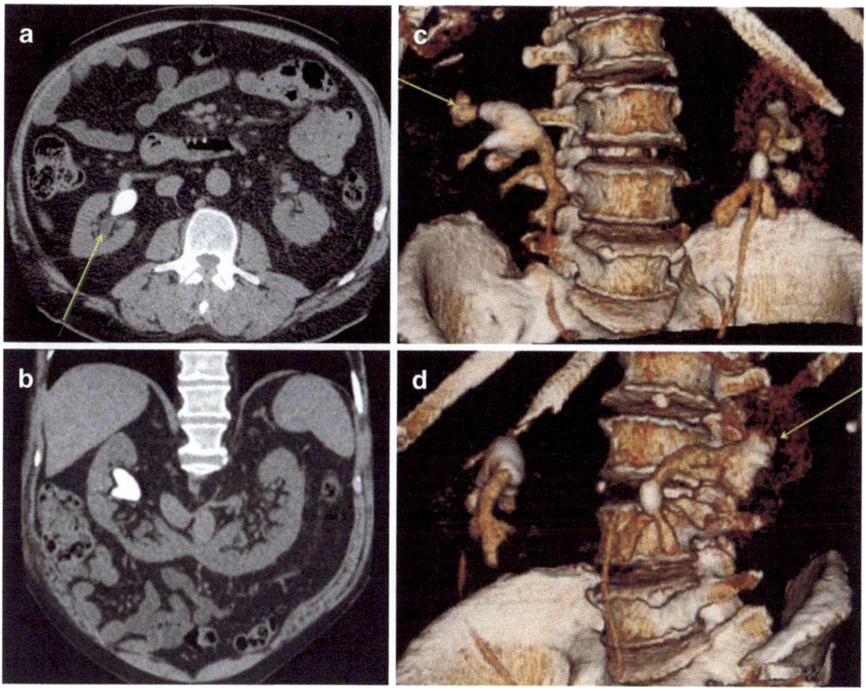

Fig. 7.5 (**a**) Axial non-contrast CT (NCCT) of horseshoe kidney; (**b**) coronal NCCT of horseshoe kidney; (**c, d**) 3-D reconstruction at different angles. *Arrows* pointing at preferred access, which in horseshoe kidneys most often is the upper posterior calyx pointing directly backwards

7.2.2 Relationship of the Kidney to Adjacent Organs

In a comparative study of CTs performed in supine and prone position, particular attention was given to bowel found posteriorly to the kidneys (retrorenal colon): its frequency of occurrence on 500 scans of supine patients was 1.9 %, but 10.0 % in the 90 prone patients [16], suggesting that supine PNL bears a lower risk of colon injury. This rather high frequency of retrorenal colon in prone position was confirmed in another study, in which the prevalence of colon lying posterior to the kidney was 13.6 % on the right and 11.9 % on the left side in males, whilst in females it was 13.4 % on the right and as high as 26.2 % on the left side [17]. Based on these data it may be argued that the supine position appears to be favourable with regard to risk of colon injury. This is supported by the fact that no colon injuries have been reported in the literature with supine PNL and that visceral organ-to-percutaneous tract distance has been found to be shorter when patients are placed in the prone position on bolsters compared with the supine position [18]. These observations were made using axial images of NCCT studies, however, and it has been shown that the risk of colon injury is overestimated by evaluation of axial CT images compared with multiplanar reformatted images (3-D CT) [19]. It is unquestionable, however, that the supine position for PNL has the advantage that the relative orientation of the

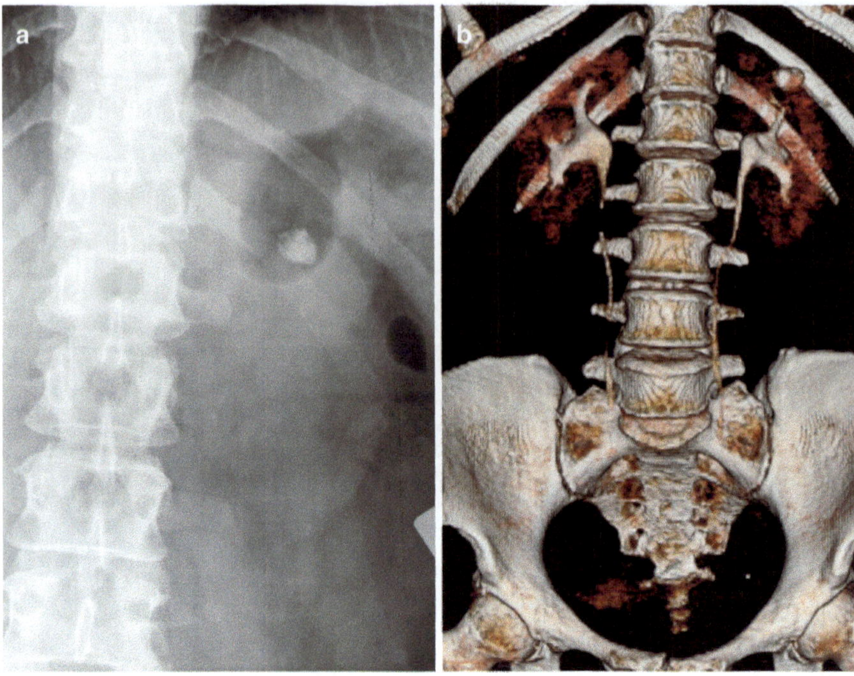

Fig. 7.6 Left calyceal diverticulum stone on (**a**) KUB and (**b**) 3-D CT. The latter showing the exact relation of the diverticulum to the collecting system and the ribs

anterior and posterior calyces as well as the interrelations of the perirenal organs to the kidney on the CT image may be transferred directly to surgery, since preoperative CT is most often performed in the same position. Whether CT before prone PNL should be done in the prone position is still a matter of debate [1].

Upper pole punctures are rarely needed in supine PNL, since most complex calculi can be dealt using ECIRS with lower pole punctures [11]. If an upper pole supracostal puncture is planned, the relation of the percutaneous tract to the pleura and the lung has to be considered. A 3-D CT in inspiratory and expiratory phases may be helpful in demonstrating the anatomical relationships among the kidney, calculi, pleura, diaphragm and ribs [20]. Although the reported incidence of pleural transgression during supracostal access is variable, most investigators recommend percutaneous puncture while the patient is in expiration [1].

7.2.3 Estimate of Renal Function

In case of severely reduced overall renal function, contrast-enhanced imaging is contraindicated, due to risk of further worsening of renal function. Both IVU and contrast-enhanced CT, together with knowledge of plasma creatinine, give a rough estimate of renal function. If these examinations give suspicion of severely reduced

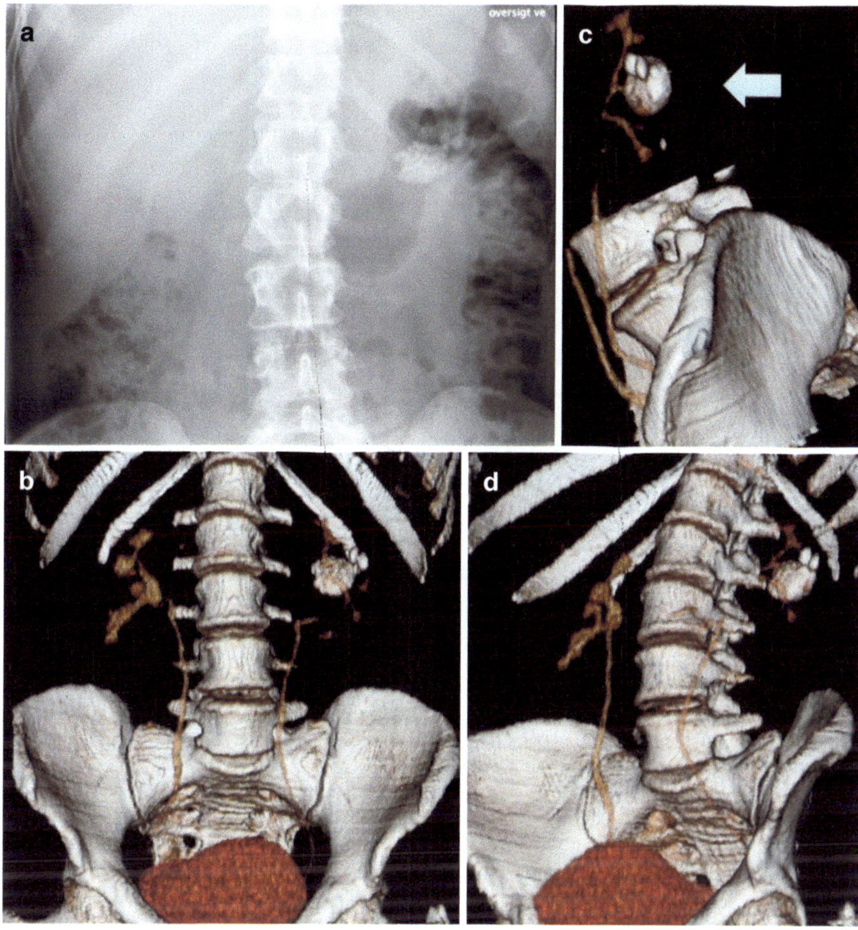

Fig. 7.7 Stones in a very large calyceal diverticulum demonstrated on (**a**) KUB, (**b–d**) in 3-D reconstructions at different angles delineating the narrow collecting system and its relation to the diverticulum at the middle calyx, as well as diverticulum size and stone burden. Access was performed by a direct puncture to the diverticulum straight from behind as indicated by the *arrow* (**c**)

function of the stone bearing kidney, a renogram/scintigraphy is mandatory for exact evaluation of the renal split function. The split function threshold deciding whether the patient should undergo PNL or nephrectomy is depending on the total renal function, which must be measured by a clearance estimate (Fig. 7.8).

7.2.4 Estimate of Stone Fragility and Patient Selection

Traditionally, smaller kidney stones (<2 cm) may be approached by SWL. Numerous factors affect SWL outcome including obesity, anatomical anomalies of the patient in general and the urinary tract in particular, size and number of stones and stone

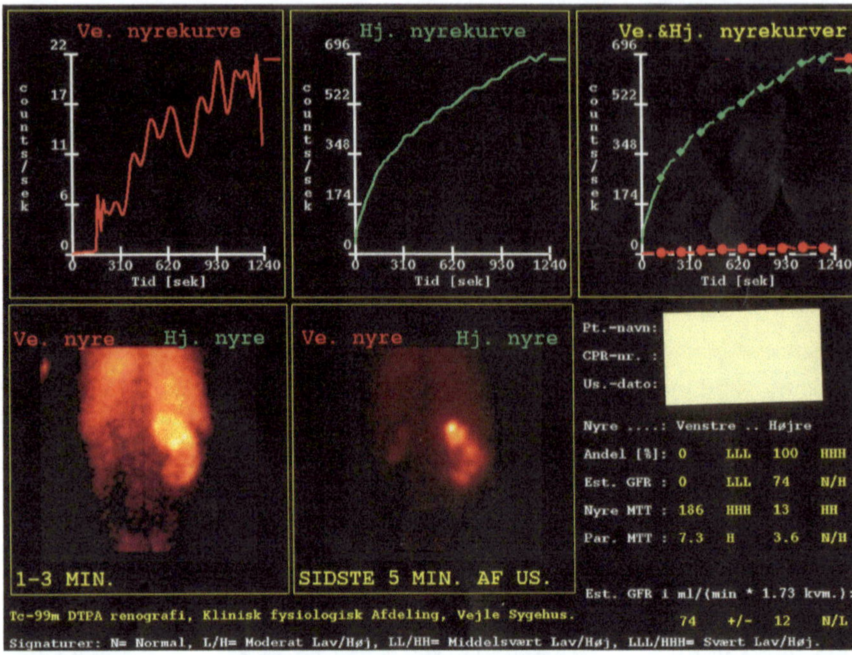

Fig. 7.8 Renogram in a patient with bilateral infection staghorn stones showing a nonfunctioning left kidney (*red line*) and compromised drainage of the right kidney (*green line*). The patient was treated by right-sided percutaneous nephrolithotomy (PNL) and left-sided laparoscopic nephrectomy

location and composition. Several authors have studied the role of measuring Hounsfield units (HU) in order to predict crystalline composition of the stone as well as stone fragility in ESWL. Zarse et al. have addressed this elegantly by using high-resolution detection of internal structure of renal calculi by helical CT [21]. They found that by using a narrow slice width and bone windows greatly improved the visualization of kidney stone structure on helical CT. These results opened up for new possibilities for determining the relationship of stone structure and fragility for ESWL. They interestingly found that CT visible internal structure rather than HU of COM stones predicted lithotripsy fragility in vitro. COM stones of homogeneous structure required almost twice as many shock waves (SWs) to comminute than stones of similar mineral composition that exhibit internal structural features that were visible by CT. HU values of COM stones did not correlate with stone fragility. Thus, it seems that it is stone morphology, rather than X-ray attenuation, which correlates with fragility to SWs in this common stone type. This simple technique has proven to be an important clinical tool for the primary selection of patients to either ESWL or endoscopic treatment. This was further indicated in a study of cystine stones in which it was found that CT visibility of void regions in cystine stones was an indicator of fragility during ESWL. Conversely, cystine stones that appeared to be homogeneous by CT were likely to be resistant to SWs [22]. Thus,

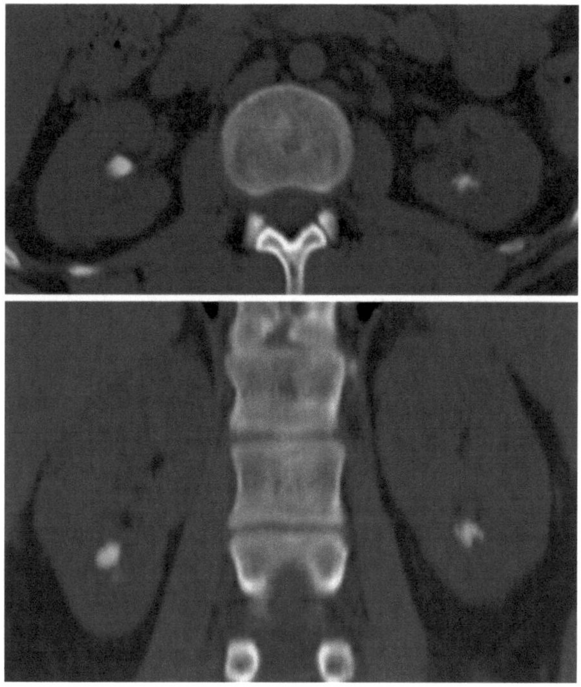

Fig. 7.9 Inhomogeneous stones in the lower calyces of a cystinuric patient. Traditionally, cystine stones are ESWL resistant; however, these inhomogeneous stones containing void regions were successfully treated by ESWL in two single sessions

these findings may be used in the clinical setting for selecting patients for primary ESWL or primary endourological treatment such as PNL and thereby increasing efficacy of both treatment approaches (Fig. 7.9).

7.3 Intraoperative Imaging

Intraoperative imaging is needed both for access and guidance of the endoscopic inspection of the collecting system [1]. The percutaneous puncture may be guided by biplanar fluoroscopy, ultrasound (US) and/or CT. Open configuration MRI may be used for nephrostomy placement in extraordinary cases such as very complex calculi in pregnancy in which ultrasound has failed or is considered unsuitable [23, 24].

It is important that whenever possible the access is carried out in the operating room (OR) at time of surgery, in order to eliminate transfer of the patient between different departments. The urologist alone can do the access. If the access is performed by an interventional uroradiologist, it should preferably be done in collaboration with the endourologist in a one-stage setting in the OR for selection of the optimal tract based on intrarenal anatomy and the ability to make secondary tracts [25]. Also placement of a ureteral catheter for contrast injection provides the ability to create a dilated system and presents intrarenal anatomic details, which improves the chances of getting 'the perfect puncture' through the cup of the desired calyx. Fewer access-related complications and higher stone-free rates can be achieved in this manner.

7.3.1 Fluoroscopy

Traditionally, biplanar fluoroscopy with a rotating C-arm has been the most common imaging modality for obtaining percutaneous access in PNL, and regardless the imaging modality used for access guidance, intraoperative fluoroscopy complementary to endoscopy is considered indispensable for successful and safe stone removal [1, 25]. Usually, a retrograde pyelography using a ureteral catheter with the C-arm in the vertical position in prone PNL and in the supine position with the C-arm tilted in accordance with degree of patient rotation is performed to delineate collecting system and locate stone(s) [25, 26]. Tilting the C-arm towards the surgeon (20°–30°) and in the caudal or cranial direction depending on whether the lower or upper pole is being accessed presents the desired posterior calyx – usually the posterior one – for end-on puncture [25]. In the prone position air instead of contrast may be instilled into the collecting system to present the posterior calyx without obscuring the stone [1]. When using contrast for puncture guidance, the posterior calyx will be less contrast enhanced in the prone position and more contrast enhanced in the supine position compared to the anterior calyces due to gravity [27].

During rigid and flexible nephroscopy, fluoroscopy injection of diluted contrast through the scope, when needed, enhances complete inspection/visualization of the collecting system including the ureter, thereby increasing stone-free rate [1].

7.3.2 Ultrasonography (US)

The limitations of using US alone for percutaneous puncture include difficulties in appropriate targeting of a non-distended calyx, poor image quality in obese patients, limited ability to identify anatomic details such a narrow infundibulum and difficulties in differentiating nephrocalcinosis from nephrolithiasis [1]. On the other hand, in combination with fluoroscopy US offers clear advantages. US permits direct real-time inspection of the intended percutaneous tract avoiding injury to any major intrarenal vessels or perirenal organs, while at the same time securing exact end-on puncture of the calyx [28]. The fact that fewer colon injuries have been reported with supine PNL may also in part be attributable to the combined US/fluoroscopy-guided puncture, which is a golden standard in this procedure [11, 26]. This combined access guidance approach also has been shown to eliminate organ perforation risk in prone PNL [28]. Indisputably, US is the preferred initial access guidance for pregnant and renal transplant patients and in patients in which a retrograde passage of a ureteral catheter for opacification of the collecting system is precluded [1].

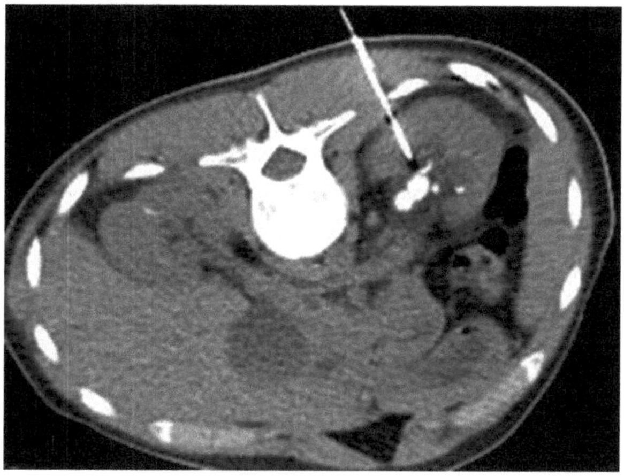

Fig. 7.10 CT-guided supra-11th rib puncture

7.3.3 Computerized Tomography (CT)

CT-guided access is reserved to very complex cases in which access has failed using standard fluoroscopy/US or in which special access difficulties are anticipated. Such indications may include spinal dysraphism, morbid obesity, abnormal visceral anatomy (retrorenal colon or spleen), urinary diversions, ectopic kidney, horseshoe kidney and transplant kidney [29]. Percutaneous renal access may be guided by CT using real-time CT or in combination with CT pyelography [28] (Fig. 7.10). Interventional CT suites are available but not yet in widespread use for PNL [24]. CT-guided puncture feasibly can be performed in a conventional CT room without radiation exposure to the interventionist. A laser guide and adjunctive guidance devices may ease the procedure [29, 30]. The major advantage of CT-guided puncture is the ability for excellent real-time imaging of perirenal organs, avoiding organ injury in patients with very complex anatomy. Also, performing PNL in interventional CT suites will enable you to evaluate presence of residual fragments with the best available imaging modality, which potentially will increase stone-free rate.

7.3.4 Radiation Safety

All imaging involving ionized radiation must be conducted according the ALARA principle. ALARA is the acronym for As Low As Reasonable Achievable. The X-ray tube should always be placed under table, and the patient should be placed as close to the image intensifier as possible in order to reduce scattered radiation to the patient, the surgeon and the OR staff. Use of collimation will further reduce scattered radiation and avoid direct exposure of the surgeon and areas of the patient adjacent to the area of interest [1]. All personnel should of course wear lead aprons, and those close to the X-ray source collar guards as well. Regarding the safety distance, the inverse-square law may be applied: radiation dose is reduced by the square of the distance to the X-ray source. This means by doubling or tripling the distance to the source, the dose is reduced by one quarter and one ninth, respectively. In other words, by backing away from the patient during fluoroscopy, the surgeon and the assistants will dramatically reduce radiation exposure. In a study of radiation exposure during ureteroscopy and PNL, average fluoroscopy time was found to be 1.3 and 10.7 min, respectively [31]. The highest scattered radiation was recorded at the lower extremities and the lowest at the level of the eyes. The estimate of maximum scatter radiation exposure to the surgeon for 50 PNL procedures did not exceed 10 mGy, which is below 2 % of the established allowable dose limit for radiation exposure in Great Britain [1, 31]. Nevertheless, medical personnel involved in PNL should be aware of scattered radiation risks and always minimize radiation exposure according to the ALARA principle.

7.4 Postoperative Imaging

7.4.1 Evaluation of Complications

A high index of suspicion postoperatively should prompt immediate imaging according to the specific clinical symptoms to limit serious sequelae.

Supracostal access is associated with a high risk of pleural injury. The frequency of hydropneumothorax has been reported up to 12 and 35 % in supra-12th and supra-11th rib, respectively [1]. Intraoperative chest fluoroscopy seems to be sufficient to detect clinically significant pleural complications during PNL [32]. This simple technique also allows for intraoperative drainage, while the patient is still anaesthetized [1]. If intraoperative fluoroscopy is normal, this of course should not delay postoperative imaging (i.e. chest CT), if the patient develops symptoms indicative of a pleural complication.

Colonic injury in PNL is very rare (<0.1 %). As mentioned previously the colon is more often located retrorenally in the prone compared to the supine position [16], thus theoretically this favours supine PNL with regard to patient safety. Colonic perforation should be suspected if the patient has intraoperative or immediate postoperative diarrhoea or hematochezia, signs of peritonitis, or passage of gas or faeces through the nephrostomy tract [33]. Usually, an abdominal CT with contrast injection into the nephrostomy tube will reveal the diagnosis and its extent. Due to the fact that the perforation is most often retroperitoneal, colonic injury following PNL is often asymptomatic, and in these situations an antegrade nephrostogram before nephrostomy removal may reveal the presence of contrast in the colon [34] (Fig. 7.11). Management most often can be done with conservative measures such as antibiotics, placement of a JJ stent and withdrawal of the nephrostomy tube into the colon under fluoroscopic guidance, creating a controlled colonic-cutaneous

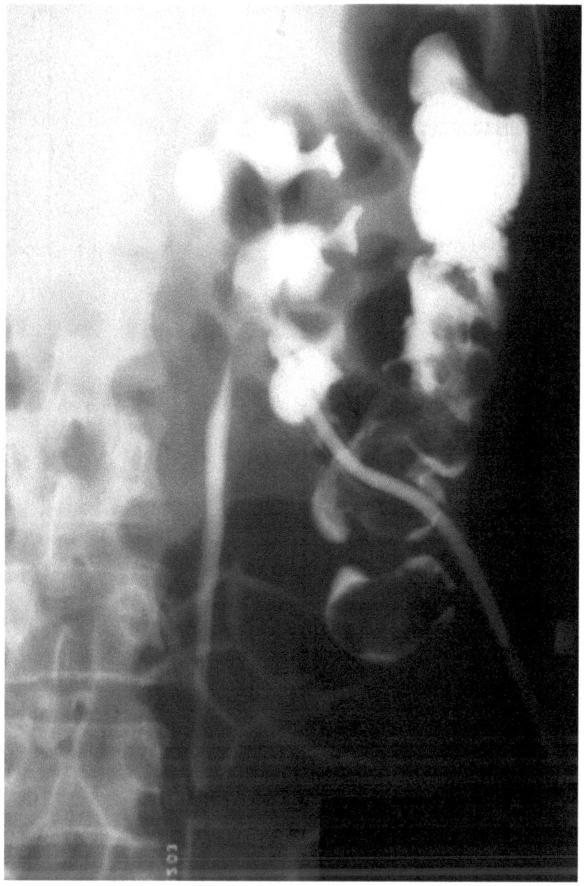

Fig. 7.11 Antegrade nephrostogram with contrast filling the descending colon. The patient was treated with antibiotics, a JJ stent and retraction of the nephrostomy tube to the colon under fluoroscopy guidance, creating a controlled fistula. The tube was later removed and the fistula closed spontaneously (The X-ray picture was kindly provided by Dr. Robert Swartz, Department of Urology, Örebro University Hospital, Örebro, Sweden)

fistula that usually closes spontaneously [33]. It is likely that minor retroperitoneal colonic injuries are never clinically diagnosed just presenting as fever and successfully treated by antibiotics alone. The fact that the occurrence of fever after PNL in the large CROES PCNL Global Study was significantly higher in prone PNL (11.1 %) compared to supine PNL (7.6 %) may in part be indicative of such a speculation [35].

Haemorrhage during and after PNL is usually venous and most often self-limiting. The most common causes of severe postprocedural renal haemorrhage are arteriovenous fistulas and pseudoaneurysms [36]. Often the bleeding presents as severe intermittent haemorrhage through the nephrostomy. In such instances the patient should undergo angiography with transarterial superselective embolization. This intervention should be considered early in the management of these cases because it is not only a life-saving but also ultimately a nephron-/kidney-sparing procedure [36]. The use of B-mode combined with

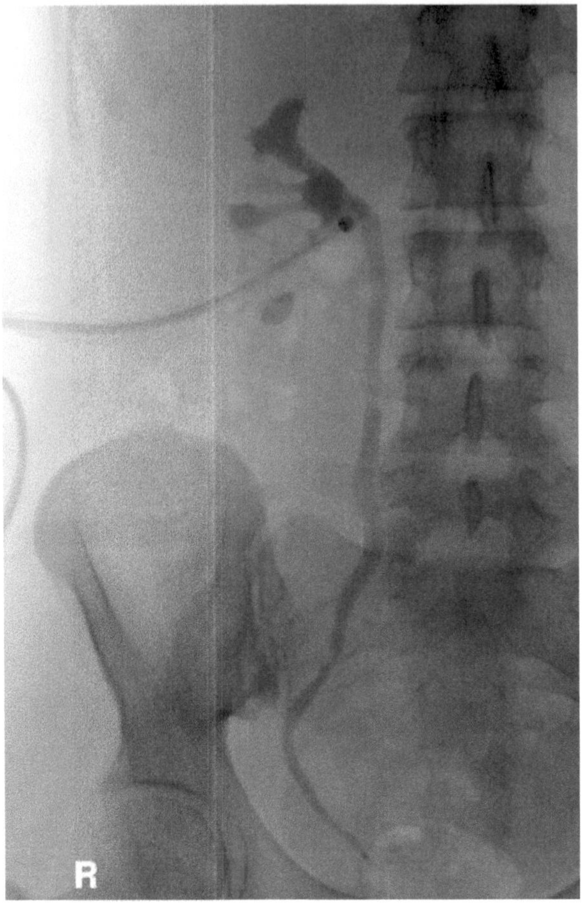

Fig. 7.12 Antegrade nephrostogram showing filling of the collecting system without filling defects and drainage to the bladder. The nephrostomy tube can be safely removed

colour Doppler ultrasound access guidance may avoid renal blood vessel injury during PNL [37].

7.4.2 Evaluation of Antegrade Drainage

Oedema of the ureteropelvic junction and the ureter may occur after stone removal in PNL. In most cases it is recommended that an antegrade nephrostogram (pyelography) is performed to assure adequate drainage before removal of the nephrostomy tube [1]. Furthermore, this examination potentially will localize residual stone fragments, thereby facilitating second-look flexible nephroscopy, and diagnose severe lesions of the collecting system as well as colon injuries (see above) [1]. Safe removal of the nephrostomy tube may be performed, when antegrade drainage has been confirmed [1] (Fig. 7.12).

7.4.3 Evaluation of Residual Stones

7.4.3.1 Intraoperative Imaging

Intraoperatively fluoroscopy is used for guidance of nephroscopy for detection of residual calculi. As outlined previously you may rely on the preoperative CT planning image (CTI) to determine whether the stone fragments are fluoroscopy positive [14]. Suspicion of residual radiolucent stones is aroused when filling defects are observed during contrast injection through the scope or through the retrogradely placed ureteral catheter. Aggressive nephroscopy in combination with high-magnification rotational fluoroscopy has been shown to be sensitive and specific with regard to intraoperative detection of residual fragments, enabling immediate removal of residuals, thereby potentially reducing the need for second-look nephroscopy [38].

7.4.3.2 Postoperative Imaging

Postoperative imaging for residual stone material is aimed at deciding whether the patient needs repeated nephroscopy, adjunctive ESWL or subsequent ureteroscopy. Also, decisions on the need for metaphylaxis may include postoperative image findings. Although medical therapy has been shown to reduce stone recurrence after ESWL, patients with residual fragments remain at higher risk for recurrence compared with patients rendered stone free, highlighting the importance of exact image studies [39].

Traditionally, KUB and/or nephrotomograms were used to determine whether the patient was stone free after a PNL. Subsequently, antegrade nephrostograms and/or second-look nephroscopy was used to better determine the stone-free status [40]. Since KUB and nephrotomograms have been found to overestimate stone-free status by 35 and 17 % [41], respectively, this evaluation scheme has been challenged. Pearle et al. prospectively evaluated 36 patients undergoing PNL for large or staghorn calculi [42]. All patients underwent KUB, NCCT and flexible nephroscopy on postoperative days 2 and 3. Using flexible nephroscopy as gold standard reference, NCCT had a sensitivity of 100 % and a specificity of 62 % compared with 46 and 82 %, respectively, for KUB [1, 42]. They concluded that selective use of flexible second-look nephroscopy after PNL based on CT-positive findings could avoid unnecessary operations and morbidity in 20 % of patients, corresponding to cost savings of over $100,000 per 100 patients [42]. The effectiveness of NCCT for detection of residual stones after PNL has subsequently been confirmed in other prospective studies [43, 44].

When addressing the importance of retained fragments following PNL, one has to remember that CT seems to overestimate the craniocaudal size of a stone by an average of 0.8 mm, whereas the transverse diameter measured on CT is accurate [45, 46].

Fowler et al. investigated the specificity and sensitivity of US in detecting renal calculi [47]. They found an overall sensitivity of 24 % and a specificity of 93 %. The sensitivity was size dependant with the highest sensitivity (71 %) in stone sizes above 7 mm. The poor sensitivity of US in detecting renal stones was confirmed in another study, in which it was additionally demonstrated that the sensitivity was poorer in the left kidney compared to the right kidney [48]. Although US – from the point of view of ionized radiation risk – is an appealing alternative, it does not seem to be accurate enough for residual fragment detection post-PNL.

Ionized radiation risk should be thoroughly considered, when planning follow-up regimen for kidney stone patients. In an evaluation of radiation exposure in acute and short-term management of urolithiasis at two large academic centres in the USA, it was found that a fifth of kidney stone patients received potentially harmful radiation doses in the short-term follow-up of an acute stone event [49]. This does not suggest that we as clinicians should avoid CT technology with its entire well-documented benefits in stone disease; rather, we should be well aware of the benefits and risks of all diagnostic procedures. In the case of evaluating residual stones following PNL, the risks of having a residual stone should outweigh the risks of ionized radiation exposure. This calls for selective evaluation, in which the high-sensitivity CT evaluation should be restricted to those patients who have a high risk of residuals and in whom the residual stones make an aggressive treatment mandatory, for instance, patients with infectious stones. In other patient categories less radiation-heavy examinations (KUB, US) may be considered. Furthermore, the urologists dealing with stone disease need to have a close relation to their uroradiologists, in order to set up selective evaluation protocols based on the population in question. For instance, children and adolescents with stone disease and patients who have previously undergone numerous CT examinations should be offered a limited radiation exposure examination. Ultra-low-dose CT protocols with radiation doses close to KUB have been developed [50], and in our experience such protocols may be equally excellent for post-PNL residual fragment evaluation; however, this needs further evaluation.

In conclusion, it is unquestionable that the applied imaging modality has a significant impact on the detection rate of residual stones and the estimated size of the residuals, which unequivocally affects clinical decision making. Nowadays there is no agreed-upon strategy for evaluation of residual stones following PNL. According to the arguments above mentioned, a selectivve approach seems advisable. Based on these considerations we suggest the following protocol:

- *Low risk of residual stones: No need of any postoperative imaging*
  Patients in whom the operation was uneventful and in whom residual stone fragments are unlikely, such as cases in which stone fragmentation was not needed (stones removed in toto) or only to a very limited extent. This patient category often could undergo a tubeless PNL.
- *Moderate risk of residual stones: KUB and antegrade nephrostogram on the first or second postoperative day*
  Patients with a large unbranched clearly radiopaque stone burden in whom significant stone fragmentation was needed, however, in whom endoscopic vision was unblurred.

– *High risk of residual stones: Low-dose NCCT and antegrade nephrostogram on the first or second postoperative day*
  Branched or multiple stones demanding significant fragmentation and multiple extractions, and patients in whom vision was blurred and intraoperative evaluation of residuals was unsatisfactory, including patients with large radiolucent and weak radiopaque stones.

Based on this evaluation scheme, the amount of ionized radiation is stratified according to the risk of the residual fragments, and safe removal of the nephrostomy tube can be assured. Patients subsequently could undergo flexible nephroscopy, ureteroscopy, ESWL, medical therapy and/or observation, depending on residual stone burden and location and other risk factors.

7.5 Future Imaging Scenarios

Percutaneous access to the renal collecting system continues to be a challenge, which is reflected in constant testing of new image modalities and puncture techniques [24]. Rotational fluoroscopy with in-OR high-quality reconstructed 3-D images for calculi localization and puncture guidance has been developed and shown to be an effective tool [38]. A 3-D US seems promising avoiding ionized radiation, and using this novel technique even US-guided robotic needle placement has been designed and tested experimentally [51]. Remaining future challenges with this technique include target motion compensation. Virtual projection of the ultrasound puncture tract onto fluoroscopic images as an aid to percutaneous renal access also has been introduced and evaluated clinically [52]. The system seems reliable and may prove to be of special value in the training setting [53]. Flat-panel volume CT has been shown to be applicable in other clinical interventional settings [54]. The major disadvantage of CT fluoroscopy is radiation exposure to the surgeon. This may in the future be overcome by robotic needle placement, which already has been developed for traditional fluoroscopic access [55]. Using a validated kidney model, this robot device even proved to be applicable as a telerobotic tool [56], which may be of value in a world with lack of experienced surgeons. Finally, a special needle system has been designed to assure successful entry into the collecting system [57]. The needle measures bioimpedance and a sharp drop in impedance means successful entry. However the needle does not assure a correct entry into the collecting system, which needs to be assured by imaging.

References

1. Park S, Pearle MS (2006) Imaging for percutaneous renal access and management of renal calculi. Urol Clin North Am 33:353–364
2. Jackman SV, Potter SR, Regan F, Jarrett TW (2000) Plain abdominal X-ray versus computerized tomography screening: sensitivity for stone localization after non-enhanced spiral computerized tomography. J Urol 164:308–310

3. Ray AA, Chung D-G, Honey JD (2009) Percutaneous nephrolithotomy in prone and prone-flexed positions: anatomic considerations. J Endourol 23:1607–1614
4. Honey JD, Wiesenthal JD, Ghiculette D, Pace SP, Ray AA, Pace KT (2011) Comparison of supracostal versus infracostal percutaneous nephrolithotomy using the novel prone-flexed position. J Endourol 25:947–954
5. Miller OF, Rineer SK, Reichard SR, Buckley RG, Donovan SM, Graham IR, Goff WB, Kane CJ (1998) Prospective comparison of unenhanced spiral computed tomography and intravenous urogram in the evaluation of acute flank pain. Urology 52:982–987
6. Pfister SA, Deckhart A, Laschke S, Dellas S, Otto U, Buitrago C, Roth J, Wiesner W, Bontgartz G, Gasser TC (2003) Unenhanced helical computed tomography vs intravenous urography in patients with acute flank pain: accuracy and economic impact in a randomized prospective trial. Eur Radiol 13:2513–2520
7. Shine S (2008) Urinary calculus IVU vs. CT renal stone? A critical appraised topic. Comput Biol Med 33:41–43
8. Patel U, Walkden RM, Ghani KR, Anson K (2009) Three-dimensional CT pyelography for planning of percutaneous nephrolithotomy: accuracy of stone measurement, stone depiction and pelvicalyceal reconstruction. Eur Radiol 19:1280–1288
9. Nolte-Emsting C, Cowan N (2006) Understanding multislice CT urography techniques: many roads lead to Rome. Eur Radiol 16:2670–2686
10. Thiruchelvam N, Mostafid H, Ubhayakar G (2005) Planning percutaneous nephrolithotomy using multidetector computed tomography urography, multiplanar reconstruction and three-dimensional reformatting. BJU Int 95:1280–1284
11. Scoffone CM, Cracco CM, Cossu M, Grande S, Poggio M, Scarpa RM (2008) Endoscopic combined intrarenal surgery in Galdakao-modified supine Valdivia position: a new standard for percutaneous nephrolithotomy? Eur Urol 54:1393–1403
12. Heyns CF, van Geldern WF (1990) 3-dimensional imaging of the pelvicalyceal system by computerized tomographic reconstruction. J Urol 144:1335–1338
13. Osther PJ, Razvi H, Liatsikos E, Averch T, Crisci A, Garcia JL, Mandal A, de la Rosette JJ (2011) Percutaneous nephrolithotomy among patients with renal anomalies: patient characteristics and outcomes; a subgroup analysis of the clinical research office of the endourological society global percutaneous nephrolithotomy study. J Endourol 25:1627–1632
14. Graumann O, Osther SS, Spasojevic D, Osther PJ (2012) Can the CT planning image determine whether a kidney stone is radiopaque on a plain KUB? Urol Res 40:333–337
15. Kalb B, Sharma P, Salman K, Ogan K, Martin DR (2010) Acute abdominal pain: is there a potential role for MRI in the setting of the emergency department in a patient with renal calculi? J Magn Reson Imaging 32:1012–1023
16. Hopper KD, Sherman JL, Lurthke JM, Ghaed N (1987) The retrorenal colon in the supine and prone patient. Radiology 162:443–446
17. Chalasani V, Bissoon D, Bhuvanagir AK, Mizzi A, Dunn IB (2010) Should PCNL patients have a CT in the prone position preoperatively? Can J Urol 17:5082–5086
18. Azhar RA, Szymanski KM, Lemercier E, Valenti D, Andonian S, Anidjar M (2011) Visceral organ-to-percutaneous tract distance is shorter when patients are placed in the prone position on bolsters compared with the supine position. J Endourol 25:687–690
19. Tuttle DN, Yeh BM, Meng MV, Breiman RS, Stoller ML, Coakley FV (2005) Risk of injury to adjacent organs with lower-pole fluoroscopically guided percutaneous nephrostomy: evaluation with prone, supine, and multiplanar reformatted CT. J Vasc Interv Radiol 16:1489–1492
20. Ng CS, Herts BR, Streem SB (2005) Percutaneous access to upper pole renal stones: role of prone 3-dimensional computerized tomography in inspiratory and expiratory phases. J Urol 173:124–126
21. Zarse CA, Hameed TA, Jackson ME, Pischalnikov YA, Lingemen JE, McAteer JA, Williams JC Jr (2007) CT visible internal stone structure, but not Hounsfield unit value, of calcium oxalate monohydrate (COM) calculi predicts lithotripsy fragility in vitro. Urol Res 35:201–206
22. Kim SC, Burns EK, Lingeman JE, Paterson RF, McAteer JA, Williams JC Jr (2007) Cystine calculi: correlation of CT-visible structure, CT number, and stone morphology with fragmentation by shock wave lithotripsy. Urol Res 35:319–324

23. Evans HJ, Wollin TA (2001) The management of urinary calculi in pregnancy. Curr Opin Urol 11:379–384
24. Kalogeropoulou C, Kallidonis P, Liatsikos EN (2009) Imaging in percutaneous nephrolithotomy. J Endourol 23:1571–1577
25. Ko R, Soucy F, Denstedt JD, Razvi H (2007) Percutaneous nephrolithotomy made easier: a practical guide, tips and tricks. BJU Int 101:535–539
26. Ibarluzea G, Scoffone CM, Cracco CM, Poggio M, Porpiglia F, Terrone C, Astobieta A, Camargo I, Gamarra M, Tempia A, Valdivia Uria JG, Scarpa RM (2007) Supine Valdivia and modified lithotomy position for simultaneous anterograde and retrograde endourological access. BJU Int 100:233–236
27. Eisner BH, Cloyd J, Stoller ML (2009) Lower-pole fluoroscopy-guided percutaneous renal access: which calix is posterior? J Endourol 23:1621–1625
28. Osman M, Wendt-Nordahl G, Heger K, Michel MS, Alken P, Knoll T (2005) Percutaneous nephrolithotomy with ultrasonography-guided renal access: experience from over 300 cases. BJU Int 96:875–878
29. Ghani KR, Patel U, Anson K (2009) Computed tomography for percutaneous access. J Endourol 23:1633–1639
30. Magnusson A, Radecka E, Lönnemark M, Raland H (2005) Computed-tomography-guided punctures using a new guidance device. Acta Radiol 46:505–509
31. Hellawell GO, Mutch SJ, Thevendran G, Wells E, Morgan RJ (2005) Radiation exposure and the urologist: what are the risks? J Urol 174:948–952
32. Ogan K, Corwin SC, Smith T, Watumull LM, Mullican MA, Cadeddu JA, Pearle MS (2003) Sensitivity of chest fluoroscopy compared with chest CT and chest radiography for diagnosing hydropneumothorax in association with percutaneous nephrostolithotomy. Urology 62:988–992
33. Traxer O (2009) Management of injury to the bowel during percutaneous stone removal. J Endourol 23:1777–1780
34. Goswami AK, Shrivatava P, Mukherjee A, Sharma SK (2001) Management of colonic perforation during percutaneous nephrolithotomy in horseshoe kidney. J Endourol 15:989–991
35. Valdivia JG, Scarpa RM, Duvdevani M, Gross AJ, Nadler RB, Nutahare K, de la Rosette JJ (2011) Supine versus prone position during percutaneous nephrolithotomy: a report from the Clinical Research Office of the Endourological Society Percutaneous Nephrolithotomy Global Study. J Endourol 25:1619–1625
36. Jain V, Ganpule A, Vyas J, Muthu V, Sabnis MRB, Rajapurkar MM, Desai MR (2009) Management of non-neoplastic renal hemorrhage by transarterial embolization. Urology 74:522–527
37. Lu M-H, Pu X-Y, Gao X, Zhou X-F, Qiu J-G, Si-Tu J (2010) A comparative study of clinical value of single B-mode ultrasound guidance and B-mode combined with color doppler ultrasound guidance in mini-invasive percutaneous nephrolithotomy to decrease hemorrhagic complications. Urology 76:815–820
38. Portis AJ, Laliberte MA, Drake S, Holtz C, Rosenberg MS, Bretzke CA (2006) Intraoperative fragment detection during percutaneous nephrolithotomy: evaluation of high magnification rotational fluoroscopy combined with aggressive nephroscopy. J Urol 175:162–166
39. Gettman MT, Pearle MS (2000) Evaluation of residual stones following percutaneous nephrolithotomy. Braz J Urol 26:579–583
40. Preminger GM (1999) Editorial comment. J Urol 162:314
41. Denstedt JD, Clayman RV, Picus DD (1991) Comparison of endoscopic and radiological residual fragment rate following percutaneous nephrolithotomy. J Urol 145:703–705
42. Pearle MS, Watamull LM, Mullican MA (1999) Sensitivity of noncontrast helical computerized tomography and plain film radiography compared to flexible nephroscopy for detecting residual fragments after percutaneous nephrolithotomy. J Urol 162:23–26
43. Park J, Hong B, Park T, Park HK (2007) Effectiveness of noncontrast computed tomography in evaluation of residual stones after percutaneous nephrolithotomy. J Endourol 21:684–687
44. Osman Y, El-Tabey N, Rafai H, Elnahas A, Shoma A, Eraky I, Kenwy M, El-Kapany H (2008) Detection of residual stones after percutaneous nephrolithotomy: role of nonenhanced spiral computerized tomography. J Urol 179:198–200

45. Narepalem N, Sundaram C, Boridy IC, Yan Y, Heiken JP, Clayman RV (2002) Comparison of helical computerized tomography and plain radiography for estimating urinary stone size. J Urol 167:1235–1238
46. Tisdale BE, Siemens DR, Lysack J, Nolan RL, Wilson JW (2007) Correlation of CT scan versus plain radiography for measuring urinary stone dimensions. Can J Urol 14:3489–3492
47. Fowler KAB, Locken JA, Duchesne JH, Williamson MR (2002) US for detecting renal calculi with nonenhanced CT as a reference standard. Radiology 222:109–133
48. Ulusan S, Koc Z, Tokmak N (2007) Accuracy of sonography for detecting renal stone: comparison with CT. J Clin Ultrasound 35:256–261
49. Ferrandino MN, Bagrodia A, Pierre SA, Scales CD, Rampersaud E, Pearle MS, Preminger GM (2009) Radiation exposure in the acute and short term management of urolithiasisat 2 academic centers. J Urol 181:668–673
50. Hyams ES, Shah O (2010) Evaluation and follow-up of patients with urinary lithiasis: minimizing radiation exposure. Curr Urol Rep 11:80–86
51. Boctor EM, Choti MA, Burdette EC, Webster RJ (2008) Three-dimensional ultrasound-guided robotic needle placement: an experimental evaluation. Int J Med Robot Comput Assist Surg 4:180–191
52. Mozer P, Conort P, Leroy A, Baumann M, Payan Y, Troccaz J, Chartier-Kastler E, Richard F (2007) Aid to percutaneous renal access by virtual projection of the ultrasound puncture tract onto fluoroscopic images. J Endourol 21:460–465
53. de la Rosette JJMCH, Laguna MP, Rassweiler JJ, Conort P (2008) Training in percutaneous nephrolithotomy – a critical review. Eur Urol 54:994–1003
54. Gupta R, Cheung AC, Bartling SH, Lisauskas J, Grasruck M, Leidecker C, Schmidt B, Flohr T, Brady TJ (2008) Flat-panel volume CT: fundamental principles, technology, and applications. Radiographics 28:2009–2022
55. Su L-M, Stoianovici D, Jarrett TW, Patriciu A, Roberts WW, Caddeddu JA, Ramakumar SY, Solomon SB, Kavoussi LR (2002) Robotic percutaneous access to the kidney: comparison with standard manual access. J Endourol 16:471–475
56. Challacombe B, Patriciu A, Glass J, Aron M, Jarrett T, Kim F, Pinto P, Stoianovici D, Smeeton N, Tiptaft R, Kavoussi L, Dasgupta P (2005) A randomized controlled trial versus robotic and telerobotic access to the kidney as the first step in percutaneous nephrolithotomy. Comput Aided Surg 10:165–171
57. Hernandez DJ, Sinkov VA, Roberts WW, Allaf ME, Patriciu A, Jarrett TW, Kavoussi LR, Stoianovici D (2001) Measurement of bio-impedance with a smart needle to confirm percutaneous kidney access. J Urol 166:1520–1523

Chapter 8
Anaesthesia for Supine and Modified Supine PNL

Adebanji A.B. Adeyoju and Neil Sutcliffe

Abstract Anaesthetists need to be aware of the difficulties and complications specific to PNL, a well-established endourological means of kidney stone removal. Although traditionally PNL has been performed in the semi-prone or prone position, more recently some centres have been successfully performing the procedure in a supine or modified supine position. This presents some significant advantages from the viewpoint of the anaesthetist, as well as a small number of disadvantages. However, many of the anaesthetist's concerns regarding PNL are similar whatever the position used. Patient's features and co-morbidities should be preliminarily evaluated in order to choose the best anaesthetic technique. Intraoperative management is also described, facing not only specific PNL complications such as blood loss or septic risk but also often overlooked issues including fluid balance and thermal control.

8.1 Introduction

Percutaneous nephrolithotomy (PNL) is well established as a surgical means of kidney stone removal, and anaesthetists need to be aware of the difficulties and complications specific to this surgery. Traditionally PNL has been performed in the semi-prone or prone position, more recently some centres have been successfully performing the procedure in a supine or modified supine position. This presents some significant advantages from the viewpoint of the anaesthetist, as well as a small number of disadvantages. However, many of the anaesthetist's concerns regarding PNL are similar whatever the position used.

A.A.B. Adeyoju, MB, BS, FRCS (Urol) (✉) • N. Sutcliffe, BSc, MBChB, FRCA, FFICM
Consultant Urological Surgeon, Department of Urology,
Stepping Hill Hospital NHS Foundation Trust, Stockport, SK2 7JE, UK
e-mail: banjibunmi@aol.com; neilsutcliffe@btinternet.com

C.M. Scoffone et al. (eds.), *Supine Percutaneous Nephrolithotomy and ECIRS*,
DOI 10.1007/978-2-8178-0459-0_8, © Springer-Verlag France 2014

8.2 Patient Considerations

8.2.1 Co-morbidities, Body Habitus

Naturally the anaesthetist's assessment of a patient for PNL starts preoperatively with a history and general examination of patient fitness. As always the cardiovascular, respiratory and airway status of the patient are foremost, but assessment of haemoglobin concentration, coagulation, renal function and current or recent episodes of urosepsis is also of particular interest, as are body habitus and any limitations of joint neck or spinal movement as these are of particular consideration for patient positioning and may occasionally preclude the use of the surgically preferable position.

Fortunately the majority of patients presented for PNL are reasonably fit and with little major organ dysfunction; however, renal stones are associated with a number of other conditions, and some patients present with significant co-morbidities either related or unrelated to their stone disease. There are associations with morbid obesity, paraplegia/quadriplegia and hypercalcaemia, amongst others, which may in themselves present challenges and difficulties for the anaesthetist. For surgery to be of acceptable risk, patients should be fit enough to undergo a prolonged procedure which is likely to require tracheal intubation and mechanical ventilation and has the potential for significant fluid shifts or bleeding. It should be borne in mind that stone disease is only rarely life threatening, and a very high perioperative risk of mortality or significant morbidity is not likely to be acceptable either to the operative team or to the patient.

8.2.2 Respiratory Diseases

Probably the most common important respiratory diseases presenting in such patients are chronic obstructive pulmonary disease, bronchial asthma, emphysema and bronchiectasis. Respiratory infection should be treated well before anaesthesia and surgery, and surgery delayed if required. Long-term treatment such as bronchodilators should be continued up to the time of surgery and reinstituted promptly postoperatively. As a long surgical procedure predisposes such patients to postoperative respiratory complications such as sputum retention, pneumonia, and respiratory failure, it is important that the patient's condition is at its best at the time of surgery. Respiratory physiotherapy should be readily available for such patients as required postoperatively.

If a patient's respiratory disease is felt to be too severe for general anaesthesia, it may be tempting to consider a regional anaesthetic technique. However bearing in mind the problems with this (dealt with later), and the significant risk of requiring conversion to general anaesthesia, such patients should probably be declined for surgery unless overwhelming reasons to proceed exist.

8.2.3 *Cardiovascular Diseases*

In common with other elective procedures, and as with respiratory disease, those patients with significant cardiovascular disease should be receiving optimal treatment for this prior to being presented for surgery. Although PNL in patients awaiting heart valve replacement might very occasionally be justified to reduce the risk of subsequent episodes of urosepsis and bacteraemia. Normally anti-angina, heart failure and antihypertensive medications should be continued as normal up until and on the day of surgery, with the possible exception of angiotensin-converting enzyme (ACE) inhibitors and angiotensin 2 receptor antagonists on the day of surgery. Anticoagulant drugs should be withheld prior to surgery in accordance with local guidelines. Antiplatelet agents should generally be withheld due to the risk of bleeding unless a risk-benefit assessment indicates otherwise.

Due to the risk of significant intraoperative fluid shifts, including occult bleeding, central venous pressure monitoring may be considered in patients with significant heart failure to avoid fluid overload, haemorrhagic anaemia and intraoperative ischaemia, although the difficulties of interpretation with changing patient positions should also be borne in mind. Patients with orthopnoea are unlikely to be able to tolerate such procedures under regional anaesthesia even if such techniques were otherwise being considered.

As with respiratory disease, in assessing the merits of surgery in patients with severe cardiovascular disease, it should be remembered that stone disease is not often life threatening.

8.2.4 *Renal Impairment*

Some degree of renal impairment is likely to be present in a large proportion of patients presenting for PNL, and this should obviously have been carefully considered by the surgical team during the patient's preoperative workup. Patients with borderline renal function, and especially those with a poorly or nonfunctioning kidney on the contralateral side, should be aware of the potential for being rendered dialysis dependent should rare major complications lead to significant decline in operated kidney function or the need for nephrectomy.

Perioperatively care should be taken to consider the avoidance of potentially nephrotoxic drugs, and it may sometimes be appropriate to avoid, for example, non-steroidal anti-inflammatory drugs and aminoglycosides. Severe renal impairment may change the pharmacodynamics and pharmacokinetics of some drugs, although this is less of a problem with modern anaesthetic agents. Due to possible renal parenchymal damage amongst other factors, it is possible that renal function may decline postoperatively at least initially.

8.3 Choice of Anaesthetic Technique

The choice of anaesthetic technique is a decision for the individual anaesthetist in discussion with the patient and with regard to the requirements of the surgery. Any technique considered needs to be suitable for a long surgical procedure whilst still allowing a reasonably rapid emergence. Although central neuraxial block is occasionally used in the prone position [1–4], few anaesthetists would use it for such potentially long procedures as many patients are unlikely to be able to tolerate prolonged prone positioning whilst fully conscious, and heavy sedation negates many of the advantages of regional anaesthetic techniques as well as potentially creating airway difficulties if excessive. The process of turning to prone is also likely to be frightening to many patients when conscious. The potential need for conversion to general anaesthesia is a major deterrent to regional anaesthesia in the prone position as it is likely to require the patient to be returned to the supine position for induction of general anaesthesia before returning to prone.

In contrast supine PNL appears on initial examination to be well suited to a regional anaesthetic technique with or without sedation. It is relatively comfortable for the patient and allows access to the airway for the anaesthetist if required. However the potential duration of the surgery will generally necessitate a continuous catheter technique such as epidural infusion, and accurate assessment of the level of the local anaesthetic block is difficult or impossible during the surgical procedure. Additionally many patients find it difficult to lie still for such long durations and may feel claustrophobic when surrounded by the mass of equipment required for the procedure. Furthermore some patients find high ambient temperatures around the upper body intolerable but may become hypothermic when these are reduced due to cooling at the surgical sites. Nevertheless PNL has even been performed with a simple peritubal local infiltration anaesthesia [5, 6].

General anaesthesia with tracheal intubation and controlled ventilation is probably the technique of choice in most PNL cases, whether prone or supine. General anaesthesia can ensure an immobile patient for prolonged periods, allows the maximum skin-surface availability for patient warming and facilitates core temperature probe placement in the oesophagus. Tracheal intubation provides a definitive secure airway which is unlikely to need intraoperative intervention, although supine PNL allows a selection of other airways, such as the laryngeal mask, to be considered where there is reason to avoid tracheal intubation. Controlled ventilation, as well as providing the most reliable gas exchange, has the additional benefit of a predictable (and potentially adjustable) movement of the kidney with respiration during the removal of difficult stone fragments. Despite occasionally very long operative durations, the combination of modern anaesthetic agents and the generally low opioid analgesic requirements in these patients still allows prompt emergence from anaesthesia at the end of surgery.

8.4 Intraoperative Considerations

8.4.1 Duration of the Procedure

PNL is highly variable in duration with surgical time varying from less than an hour to several hours and may indeed sometimes require more than one surgical session for complete stone clearance of just one kidney. Unfortunately so many factors influence the duration of the procedure (difficult kidney puncture, difficult dilation, stone size, location and hardness) that it becomes difficult for the anaesthetist to make accurate estimates in advance and this may influence both assessment of patient suitability and choice of anaesthetic technique. Longer procedures imply more complications, such as atelectasis, mucociliary dysfunction, sputum retention, bleeding, hypothermia, pressure injuries and prolonged recovery time [7, 8].

8.4.2 Patient Positioning

The traditional prone position as used for a number of procedures including PNL has long been known to present a number of hazards to the patient and difficulties to the anaesthetist [9]. Complications of the prone position are well described in standard anaesthetic textbooks [10, 11] and include respiratory and cardiovascular [12–15] difficulties due to abdominal compression [16], hyperextension of the arm at the shoulder and of the neck [17–20], pressure area injury including the face [21], blindness from orbital pressure and retinal vessel occlusion [22, 23] and neurological problems [24]. Inadvertent airway displacement in the prone position presents a major life-threatening emergency which may be very difficult to deal with successfully [25, 26]. The transition from a supine position to the prone one is a particular time for concern [27].

For prone PNL patients are initially placed in the lithotomy position and then are turned to the prone or semi-prone position. There is considerable potential for harm to the patient during turning, and it is essential to have adequate numbers of staff to perform this safely (at least 6 for most patients). Such staff should be familiar with the equipment to be used to support the patient in the prone position and with the normal (and the individual patient's) limitations of joint movements. The loss of normal muscle tone due to anaesthesia makes damage more likely to occur. Great care must also be taken not to displace venous, arterial or urinary catheters, and it is essential that the airway is kept secure. Care must also be taken to avoid undue pressure on vulnerable areas, especially the face and eyes. It is difficult to maintain continuous monitoring of the patient by the anaesthetist during the turn, and this may delay appropriate response to physiological changes such as hypotension or hypoxia. Once turned the patient should be positioned so that the abdomen is

Table 8.1 Anaesthesiological and urological equipment for PNL

Typical equipment for PNL	
Anaesthetic machine	X-ray C-arm and screens
Fluid warmer	Ultrasound machine
Forced-air patient warming device	Lithotripsy devices
	Nephroscope camera and screen
	Fluid irrigation
	Suction

relatively free, to avoid respiratory and cardiovascular embarrassment. This can be challenging or impossible in the very obese patient in the prone position. Exaggeration of the lumbar lordosis, which can make surgical access more difficult, is particularly difficult to achieve in the semi-prone position without undesirable pressure on the abdomen (see also Chaps. 8 and 10).

In marked contrast to the prone position [28], the supine position for PNL requires fewer personnel and presents much less opportunity for injury to the patient. Care must be taken here to avoid too localised a pressure, to avoid pressure on the sciatic nerve, and to tilt the pelvis and thorax equally to avoid stress on the lumbar spine. Additionally the thoracolumbar spine should be kept straight or with a bend away from the operative side to "open up" the renal angle. It is easy to inadvertently allow the patient's pelvis/abdomen to slide away from the operative side at this point (bending the spine concave to the operative side) which makes ultrasound and surgical access difficult. The arm on the operative side should be positioned so as to allow easy surgical and X-ray access and may be held in a gutter above the patient's upper chest or adducted across the chest with a sling. The advantages of this position compared to the prone position are many for the anaesthetist: access to the airway is still relatively easy, as is access to the neck if central venous cannulation becomes necessary; there is no pressure on the abdomen avoiding splinting of the diaphragm and vena cava compression; and it is easy to maintain proper monitoring throughout.

8.4.3 Intraoperative Anaesthetic Management

PNL is a very equipment-dependent procedure, and this can significantly impair the anaesthetist's access to the anaesthetised patient (Table 8.1); this is in addition to instrument trolleys and the surgical and scrub team. A large operating theatre is a significant advantage. Some centres perform PNL in the X-ray department, and if this is proposed careful consideration should be made as to the feasibility of positioning ancillary equipment properly, as well as the logistics for dealing with any rare major surgical complications. This should include provision to transport the anaesthetised patient to an available operating theatre at short notice. Anaesthetic equipment, staffing and support, including recovery, should be of equivalent standard to that provided in the operating theatres.

Due to the large amount of equipment required simultaneously for the procedure, it is helpful if the anaesthetist is able to work at some distance from the patient, and this may involve the use of longer ventilator tubing, intravenous fluid line extensions, longer monitoring leads, etc. Similarly access to the patient may be hindered intraoperatively, especially in the prone position. Although rarely required for this procedure, any invasive monitoring such as intra-arterial and central venous catheters should be placed before surgery and is allowed to commence, and there should be a low threshold for its use in view of the difficulty in inserting such devices intraoperatively (although the supine position minimises this difficulty).

8.4.4 Thermal Issues

In addition to standard anaesthetic monitoring, true core temperature monitoring is highly recommended, ideally with an oesophageal temperature probe (if the prone position is used, a rectal temperature probe may be placed after turning prone). The length of the procedure predisposes patients to intraoperative hypothermia [7, 8, 29] with its attendant risks, and active patient warming and temperature monitoring is mandatory; forced air or equivalent warming should be applied to as much of the body surface area as possible whilst maintaining surgical access. This can be more difficult to achieve in the supine position as continued access to the perineum is desired by the surgeon and the legs are more difficult to warm in the lithotomy position. Intravenous fluids should be warmed, as should surgical irrigation which can amount to many tens of litres. Despite these measures mild intraoperative hypothermia is common; however, occasional patients may become pyrexial, either due to overly effective warming or due to release of organisms or toxins from the stone, and may even require cooling measures. Core temperature monitoring gives effective warning of these problems.

8.4.5 Fluid Balance and Blood Loss

Fortunately major blood loss during PNL is not common, although the large proportion of cardiac output taken by the kidneys emphasises the potential for major haemorrhage on occasion. Venous access should be of sufficiently large bore to cope with this, especially as patient access to allow insertion of additional cannulae may be difficult. Serum samples should have been saved preoperatively to allow provision of cross-matched blood in a timely fashion should it be required. Blood loss is difficult to assess due to the large volumes of irrigating fluid in which lost blood is diluted. Modern point-of-care instruments allow rapid assessment of haemoglobin concentration from capillary blood obtained by fingerprick which may help guide the requirement for intraoperative transfusion. Due to the risk of significant intraoperative fluid shifts, including occult or occasional brisk bleeding and involving the inability to monitor urine output, central venous pressure monitoring may be considered in patients with significant heart failure to avoid fluid overload, haemorrhagic anaemia and intraoperative ischaemia.

8.4.6 Sepsis

Mention has already been made of the possibility of intraoperative sepsis, and it is helpful if the organisms responsible for an individual patient's previous episodes of urosepsis, and their antibiotic sensitivities, are known in order to allow the provision of rational prophylactic and therapeutic antibiotic treatments intraoperatively and postoperatively.

8.5 Postoperative Considerations

8.5.1 Pain

The surgical procedure itself produces relatively little nociceptive stimulation and hence a relatively small intraoperative analgesic requirement and the need for only light anaesthesia. However the dilatation of the access tract from skin to calyx is more stimulating, and it is helpful if the surgical team can warn the anaesthetist when this is imminent to ensure the provision of adequate analgesia/muscle relaxation to prevent patient movement at this time.

Postoperative pain is only rarely problematic, and only small or moderate doses of opioids are usually required in addition to simple analgesics such as paracetamol. Prolonged postoperative central neural blockade (i.e. epidural analgesia) is generally not warranted.

Again, fluid balance, renal function, rewarming and sepsis are central issues in the postoperative phase.

8.6 Conclusions

In summary the supine position for PNL has many advantages for the anaesthetist. It allows a potentially greater range of anaesthetic techniques to be used, it allows access to the airway and neck veins and it allows the positioning of some patients who could not be safely managed in the prone position (e.g. the particularly obese). By avoiding a hazardous turn to prone, it presents fewer opportunities for inadvertent harm to come to the patient. Due to the considerable time taken to properly position patients prone, the supine position for PNL is also likely to result in shorter anaesthetic times once the theatre teams are familiar with the procedure. Anaesthetists providing anaesthesia for PNL in the traditional positions are encouraged to discuss with their surgical colleagues the merits of the supine procedure.

References

1. Karacalar S, Bilen CY, Sarihasan B, Sarikaya S (2009) Spinal-epidural anesthesia versus general anesthesia in the management of percutaneous nephrolithotripsy. J Endourol 23:1591–1597
2. Kuzgunbay B, Turunc T, Akin S et al (2009) Percutaneous nephrolithotomy under general versus combined spinal-epidural anesthesia. J Endourol 23:1835–1838
3. Singh V, Sinha RJ, Sankhwar SN, Malik A (2011) A prospective randomized study comparing percutaneous nephrolithotomy under combined spinal-epidural anesthesia with percutaneous nephrolithotomy under general anesthesia. Urol Int 87:293–298
4. Tangpaitoon T, Nisoog C, Lojanapiwat B (2012) Efficacy and safety of percutaneous nephrolithotomy (PCNL): a prospective and randomized study comparing regional epidural anesthesia with general anesthesia. Int Braz J Urol 38:504–511
5. Chen Y, Zhou Z, Sun W et al (2011) Minimally invasive percutaneous nephrolithotomy under peritubal local infiltration anesthesia. World J Urol 29:773–777
6. Parikh GP, Shah VR, Modi MP, Chauchan NC (2011) The analgesic efficacy of peritubal infiltration of 0.25 % bupivacaine in percutaneous nephrolithotomy – a prospective randomized study. J Anasesthesiol Clin Pharmacol 27:481–484
7. Rozentsveig V, Neulander EZ, Roussabrov E et al (2007) Anesthetic considerations during percutaneous nephrolithotomy. J Clin Anesth 19:351–355
8. Vorrakitpokatorn P, Permtongchuchai K, Raksamani EO, Phettongkam A (2006) Perioperative complications and risk factors of percutaneous nephrolithotomy. J Med Assoc Thai 89:826–833
9. Akhavan A, Gainsburg DM, Stock JA (2010) Complications associated with patient positioning in urologic surgery. Urology 76:1309–1316
10. Anderton J (1991) The prone position for the surgical patient: a historical review of the principles and hazards. Br J Anaesth 67:452–463
11. Edgecombe H, Carter K, Yarrow S (2008) Anaesthesia in the prone position. Br J Anaesth 100:165–183
12. Borthakur B, Garg R (2011) Arrhythmias in prone position. J Anaesthesiol Clin Pharmacol 27:420
13. Dube SK, Bharti SJ, Rath GP (2011) Frequent ventricular contractions under anaesthesia in prone position. J Anaesthesiol Clin Pharmacol 27:142–143
14. Ho JD, Dawes DM, Moore JC et al (2011) Effect of position and weight force on inferior vena cava diameter – implications for arrest-related death. Forensic Sci Int 212:256–259
15. Leslie K, Wu CY, Bjorksten AR et al (2011) Cardiac output and propofol concentrations in prone surgical patients. Anaesth Intensive Care 39:868–874
16. Yu M, Leng Y, Bai Y et al (2011) The evaluation of the effect of body positioning on intra-abdominal pressure measurement and the effect of intra-abdominal pressure at different body positioning on organ function and prognosis in critically ill patients. J Crit Care 27:222.e1–222.e6
17. Anusionwu IM, Wright EJ (2011) Compartment syndrome after positioning in lithotomy: what a urologist needs to know. BJU Int 108:477–481
18. Anderton J, Schady W, Markham D (1994) An unusual cause of postoperative brachial plexus palsy. J Anaesth 72:605–607
19. Schwartz D, Drummond D, Hahn M et al (2000) Prevention of positional brachial plexopathy during surgical correction of scoliosis. Spinal Disord 13:178–182

20. Winfree C, Kline D (2005) Intraoperative positioning nerve injuries. Surg Neurol 63:5–18
21. Addla SK, Rajpal S, Sutcliffe N, Adeyoju A (2008) A simple aid to improve patient positioning during percutaneous nephrolithotomy. Ann R Coll Surg Engl 90:433–434
22. Agah M, Ghasemi M, Roodneshin F et al (2011) Prone position in percutaneous nephrolithotomy and postoperative visual loss. Urol J 8:191–198
23. Tempelhoff R (2008) An optic nerve at risk and a prolonged surgery in the prone position. Anaesthesiology 108:775–776
24. Langmayr J, Ortler M, Obwegeser A, Felber S (1996) Quadriplegia after lumbar disc surgery. Spine 21:1932–1935
25. Barak M, Putilov V, Meretyk S, Halachmi S (2010) ETView tracheoscopic ventilation tube for surveillance after tube position in patients undergoing percutaneous nephrolithotomy. Br J Anaesth 104:501–504
26. Singh G, Manikandan S, Neema PK (2011) Endotracheal tube fixation in neurosurgical procedure operated in prone position. J Anaesthesiol Clin Pharmacol 27:574–575
27. Wu SD, Yilmaz M, Tamul PC et al (2009) Awake endotracheal intubation and prone patient self-positioning: anesthetic and positioning considerations during percutaneous nephrolithotomy in obese patients. J Endourol 23:1599–1602
28. Atkinson CJ, Turney BW, Noble JG et al (2011) Supine vs prone percutaneous nephrolithotomy: an anaesthetist's view. BJU Int 108:306–309
29. Roberts S, Bolton DM, Stoller ML (1994) Hypothermia associated with percutaneous nephrolithotomy. Urology 44:832–835

Chapter 9
Prone PNL: Is It Still the Gold Standard? Review and Results

Thomas Knoll

Abstract Conventionally PNL is performed with the patient in the prone position, and the present chapter reviews the "classic" standard technique in this position. Prone PNL has proven to be effective and safe in all situations, in spite of the potential advantages of the supine PNL. Its indications are identical in any position and can also be expanded, exploiting the advent of the mini-PNL approach. The option of simultaneous retrograde access makes supine position an interesting alternative for selected cases, although nowadays prone PNL can still be considered the gold standard.

9.1 Introduction

The introduction of percutaneous nephrolithotomy (PNL) in the 1970s marked a turning point in the interventional treatment of nephrolithiasis. For the first time minimally invasive removal of larger kidney stones, which had hitherto required open surgery, became possible [1, 2].

However, the advent of Extracorporeal Shock Wave Lithotripsy (ESWL) during the 1980s led to the decline in the use of PNL, due in part to the former's perceived lack of associated complications. The situation changed again when both patients' preferences and economic demands required a faster stone removal. Improvements in instruments and lithotripsy technology (including flexible and digital nephroscopes) have expanded the indications and efficacy of percutaneous stone removal with stone-free rates up to >90 % [3].

T. Knoll
Department of Urology, Klinikum Sindelfingen-Boeblingen,
Arthur-Gruber-Street 70, 71065 Sindelfingen, Germany
e-mail: t.knoll@klinikverbund-suedwest.de

C.M. Scoffone et al. (eds.), *Supine Percutaneous Nephrolithotomy and ECIRS*,
DOI 10.1007/978-2-8178-0459-0_9, © Springer-Verlag France 2014

Conventionally PNL is performed with the patient in the prone position. In a bid to improve patients' outcome, several surgeons have experimented with different aspects of PNL. The commonest of these has been the positioning of the patient, with increasing authors reporting favorable results using the supine position [4–8]. This chapter reviews the "classic" standard technique with the patient in prone position. The indications of prone and supine PNL, extensively discussed in Chap. 3, are principally identical, with some pros and cons for each position depending on the individual cases which are mentioned later in this chapter.

9.2 Renal Access

The success of PNL depends on the ability of achieving an optimal access tract. A subcostal tract through the posterior middle or the inferior calyx is considered ideal for most stone localizations. This part of the kidney has the lowest vessel density and is therefore the safest approach [9–11]. A more detailed discussion of the renal spatial and vascular anatomy is presented in Chap. 4. In some situations an upper pole or even a multi-tract access might be required to achieve best stone clearance [12–14]. However, multiple tracts are associated with significantly increased complication rate (25 % vs. 45 %), in particular of the hemorrhagic ones [13, 14], and are only used in special circumstances. The use of simultaneous antegrade and retrograde stone manipulation, discussed in Chap. 9, associated or not with the use of flexible endoscopes, has been shown to reduce the need of multiple punctures without compromising stone-free rates [15, 16]. As mentioned above, an upper pole puncture in some cases is the best access. It is however associated with increased complications including bleeding and injury to adjacent viscera (liver, spleen, or pleura) [17–19]. In our opinion, simultaneous fluoroscopy- and ultrasound-guided access provides maximum safety by visualizing all these surrounding structures of the kidney [20–23]. In a large consecutive series, we did not observe any injury to neighboring structures [23]. Of equal importance is that the percutaneous surgeon establishes the renal access by himself. Watterson et al. demonstrated in a nice comparative series that this leads to both a higher stone-free and reduced complication rate when compared to access by a radiologist [24]. The different dilation and stone disintegration systems as well as the placement of nephrostomies after stone removal are not related to patient positioning and are discussed elsewhere.

9.3 Expanding Indications: Mini-PNL

While PNL is the treatment of choice for renal calculi larger than 20 mm [25], ESWL is recommended for smaller renal calculi by most urolithiasis guidelines [25, 26]. However, ESWL regularly requires repeated treatment sessions, and therefore, patient and urologist often require investing a lot of time before stone clearance is achieved. Furthermore, in a substantial number of patients, residual fragments remain within the kidney [27, 28], and the success rates of ESWL treatment for lower-pole stones are often unsatisfying [29, 30]. On the other hand, several authors have demonstrated that PNL achieves excellent stone-free rates irrespective of stone burden and has reasonable low complication rates [23, 30, 31]. This has led to expanded indications for PNL in many centers, even for smaller calculi [32].

The so-called mini-PERC or mini-PNL (mPNL) was first described by Jackman et al. for percutaneous nephrolithotomy in infants [33]. The use in adults has subsequently been described by several groups during the last years [34–36]. To date, the term mini-PNL has not been standardized and in general sheath diameters below 20 F are considered miniaturized. Nagele et al. and Lahme et al. have used 18 and 15 F access tracts, respectively, while Jackman et al. has used one as small as 11 F [32, 34, 36 F]. The potential reduction in PNL-associated morbidity is the main advantage of miniaturized instruments, requiring a reduced tract dilation and less renal trauma. This is desirable in all patients, especially in the infant [37]. Very recently, the very experienced group of Desai demonstrated a higher hemoglobin drop after conventional PNL compared to mPNL [38]. This is confirmed by the series of Giusti who reported lower hematocrit drop and lack of blood transfusions after mPNL [39]. The main drawback of reduced sheaths diameters is the increased operative time due to reduced irrigation flow and the need for more extensive stone disintegration [35, 39]. Finally, Li and coworkers prospectively evaluated the systemic response to PNL (30 F) and mPNL (14–18 F) without noticing differences between both techniques [40]. In our own series, both conventional PNL and tubeless mPNL were effective and safe procedures [35]. The efficacy of stone removal and complication rates did not show significant differences. As expected, there was a tendency to longer operating times despite the smaller stone mass for mPNL due to the required extensive stone fragmentation. In conclusion, the benefit of mPNL remains undefined and will be subject of further studies.

9.4 Results of PNL in Prone Position

The success rate of PNL depends on stone mass, stone localization, and the individual anatomic situation [41]. The overall stone-free rate after PNL ranges from 71 to 95 %, depending on stone size and localization, which corresponds to our own results [23, 25, 41–43]. We achieved a total stone-free rate of 96.5 % after 4 weeks; 67 % of our patients were stone-free or had insignificant residual stones after one single PNL procedure, while 33 % needed supplementary operations (second-look PNL, ESWL, or ureterorenoscopy).

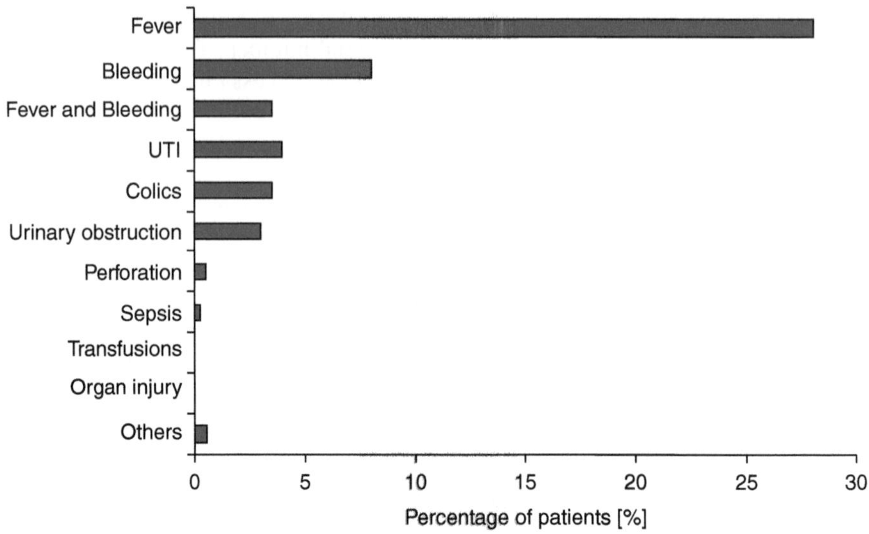

Fig. 9.1 Complications after percutaneous stone removal, data shown as percentage of patients [23]

While PNL is recommended for renal stones of more than 2 cm, the situation is different for the lower pole [44, 45]. Stone-free rate of ESWL for lower-pole stones is poor because disintegrated fragments do not pass [46]. The Lower Pole Study Group demonstrated that for a mean stone size of 1.4 cm, PNL achieved a stone-free rate of 95 % compared to only 37 % after ESWL [30]. A Cochrane analysis, based on only three studies with sufficient data quality, confirmed the superiority of PNL versus ESWL for the lower pole [47]. Therefore, for this location PNL is recommended even for smaller fragments of about 1.5 cm [26].

Several studies have shown excellent results of PNL even for difficult anatomic situations, such as horseshoe kidneys and ectopic or even transplant kidneys [48–51]. Obesity may increase the challenge to the surgeon but usually does not significantly limit treatment outcome [52].

PNL-related complications have been reported to be as high as 83 %, though in our own series, we observed complications in only 50.8 % of the procedures [23, 41, 53]. Most of them were clinically insignificant and could be managed conservatively; no blood transfusions or open surgery was required (Fig. 9.1). We believe the reasons for this are twofold: firstly the appropriate choice and positioning of the puncture into the desired calyx under ultrasound and fluoroscopic guidance and secondly the procedures were performed by a well-trained surgeon. Moreover, we performed most of our procedures using a subcostal approach, which may – apart from the use of ultrasound – further explain the absence of intrathoracic complications in our series. These excellent results, demonstrated in Table 9.1, illustrate that PNL in prone position remains the gold standard, with which alternatives have to compete with.

Table 9.1 Indications success and complication rates for PNL

	Mean stone size (cm)	% Stone free rate	% of ancillary procedures needed[a]	Hospital stay (days)	% Complication rate
Lower pole stones	0.5–10	70–100	4–62.5	3–6	13–38
Calyceal diverticula	0.2–3	76–100	0.04–18	2–15	0–30
Horseshoe kidneys	All sizes	72–87.5	8.3–33	3–10	8–29
Children	All sizes	67–100	0–32	1–11	0–28
Bilateral PNL	All sizes	76–100	3–81	11–21	3–25
Obesity	All sizes	60–100	14–45	2–10	0–37
Previous surgery	Up to 3	51–92	27–78	3–7	13.6–24
Lateral decubitus and supine position	All sizes	66.6–89	7.5–33.3	2.5[b]	0–17
Mini–PNL	0.1–10.62[c]	62.5–100	9–68	1–5	0–17.5

Adapted from 2nd International Consultation on Stone Disease 2008
[a]% of more than one PNL or additional ESWL/URS procedures needed to render the patients stone free
[b]Average hospital stay
[c]Stone size in cm^2

9.5 Is Prone PNL Still the Gold Standard?

PNL has been performed successfully with the patient in prone position for decades. Increasingly, though, authors are reporting impressive results with different variations of the supine position [7, 8, 54, 55]. What are the potential advantages of PNL in supine or modified lithotomy position? A ureteral catheter is usually placed prior to PNL for better visualization of the renal collecting system. As this procedure is performed in lithotomy position, the patient has to be turned on the operation table into prone position. Apart from this potentially time-consuming maneuver, other limitations include the placement in prone could be limited in patients with difficult anatomy (as severe kyphosis or lordosis), the anesthesiological risk might be higher and management of anesthesia problems could be demanding, and lastly surgeons have a higher radiation exposure [7].

The major advantage of supine PNL that has contributed to the wide spread of this technique is the option of simultaneous retrograde and antegrade stone management. This technique has been established in a modified supine lithotomy position [6, 56].

Apart from this true advantage, other potential benefits of supine PNL such as decreased operating time and less anaesthesiological problems are yet to be confirmed. In contrast, de la Rosette et al. demonstrated in a meta-analysis that most peri- and postoperative parameters were comparable between prone and supine PNL [5]. For obese patients, their analysis indicates even an advantage for prone positioning. This is important, because obese patients usually have a higher ASA score and would therefore probably benefit of supine positioning and a significant portion of PNL patients is obese. Furthermore, as large renal stone burden seems to be related to obesity and the metabolic syndrome complex, these patients may be candidates for upper pole or multi-tract PNL. However, several authors have demonstrated that supracostal accesses are difficult (and often impossible) to establish in supine position [5, 57]. Another important issue to consider is the higher learning curve associated with supine PNL [7, 58].

The meta-analysis of de la Rosette et al. is in accordance to the results of the Clinical Research Office of the Endourological Society (CROES). The CROES study is the largest published database including more than 5,700 patients [41]. Very recently, Valdivia et al. have published a subanalysis investigating the impact of patient positioning on outcome and complication rate [59]. In this series, the majority of procedures were performed in prone position (80.3 %). The mean operating time was significantly lower for prone versus supine position (82.7 vs. 90.1 min.). It is important to note that the method of tract dilation had not impact on operating time. Stone-free rate was higher for prone position (77.0 % vs. 70.2 %, $p<0.0001$). On the other hand, more patients received blood transfusions (6.1 % vs. 4.3 %, $p=0.026$) and developed fever (11.1 % vs. 7.6 %, $p=0.001$) in the prone group. Slightly more treatment attempts failed in prone position (2.7 % vs. 1.5 %, $p=0.01$). Although this series impresses with the very high number patients, it is questionable whether the described differences reflect clinical reality. The data was collected in 96 global centers, with each of them having its own standards. This includes important parameters as methods to assess stone-free rates and calculating operating times. More importantly, the term supine was used for different positions, from flat supine to elevated lithotomy positions.

This underlines that the discussion on the best patient positioning is still open and further studies have to identify advantages and disadvantages of both options.

9.6 Conclusions

PNL in prone position has proven to be effective and safe in all situations, while supine positioning has limitations that may negate its potential advantages. While the option of simultaneous retrograde access makes supine position an interesting alternative for selected cases, no study has yet demonstrated its overall advantage to prone. Considering this lack of evidence, PNL in prone position remains the gold standard.

References

1. Alken P, Hutschenreiter G, Günther R et al (1981) Percutaneous stone manipulation. J Urol 125:463–466
2. Fernstrom I, Johansson B (1976) Percutaneous pyelolithotomy. A new extraction technique. Scand J Urol Nephrol 10:257–259
3. Kim SC, Kuo RL, Lingeman JE (2003) Percutaneous nephrolithotomy: an update. Curr Opin Urol 13:235–241

4. Cracco CM, Scoffone CM, Poggio M et al (2010) The patient position for PNL: does it matter? Arch Ital Urol Androl 82:30–31
5. de la Rosette JJ, Tsakiris P, Ferrandino MN et al (2008) Beyond prone position in percutaneous nephrolithotomy: a comprehensive review. Eur Urol 54:1262–1269
6. Scoffone CM, Cracco CM, Cossu M et al (2008) Endoscopic combined intrarenal surgery in Galdakao-modified supine Valdivia position: a new standard for percutaneous nephrolithotomy? Eur Urol 54:1393–1403
7. Cormio L, Annese P, Corvasce T et al (2007) Percutaneous nephrostomy in supine position. Urology 69:377–380
8. Manohar T, Jain P, Desai M (2007) Supine percutaneous nephrolithotomy: effective approach to high-risk and morbidly obese patients. J Endourol 21:44–49
9. Sampaio FJ (2000) Renal anatomy. Endourologic considerations. Urol Clin North Am 27:585–607
10. Sampaio FJ, Passos MA (1992) Renal arteries: anatomic study for surgical and radiological practice. Surg Radiol Anat 14:113–117
11. Sampaio FJ, Aragao AH (1990) Anatomical relationship between the intrarenal arteries and the kidney collecting system. J Urol 143:679–681
12. Aron M, Yadav R, Goel R et al (2005) Multi-tract percutaneous nephrolithotomy for large complete staghorn calculi. Urol Int 75:327–332
13. Netto NR Jr, Ikonomidis J, Ikari O et al (2005) Comparative study of percutaneous access for staghorn calculi. Urology 65:659–662
14. Muslumanoglu AY, Tefekli A, Karadag MA et al (2006) Impact of percutaneous access point number and location on complication and success rates in percutaneous nephrolithotomy. Urol Int 77:340–346
15. Ganpule AP, Mishra S, Desai MR (2009) Multiperc versus single perc with flexible instrumentation for staghorn calculi. J Endourol 23:1675–1678
16. Lahme S, Zimmermanns V, Hochmuth A et al (2008) Stones of the upper urinary tract. Update on minimal-invasive endourological treatment. Arch Ital Urol Androl 80:13–17
17. Lang E, Thomas R, Davis R et al (2009) Risks, advantages, and complications of intercostal vs subcostal approach for percutaneous nephrolithotripsy. Urology 74:751–755
18. Schaeffer AJ, Handa SE, Lingeman JE et al (2008) Transsplenic percutaneous nephrolithotomy. J Endourol 22:2481–2484
19. Lojanapiwat B, Prasopsuk S (2006) Upper-pole access for percutaneous nephrolithotomy: comparison of supracostal and infracostal approaches. J Endourol 20:491–494
20. Fu YM, Chen QY, Zhao ZS et al (2011) Ultrasound-guided minimally invasive percutaneous nephrolithotomy in flank position for management of complex renal calculi. Urology 77:40–44
21. Basiri A, Ziaee AM, Kianian HR et al (2008) Ultrasonographic versus fluoroscopic access for percutaneous nephrolithotomy: a randomized clinical trial. J Endourol 22:281–284
22. Knoll TM, Michel MS, Alken P (2007) Surgical Atlas. Percutaneous nephrolithotomy: the Mannheim technique. BJU Int 99:213–231
23. Osman M, Wendt-Nordahl G, Heger K et al (2005) Percutaneous nephrolithotomy with ultrasonography-guided renal access: experience from over 300 cases. BJU Int 96:875–878
24. Watterson JD, Soon S, Jana K (2006) Access related complications during percutaneous nephrolithotomy: urology versus radiology at a single academic institution. J Urol 176:142–145
25. Preminger GM, Assimos DG, Lingeman JE et al (2005) Chapter 1: AUA guideline on management of staghorn calculi: diagnosis and treatment recommendations. J Urol 173:1991–2000
26. Tiselius HG, Ackermann D, Alken P et al (2001) Guidelines on urolithiasis. Eur Urol 40:362–371
27. El-Assmy A, El-Nahas AR, Madbouly K et al (2006) Extracorporeal shock-wave lithotripsy monotherapy of partial staghorn calculi. Prognostic factors and long-term results. Scand J Urol Nephrol 40:320–325
28. Osman MM, Alfano Y, Kamp S et al (2005) 5-year-follow-up of patients with clinically insignificant residual fragments after extracorporeal shockwave lithotripsy. Eur Urol 47:860–864

29. Pearle MS, Lingeman JE, Leveillee R et al (2005) Prospective, randomized trial comparing shock wave lithotripsy and ureteroscopy for lower pole caliceal calculi 1 cm or less. J Urol 173:2005–2009
30. Albala DM, Assimos DG, Clayman RV et al (2001) Lower pole I: a prospective randomized trial of extracorporeal shock wave lithotripsy and percutaneous nephrostolithotomy for lower pole nephrolithiasis-initial results. J Urol 166:2072–2080
31. Lingeman JE, Siegel YI, Steele B et al (1994) Management of lower pole nephrolithiasis: a critical analysis. J Urol 151:663–667
32. Nagele U, Schilling D, Sievert KD et al (2008) Management of lower-pole stones of 0.8 to 1.5 cm maximal diameter by the minimally invasive percutaneous approach. J Endourol 22: 1851–1853
33. Jackman SV, Hedican SP, Peters CA et al (1998) Percutaneous nephrolithotomy in infants and preschool age children: experience with a new technique. Urology 52:697–701
34. Nagele U, Horstmann M, Sievert KD et al (2007) A newly designed Amplatz sheath decreases intrapelvic irrigation pressure during mini-percutaneous nephrolitholapaxy: an in-vitro pressure-measurement and microscopic study. J Endourol 21:1113–1116
35. Knoll T, Wezel F, Michel MS et al (2010) Do patients benefit from miniaturized tubeless percutaneous nephrolithotomy? A comparative prospective study. J Endourol 24:1075–1079
36. Lahme S, Bichler KH, Strohmaier WL et al (2001) Minimally invasive PCNL in patients with renal pelvic and calyceal stones. Eur Urol 40:619–624
37. Bilen CY, Kocak B, Kitirci G et al (2007) Percutaneous nephrolithotomy in children: lessons learned in 5 years at a single institution. J Urol 177:1867–1871
38. Mishra S, Sharma R, Garg C et al (2011) Prospective comparative study of Miniperc and standard PNL for treatment of 1 to 2 cm size renal stone. BJU Int 108:896–899
39. Giusti G, Piccinelli A, Taverna G et al (2007) Miniperc? No, thank you! Eur Urol 51: 810–814
40. Li LY, Gao X, Yang M et al (2010) Does a smaller tract in percutaneous nephrolithotomy contribute to less invasiveness? A prospective comparative study. Urology 75:56–61
41. de la Rosette J, Assimos D, Desai M et al (2011) The Clinical Research Office of the Endourological Society Percutaneous Nephrolithotomy Global Study: indications, complications, and outcomes in 5803 patients. J Endourol 25:11–17
42. Segura JW, Patterson DE, LeRoy AJ et al (1985) Percutaneous removal of kidney stones: review of 1,000 cases. J Urol 134:1077–1081
43. Preminger GM (2010) High burden and complex renal calculi: aggressive percutaneous nephrolithotomy versus multi-modal approaches. Arch Ital Urol Androl 82:37–40
44. Knoll T, Tasca A, Buchholz NP (2011) Treatment of small lower pole calculi–SWL vs. URS vs. PNL? Arch Ital Urol Androl 83:6–9
45. Preminger GM (2006) Management of lower pole renal calculi: shock wave lithotripsy versus percutaneous nephrolithotomy versus flexible ureteroscopy. Urol Res 34:108–111
46. Elbahnasy AM, Clayman RV, Shalhav AL et al (1998) Lower-pole caliceal stone clearance after shockwave lithotripsy, percutaneous nephrolithotomy, and flexible ureteroscopy: impact of radiographic spatial anatomy. J Endourol 12:113–119
47. Srisubat A, Potisat S, Lojanapiwat B et al (2009) Extracorporeal shock wave lithotripsy (ESWL) versus percutaneous nephrolithotomy (PCNL) or retrograde intrarenal surgery (RIRS) for kidney stones. Cochrane Database Syst Rev: CD007044
48. Rana AM, Bhojwani JP (2009) Percutaneous nephrolithotomy in renal anomalies of fusion, ectopia, rotation, hypoplasia, and pelvicalyceal aberration: uniformity in heterogeneity. J Endourol 23:609–614
49. Liatsikos EN, Kallidonis P, Stolzenburg JU et al (2010) Percutaneous management of staghorn calculi in horseshoe kidneys: a multi-institutional experience. J Endourol 24:531–536
50. Stein RJ, Desai MM (2007) Management of urolithiasis in the congenitally abnormal kidney (horseshoe and ectopic). Curr Opin Urol 17:125–131
51. Gross AJ, Fisher M (2006) Management of stones in patients with anomalously sited kidneys. Curr Opin Urol 16:100–105

52. Bagrodia A, Gupta A, Raman JD et al (2008) Impact of body mass index on cost and clinical outcomes after percutaneous nephrostolithotomy. Urology 72:756–760
53. Michel MS, Trojan L, Rassweiler JJ (2007) Complications in percutaneous nephrolithotomy. Eur Urol 51:899–906
54. Clayman RV (2005) Supine position is safe and effective for percutaneous nephrolithotomy. J Urol 174:601–602
55. Shoma AM, Eraky I, El-Kenawy MR et al (2002) Percutaneous nephrolithotomy in the supine position: technical aspects and functional outcome compared with the prone technique. Urology 60:388–392
56. Scoffone CM, Cracco CM, Poggio M et al (2010) Endoscopic combined intrarenal surgery for high burden renal stones. Arch Ital Urol Androl 82:41–42
57. De Sio M, Autorino R, Quarto G et al (2008) Modified supine versus prone position in percutaneous nephrolithotomy for renal stones treatable with a single percutaneous access: a prospective randomized trial. Eur Urol 54:196–202
58. Tanriverdi O, Boylu U, Kendirci M et al (2007) The learning curve in the training of percutaneous nephrolithotomy. Eur Urol 52:206–211
59. Valdivia JG, Scarpa RM, Duvdevani M et al (2011) Supine versus prone position during percutaneous nephrolithotomy: a report from the Clinical Research Office of the Endourological Society Percutaneous Nephrolithotomy Global Study. J Endourol 25:1619–1625

Chapter 10
Endoscopic Combined IntraRenal Surgery (ECIRS): Rationale

Cesare Marco Scoffone, Cecilia Maria Cracco, and Roberto Mario Scarpa

Abstract The present chapter reviews the rationale of ECIRS (Endoscopic Combined IntraRenal Surgery), the logical evolution of PNL and of the old prone split-leg position. ECIRS would not exist without the Galdakao-modified supine Valdivia position, specifically supporting this versatile antero-retrograde approach to the upper urinary tract. ECIRS is a synergic approach in all its aspects, being a combination of retrograde intrarenal surgery (RIRS) and antegrade PNL and including essential intraoperative interactions among all operators (urologists, anaesthesiologists, nurses, scrub nurse, radiology technician, with the respective armamentaria), rigid and flexible instruments, endoscopes and accessories, intraoperative imaging techniques for renal puncture, ECIRS itself, and other surgical techniques. The anesthesiological, urological, and management advantages of ECIRS are described in detail.

10.1 Introduction

Percutaneous nephrolithotomy (PNL) has been practiced for more than 35 years and is still considered the treatment of choice for the management of large volume and/or otherwise complex renal stones [1]. From its introduction in the 1970s [2, 3],

C.M. Scoffone, MD (✉) • C.M. Cracco, MD, PhD
Department of Urology, Cottolengo Hospital,
Via Cottolengo 9, 10152 Torino, Italy
e-mail: scoof@libero.it; cecilia.cracco@libero.it

R.M. Scarpa
Department of Urology, San Luigi Hospital, University of Torino,
Regione Gonzole, 10, 10043 Orbassano, Torino, Italy
e-mail: romasca@tiscali.it

C.M. Scoffone et al. (eds.), *Supine Percutaneous Nephrolithotomy and ECIRS*,
DOI 10.1007/978-2-8178-0459-0_10, © Springer-Verlag France 2014

PNL procedure has undergone considerable evolution, mainly driven by the improvement in access techniques, endoscopic instrumentation technology, lithotripsy devices, and drainage management [4]. The consequent progressive improvement in PNL outcomes confirmed its essence of minimally invasive approach.

All the same, although considered safe and effective in expert hands, PNL requires experience and permanent training and is not exempt from specific intra- and postoperative complications including visceral injury, hemorrhage requiring blood transfusions, and infectious events. Efforts have been made to decrease PNL perioperative morbidity, starting from the issue of patient positioning, often overlooked in the past and only recently recognized as a critical part of this as of any other surgical procedure, thus a real matter of discussion.

10.2 The Conventional Prone Position for PNL

The conventional position for PNL has always been the prone one in the past, because – as explained in Chap. 1 – initially the radiologists aimed at the direct puncture of the renal pelvis without passing through the renal parenchyma. Also when puncturing the kidney via the calyceal papilla became the habit, it was not considered necessary to modify the patient's position.

The traditional prone position (Figs. 10.1 and 10.2) presents some advantages but also a number of disadvantages [5, 6], mainly anaesthesiological and related to the difficulties of performing a simultaneous retrograde access to the kidney (Tables 10.1 and 10.2).

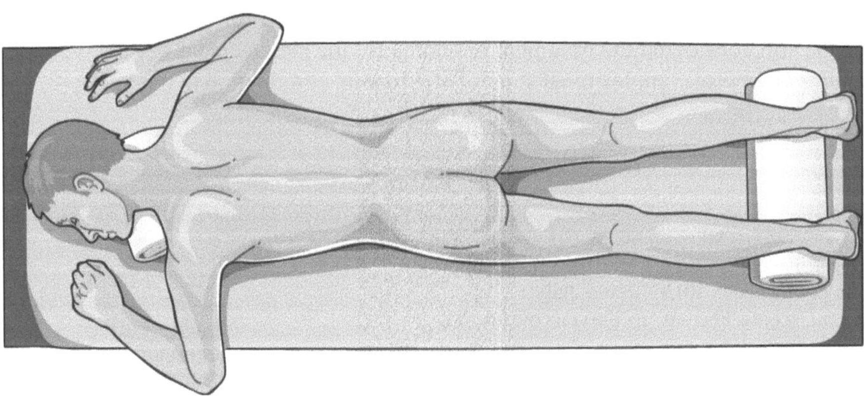

Fig. 10.1 Prone decubitus – frontal view (© Carole Fumat)

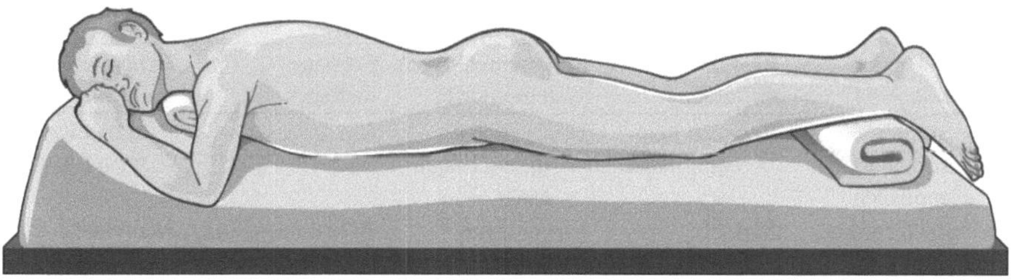

Fig. 10.2 Prone decubitus – lateral view (© Carole Fumat)

Table 10.1 Advantages and disadvantages of the prone position

Advantages	Disadvantages
Wide surgical field for renal puncture	Patient discomfort
Easier upper calyceal puncture	Difficult retrograde access if needed
Enough room for nephroscopic manipulation	Need of several nurses for intraoperative change of the decubitus from lithotomic to prone
Feasibility of bilateral procedures	Increased radiological hazard to the urologist's hands operating within the fluoroscopic field
Lower risk of lung, liver, and spleen injury with an upper pole puncture	Anesthesiological difficulties (especially in obese, kyphotic, and debilitated patients)
Good distension of the collecting system	A more evident risk of iatrogenic injuries (mainly peripheral nerve damage and compartment syndrome)

10.3 Modifications of the Prone Position for PNL

Several modifications of the prone position have been proposed during the years, mainly in order to gain the possibility of a working retrograde access to the renal cavities, and only recently to obviate the recognized anesthesiological problems. This trend is going on in the recent surgical practice and literature, with urologists from all over the world reporting their experience with alternative positions for PNL:

- The reverse lithotomy position [7];
- The lateral decubitus [8–10];
- The prone split-leg position [1–12];
- The flank position [13, 14];
- The prone-flexed position [15, 16];
- The split-leg modified lateral position [17];
- The complete supine position [18–21];
- The modified supine position [22];
- The Valdivia supine position [23–25];
- The supine-oblique position [26];
- The semisupine position [27];
- The Galdakao-modified supine Valdivia position [4–6, 28–31].

Table 10.2 Anaesthesiological problems in the prone position

Cardiovascular problems	Respiratory difficulties	Peripheral nervous system injuries	Pressure damages	Ischemic accidents
Reduced left ventricular compliance	Reduced lung compliance	Upper limbs (ulnar, radial, etc.)	Lip necrosis	Partial or total visual loss
Decreased cardiac output	Risk of endotracheal tube kinking	Lower limbs (peroneal, sciatic, saphenous, etc.)	Breast necrosis	Hemiparesis
Reduced venous return and venous stasis	Reduced thorax expansion for ribs compression by the body weight	Compartment syndromes	Liver necrosis	Quadriplegia
Increased risk of thromboembolic complications			Rhabdomyolysis	Aphasia
Poor access in case of unforeseen cardiovascular complications				
Increased heart rate and total peripheral vascular resistance				

10.4 The Supine and the Modified Supine Positions for PNL

As already mentioned in previous chapters, the supine position – conceived in the late 1980s and pioneered by Gabriel Valdivia Urìa – only recently started to gain acceptance and diffusion among urologists (Figs. 10.3 and 10.4).

In particular, we appreciated from the very beginning the modification of the supine Valdivia position proposed by Gaspar Ibarluzea, called the Galdakao-modified supine Valdivia (GMSV) position (Figs. 10.5 and 10.6), which we found extremely innovative, versatile, and handy. This position (see Chap. 11) combines the supine decubitus with a modified lithotomy position of the legs, presents few disadvantages, and optimally supports a versatile combined approach to the upper urinary tract, being safe, effective, ergonomic, and extremely appreciated by anesthesiologists as well (Table 10.3) [32–38].

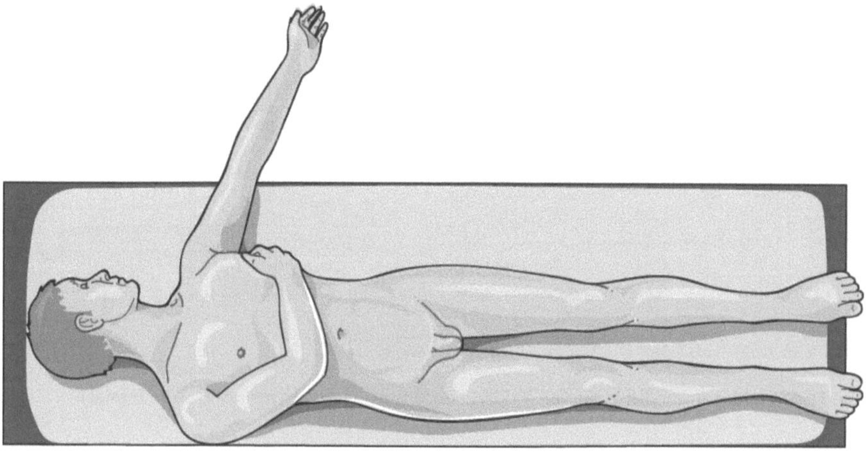

Fig. 10.3 Supine decubitus (Valdivia position) – frontal view (© Carole Fumat)

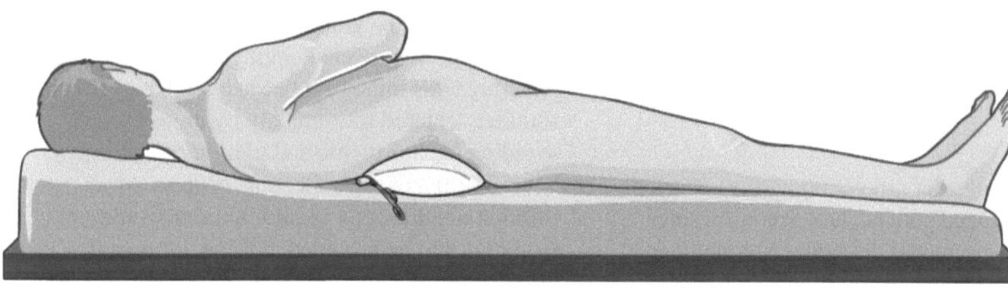

Fig. 10.4 Supine decubitus (Valdivia position) – lateral view (© Carole Fumat)

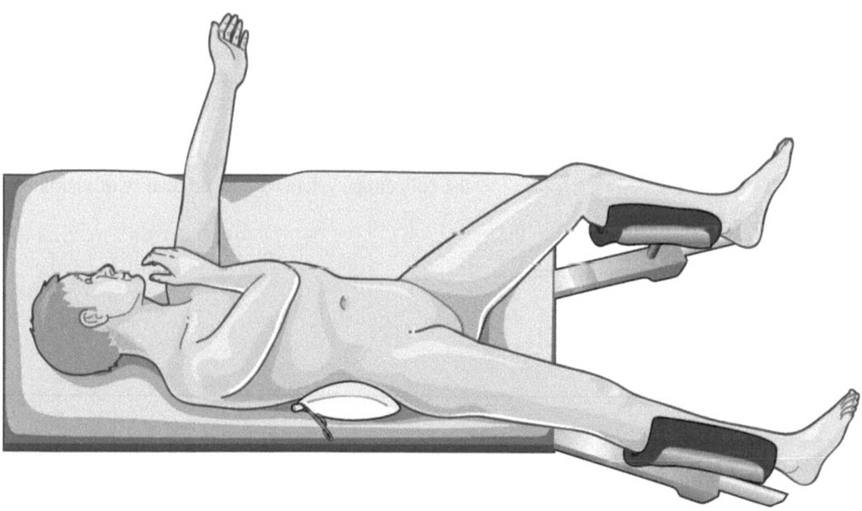

Fig. 10.5 Galdakao-modified supine Valdivia decubitus – frontal view (© Carole Fumat)

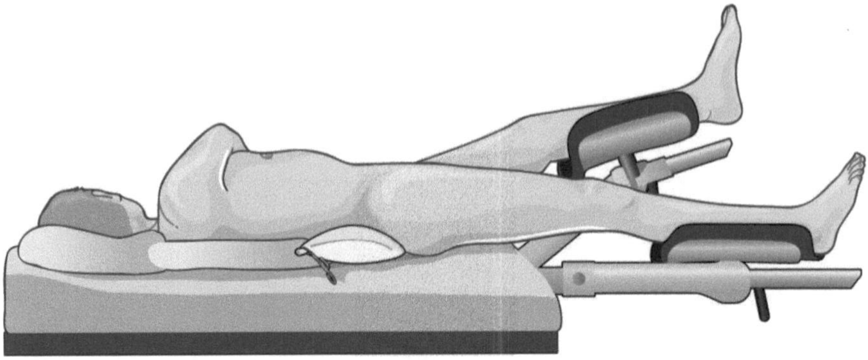

Fig. 10.6 Galdakao-modified supine Valdivia decubitus – lateral view (© Carole Fumat)

Table 10.3 Advantages and disadvantages of the supine and supine-derived positions

Advantages	Disadvantages
Easy and comfortable patient positioning	The upper pole of the kidney is deeply located within the rib cage = More challenging superior calyceal puncture (less important because such calyces are routinely entered retrogradely by ureteroscopy, avoiding hepatosplenic and pleuric risk of injury)
No need of repositioning the anaesthetized patient (less need of trained personnel, less occupational load due to shifting of heavy loads, a single sterile draping)	Decreased filling of the collecting system = More difficult nephroscopy (additional retrograde irrigation can be provided, but low intrarenal pressures imply less risk of pyelovenous back flow and septic risk)
The surgeon works sitting and with the hands outside the fluoroscopic field	More mobile kidney = More difficult puncture (constant counterpressure on the abdomen has been suggested during the access)
Combined retrograde approach (with all implications)	Longer tract length = Need of extralong equipment in obese patients, decreased nephroscope mobility, more torque on renal parenchyma meaning more bleeding risk
Optimal cardiovascular and airways control	Air bubbles produced during lithotripsy accumulate in the collecting system = Reduced quality of vision
Less risk of colon injury	
Less overall X-ray exposure (for the retrograde endoscopic contribution)	
Better descending drainage and retrieval of stone fragments (the tract is horizontal or slightly inclined downwards)	

10.5 ECIRS (Endoscopic Combined IntraRenal Surgery)

ECIRS would not exist without the GMSV position [5, 28]. In fact, this position specifically and optimally supports this versatile antero-retrograde approach to the upper urinary tract.

ECIRS is a synergic approach in all its aspects, starting from the fact that it is a combination of retrograde intrarenal surgery (RIRS) and PNL and going on with the intraoperative interaction among all operators (urologists, anaesthesiologists, nurses, scrub nurse, radiology technician, with the respective armamentaria); between retrograde and antegrade access; between rigid and flexible instruments; between endoscopes and accessories; among fluoroscopy, ultrasound, and Endovision technique for renal puncture; and between ECIRS itself and other surgical techniques like open surgery; laparoscopy, for instance, in case of associated ureteropelvic junction (UPJ) stricture; and Extracorporeal Shock Wave Lithotripsy (ESWL), in very selected and particular cases.

Although versatile in itself and rather complex at a first glance, ECIRS has been from the very beginning [5, 28] a completely standardized procedure, with the final aim to critically afford each step and maximize its safety, efficacy, and repeatability. The freedom of the urologist performing ECIRS lies in the fact that he/she is not the uncritical executor of a crystallized sequence of established steps, but rather an active figure continuously exerting his/her critical mind and choosing the best strategy for an optimal outcome, constantly related to the anatomical and clinical condition of the patient.

Among the urological advantages of a combined approach to the upper urinary tract like that allowed by ECIRS, we wish to underline:

- The role of the preliminary RIRS (for a baseline endoscopic evaluation of stone hardness, position, and mobility, possibly suggesting a change of indication from PNL to RIRS, and of concomitant ureteral stones or ureteral or UPJ stenosis to be simultaneously treated);
- The importance of performing renal puncture, tract dilation, and Amplatz sheath application under visual control, when possible;
- The possibility to prepare the maximally guaranteed "kebab patient," with the guidewire entering the kidney through the percutaneous tract and exiting the external urethral meatus, in order to have the complete control of the endoscopic field;
- The chance of avoiding multiple tracts and related bleeding risk by accessing calyces parallel to the percutaneous tract, thanks to the aid of the retrograde flexible ureteroscopy and the contemporary use of flexible nephroscope;
- The final visual ureteroscopic assessment of the stone-free status (integrating flexible nephroscopy) with the visual check of all calyces, which we call "Grand Tour" (with reduced radiological exposure for both the patient and the surgeon and the possibility of completing the procedure or planning a second look);
- The final endoscopic evaluation not only of renal cavities for a tubeless procedure but also of UPJ and ureter in order to decide for a stentless PNL;
- The overall reduced radiation exposure of the patient (and in particular children and young women) during the whole procedure, thanks to the integration of the direct visual information with radiological imaging.

It should be underlined that prone and supine PNL are in any case similar in terms of feasibility, safety, and efficacy [39–43]. Nonetheless, all published works only consider classical parameters such as operation time, stone-free rate, or complication rates (bleeding, transfusions, urosepsis, visceral injury). We believe that safety should be considered from a wider point of view, including the variety of anesthesiological risks reported for the prone position [31–38], poorly perceived by urologists but very familiar to anaesthesiologists, neurosurgeons, or orthopaedics in fields of surgery in which it is unavoidable. Even one of those devastating – although rare – ischemic, cardiovascular, or neurological complications reported in the literature, sometimes implying long-term or irreversible consequences, is unacceptable for the treatment of a benign pathology such as urolithiasis, unless life threatening in itself. The precautionary principle must be the first step of all medical or surgical procedures, and we believe that the supine position for PNL fulfils this principle under all points of view.

10.6 Conclusions

Surgery should not be a dogmatic field, where the new techniques are seen like heresy or even nonsense. We have the instruments for checking the value of a new technique. ECIRS is the logical evolution of PNL and of the old prone split-leg position [10, 11], exploiting the surgeon's versatility and adherence to the patient's clinical needs, thanks to the use of a variety of technically updated instruments and accessories. In fact, new technological advancements and innovative instruments and accessories require the urologist to make the effort to consensually evolve his surgical technique, in order to fully exploit such progresses. ECIRS proposal has the additional merit of having triggered a large amount of critical analysis of the patient's positioning and of various PNL steps.

As to ECIRS, now well known and practiced all around the world, we can conclude with the words of the late Latin poet Horace: "*maiores pinnas nido extendisse*" (Ep. 1, 20, 21), meaning "have now spread the wings larger than the nest."

References

1. Türk C, Knoll T, Koehrmann KU (2008) New guidelines for urinary stone treatment. Controversy or development? Urologe A 47:591–593
2. Guenther R, Alken P, Altwein JE (1978) Percutaneous nephro-pyelostomy applications and results. Rofo 128:720–726
3. Alken P, Hutschenreiter G, Günter R, Marberger M (1981) Percutaneous stone manipulation. J Urol 125:463–466
4. Cracco CM, Scoffone CM, Scarpa RM (2011) New developments in percutaneous techniques for simple and complex branched renal stones. Curr Opin Urol 21:154–160
5. Scoffone CM, Cracco CM, Cossu M et al (2008) Endoscopic combined intrarenal surgery in Galdakao-modified supine Valdivia position: a new standard for percutaneous nephrolithotomy? Eur Urol 54:1393–1403
6. Cracco CM, Scoffone CM (2011) ECIRS (Endoscopic Combined IntraRenal Surgery) in the Galdakao-modified supine Valdivia position: a new life for percutaneous surgery? World J Urol 29:821–827

7. Lehman T, Bagley DH (1988) Reverse lithotomy modified prone position for simultaneous nephroscopic and ureteroscopic procedures in women. Urology 32:529–531
8. Kerbl K, Clayman RV, Chandhoke PS et al (1994) Percutaneous stone removal with the patient in the flank position. J Urol 151:686–688
9. Gofrit ON, Shapiro A, Donchin A et al (2002) Lateral decubitus position for percutaneous nephrolithotripsy in the morbidly obese or kyphotic patient. J Endourol 16:383–386
10. El-Husseiny T, Moraitis K, Maan Z et al (2009) Percutaneous endourologic procedures in high-risk patients in the lateral decubitus position under regional anesthesia. J Endourol 23:1603–1606
11. Scarpa RM, Cossu FM, De Lisa A et al (1997) Severe recurrent ureteral stricture, the combined use of an anterograde and retrograde approach in the prone-split-leg position without X-rays. Eur Urol 31:254–256
12. Grasso M, Nord R, Bagley DH (1993) Prone split leg and flank roll positioning: simultaneous anterograde and retrograde access to the upper urinary tract. J Endourol 7:307–310
13. Karami H, Rezaei A, Mohammadhosseini M et al (2010) Ultrasonography-guided percutaneous nephrolithotomy in the flank position versus fluoroscopy-guided percutaneous nephrolithotomy in the prone position: a comparative study. J Endourol 24:1357–1361
14. Jang WS, Choi KH, Yang SC, Han WK (2011) The learning curve for flank percutaneous nephrolithotomy for kidney calculi: a single surgeon's experience. Korean J Urol 52: 284–288
15. Ray AA, Chung DG, Honey RJ (2009) Percutaneous nephrolithotomy in the prone and prone-flexed positions: anatomic considerations. J Endourol 23:1607–1614
16. Honey RJ, Wiesenthal JD, Ghiculete D et al (2011) Comparison of supracostal versus infracostal percutaneous nephrolithotomy using the novel prone-flexed patient position. J Endourol 25:947–954
17. Lezrek M, Ammani A, Bazine K et al (2011) The split-leg modified lateral position for percutaneous renal surgery and optimal retrograde access to the upper urinary tract. Urology 78:217–220
18. Shoma AM, Eraky I, El-Kenawy MR et al (2002) Percutaneous nephrolithotomy in the supine position: technical aspects and functional outcome compared with the prone technique. Urology 60:388–392
19. Ng MT, Sun WH, Cheng CW, Chan ES (2004) Supine position is safe and effective for percutaneous nephrolithotomy. J Endourol 18:469–474
20. Steele D, Marshall V (2007) Percutaneous nephrolithotomy in the supine position: a neglected approach? J Endourol 21:1433–1437
21. Falahaktar S, Moghaddam AA, Salhei M et al (2008) Complete supine percutaneous nephrolithotripsy comparison with the prone standard position. J Endourol 22:2513–2517
22. Chedid Neto EA, Mitre AI, Mendes Gomes C et al (2007) Percutaneous nephrolithotripsy with the patient in a modified supine position. J Urol 178:165–168
23. Valdivia Uria JG, Lanchars E, Villaroya S (1987) Percutaneous nephrolithectomy: simplified technique (preliminary report). Arch Esp Urol 40:177–180
24. Valdivia Uria JG, Valle GJ, Villaroya S (1990) Why is percutaneous nephroscopy still performed with the patient prone? J Endourol 4:269–272
25. Valdivia Uria JG, Valle GJ, Lopez Lopez JA et al (1998) Technique and complications of percutaneous nephroscopy: experience with 557 patients in the supine position. J Urol 160:1975–1978
26. Arrabal-Polo MA, Arrabal-Martin M, Saz T, Paiz P (2011) Emergency percutaneous nephrostomy in supine-oblique position without cushion. Urol Res 39:521–522
27. Xu KW, Huang J, Guo ZH et al (2011) Percutaneous nephrolithotomy in semisupine position: a modified approach for renal calculus. Urol Res 39:467–475
28. Ibarluzea G, Scoffone C, Cracco CM et al (2007) Supine Valdivia and modified lithotomy position for simultaneous anterograde and retrograde urological access. BJU Int 100:233–236
29. Daels F, Gonzalez MS, Freire FG et al (2009) Percutaneous lithotripsy in Valdivia-Galdakao decubitus position: our experience. J Endourol 23:1615–1620
30. Miano R, Scoffone C, De Nunzio C et al (2010) Position: prone or supine is the issue of percutaneous nephrolithotomy. J Endourol 24:931–938

31. Hoznek A, Rode J, Ouzaid I et al (2012) Modified supine percutaneous nephrolithotomy for large kidney and ureteral stones: technique and results. Eur Urol 61:164–170
32. Agah M, Ghasemi M, Roodneshin F et al (2011) Prone position in percutaneous nephrolithotomy and postoperative visual loss. Urol J 8:191–196
33. Akhavan A, Gainsburg DM, Stock JA (2010) Complications associated with patient positioning in urologic surgery. Urology 76:1309–1316
34. Anusionwu IM, Wright EJ (2011) Compartment syndrome after positioning in lithotomy: what a urologist needs to know. BJU Int 108:477–481
35. Edgcombe H, Carter K, Yarrow S (2008) Anaesthesia in the prone position. Br J Anaesth 100:165–183
36. Ho JD, Dawes DM, Moore JC et al (2011) Effect of position and weight force on inferior vena cava diameter – implications for arrest-related deaths. Forensic Sci Int 212:256–259
37. Rau CS, Liang CL, Lui CC et al (2002) Quadriplegia in a patient who underwent posterior fossa surgery in the prone position. J Neurosurg 96(1 Suppl):101–103
38. Tempelhoff R (2008) An optic nerve at risk and a prolonged surgery in the prone position. Anesthesiology 108:775–776
39. De Sio M, Autorino R, Quarto G et al (2008) Modified supine versus prone position in percutaneous nephrolithotomy for renal stones treatable with a single percutaneous access: a prospective randomized trial. Eur Urol 54:196–203
40. De La Rosette JJ, Tsakiris P, Ferrandino MN et al (2008) Beyond prone position in percutaneous nephrolithotomy: a comprehensive review. Eur Urol 54:1262–1269
41. Liu L, Zheng S, Xu Y, Wei Q (2010) Systematic review and meta-analysis of percutaneous nephrolithotomy for patients in supine versus prone position. J Endourol 24:1941–1946
42. Wu P, Wang L, Wang K (2011) Supine versus prone position in percutaneous nephrolithotomy for kidney calculi: a meta-analysis. Int Urol Nephrol 43:67–77
43. Arrabal-Martin M, Arrabal-Polo MA, Lopez-Leon V et al (2012) The oblique supine decubitus position: technical description and comparison of results with the prone decubitus and dorsal decubitus positions. Urol Res 40:587–592

Chapter 11
ECIRS: Patient Positioning and Organization of the Operating Room

András Hoznek, Francisco Pedro Juan Daels, Michael N'Tege Kimuli, Cecilia Maria Cracco, and Cesare Marco Scoffone

Abstract A standardized patient positioning and operating room organization are fundamental in order to perform a successful ECIRS. In particular, reference lines for the renal puncture and correct patient positioning in order to prevent pressure damages are described, as well as sterile draping and preparation of the surgical field. The operating room (OR) is very crowded and therefore it is relevant to define the right place for any operator and device. This aspect may appear time-consuming but is essential in order to optimize the cooperation of all the working team and to avoid both intraoperative problems and postoperative complications.

A. Hoznek, MD (✉)
Department of Urology, CHU Henri Mondor, 51. Av. du Ml. de Lattre de Tassigny, 94010 Créteil Cedex, France
e-mail: andras.hoznek@gmail.com

F.P.J. Daels, MD
Department of Urology, Instituto Universitario del Hospital Italiano de Buenos Aires, Buenos Aires, Argentina
e-mail: pedro.daels@hospitalitaliano.org.ar

M.N. Kimuli
Pyrah Department of Urology, St James's University Hospital, Beckett Street, Leeds LS9 7TF, UK
e-mail: nkimuli@hotmail.com

C.M. Cracco, MD, PhD • C.M. Scoffone, MD
Department of Urology, Cottolengo Hospital, Via Cottolengo 9, 10152 Torino, Italy
e-mail: cecilia.cracco@libero.it; scoof@libero.it

C.M. Scoffone et al. (eds.), *Supine Percutaneous Nephrolithotomy and ECIRS*,
DOI 10.1007/978-2-8178-0459-0_11, © Springer-Verlag France 2014

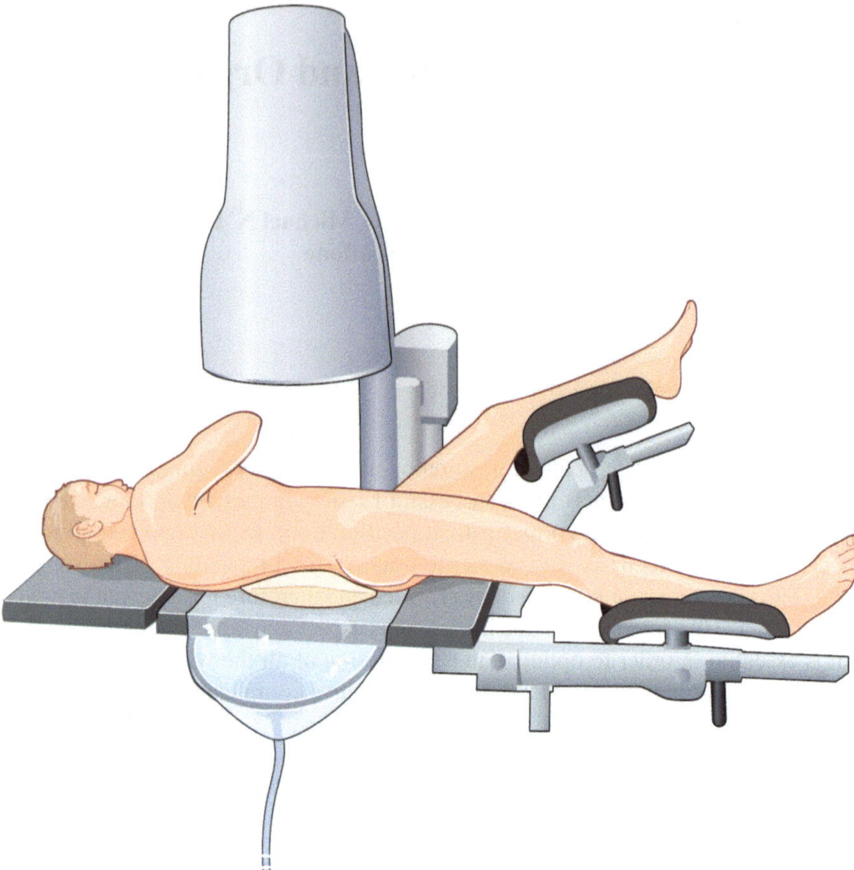

Fig. 11.1 Patient ready for ECIRS in the Galdakao-modified supine Valdivia position

11.1 Patient Positioning

The Galdakao-modified supine Valdivia (GMSV) position (Fig. 11.1) (see also Chap. 3) is simply reproducible and adaptable to most urologic centers. There is not a single universal positioning technique, and every endourological surgeon brings individual adjustments according to local specificities and personal preferences [1–8]. In this chapter we describe how we realize in our daily practice the GMSV position. Adequate antidecubitus padding, no matter which kind, is in any case fundamental to avoid inadvertent pressure damages, especially during prolonged procedures (Fig. 11.2) (see also Chap. 19):

- Check according to your internal hospital procedures the identity of the patient, the kind of procedure, and the side to be operated (that has to be correctly marked).
- Check that the operating table is radiolucent, can be sufficiently translated leaving the abdomen free of radiopaque obstacles and easily host the C-arm of the fluoroscopy for radiological control during the procedure in the areas of interest, and can be arranged with the leg stirrups for lithotomic position.

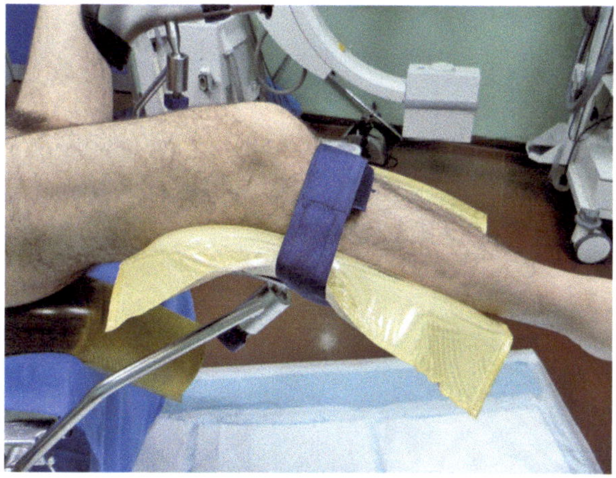

Fig. 11.2 Adequate padding of the legs' stirrups to prevent pressure damages

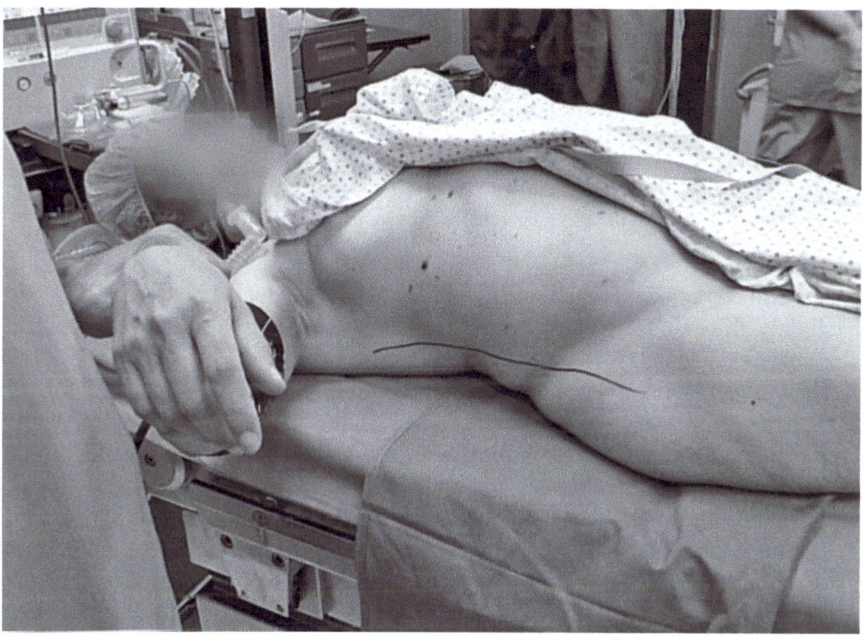

Fig. 11.3 The posterior axillary line is drawn in the simple supine position

- If the OR is too narrow, incline the operating table, leaving more space on that side to be operated; the floor may be prepared with absorbing materials, in order to avoid inadvertent spilling of irrigation fluids all around.
- The first landmark is the posterior axillary line (Fig. 11.3) that has to be drawn with an undeletable pen possibly with the patient standing, arm up, or in any case with the patient pure supine before starting the positioning maneuvers.
- The patient is then positioned supine on the operating table, near to the border of the side with the stone to be operated (this is important to increase free mobility of the nephroscope), then prepared and anaesthetized.

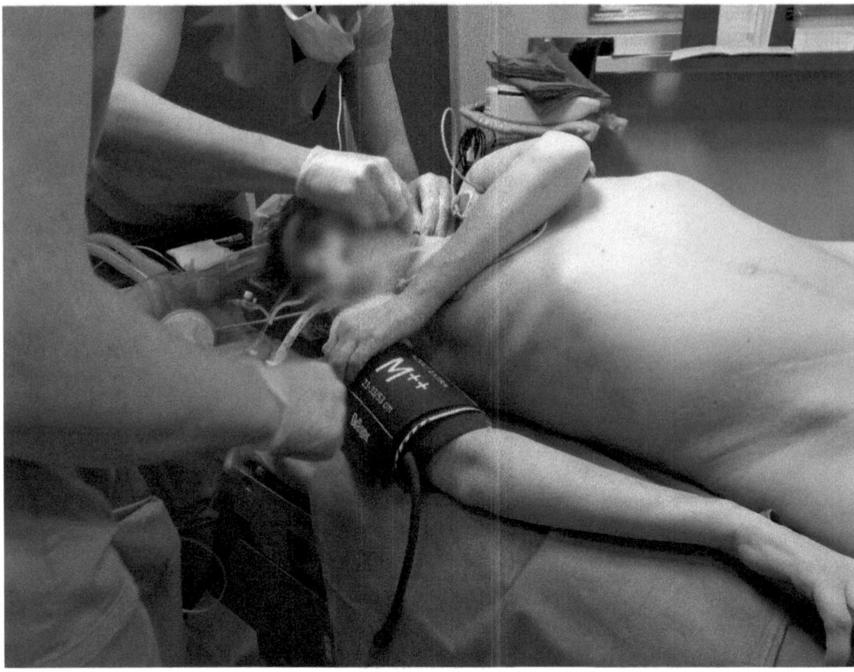

Fig. 11.4 Arrangement of the contralateral arm for venous access

- The arm contralateral to the side to be operated lies abducted of less than 90° and slightly flexed on a padded support, or along the body, for anesthesiological management (Fig. 11.4).
- The ipsilateral arm of the patient crosses the chest lying on it or supported, further elevating the posterior axillary line (Fig. 11.5). It is preferable not to use metallic arm support, because this interferes with the X-ray beam, should the C-arm be tilted cephalad, during fluoroscopic-controlled access creation. A padded support maintains the arm with an angle less than 90° with that of the operating table.
- The lumbar region is lifted approximately 20° and exposed. There are several ways to tilt the patient. Valdivia Urìa in his original description used an emptied 3 l saline irrigation bag for transurethral resection, inflating it with air and closing the outflow tube with a Kocher forceps, allowing volume control until the best position is found (Fig. 11.6a, courtesy of Dr. Gaspar Ibarluzea). Others use two silicone gel pads or two "plum cake"-shaped jelly pillows, one under the shoulder and another under the gluteal region, leaving the lumbar region free and creating a space preventing instruments collision (Fig. 11.6b). There is also an inflatable device called "Pelvic-Tilt" (OR comfort LLC, Glen Ridge, NJ, USA) (Fig. 11.6c). This device has a non-inflated flap extending from one side. The flap is placed under the lumbar region opposite to the stone, while the inflatable portion is placed under the stone side. The weight of the patient on the flap prevents the lateral shifting of the pillow.

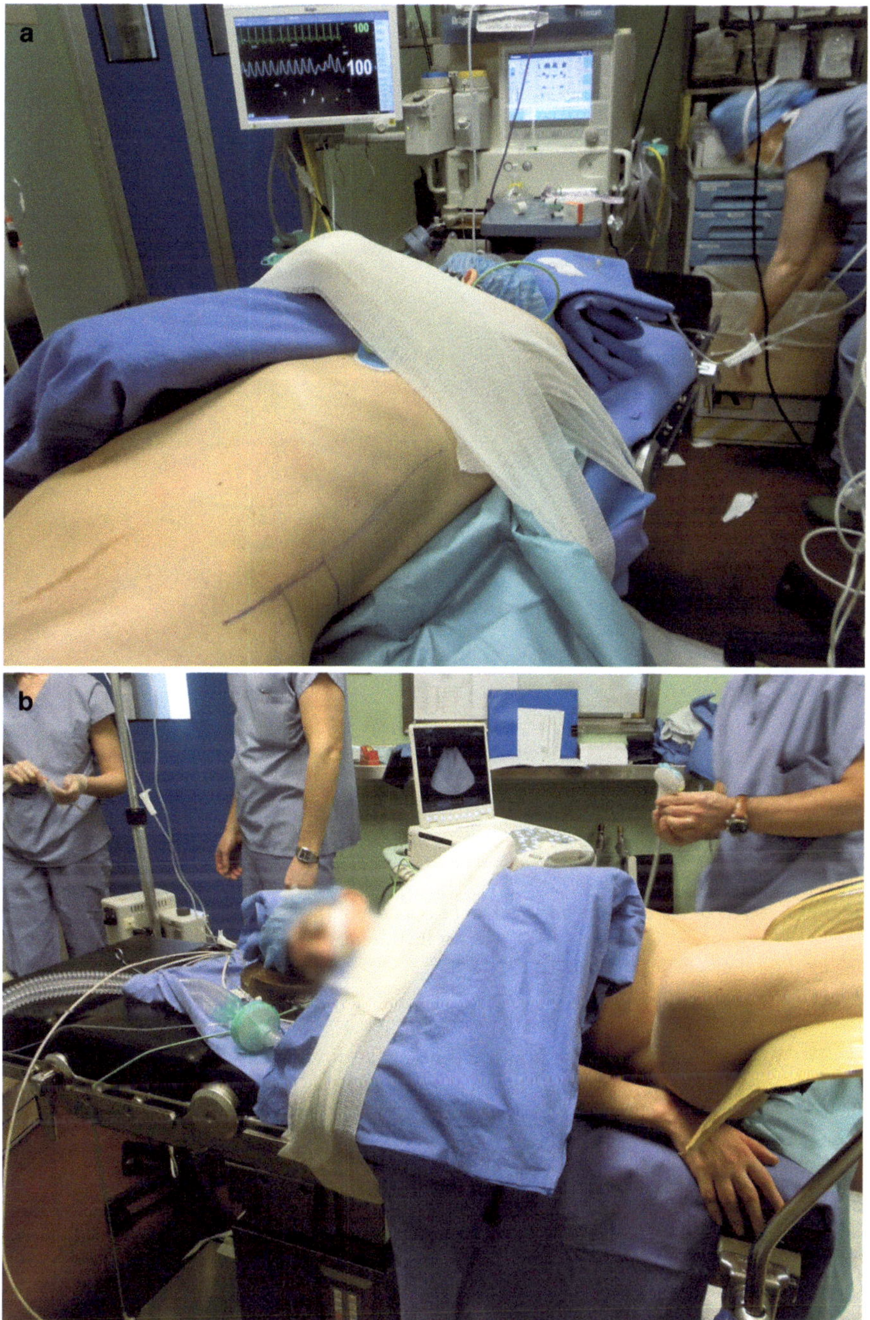

Fig. 11.5 Arrangement of the ipsilateral arm, adequately fixed (**a**) and with a cushion under it to prevent peripheral nerve damage (**b**)

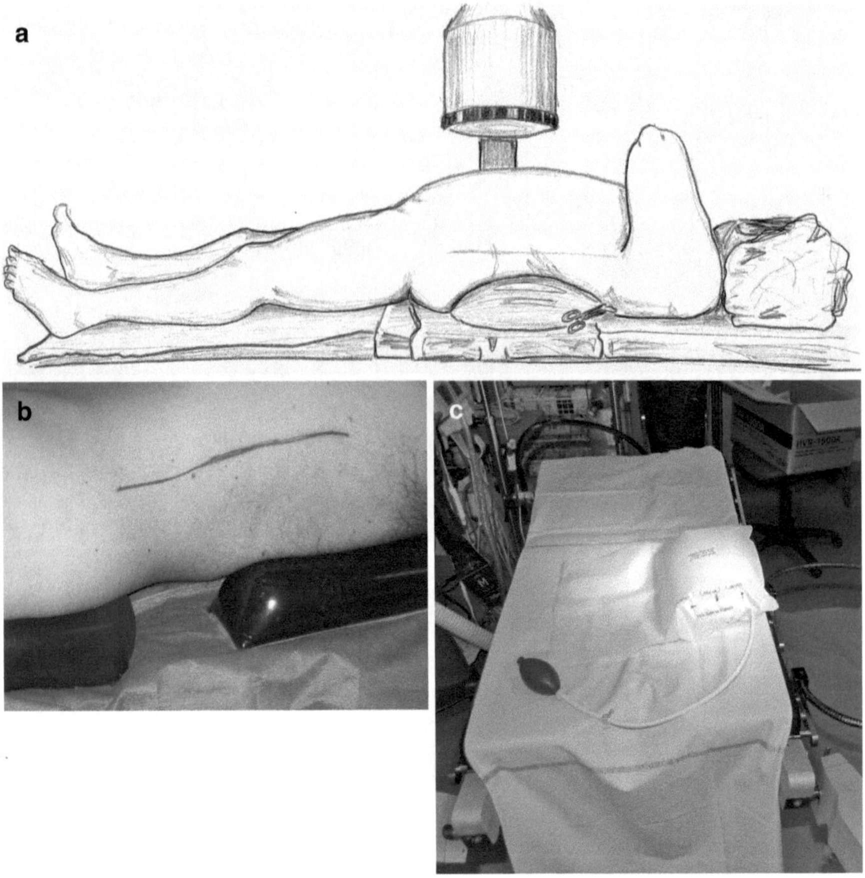

Fig. 11.6 Methods for elevating the flank to be operated: (**a**) saline bag under the flank, original method (The drawing is a courtesy of Dr. Gaspar Ibarluzea), (**b**) jelly pillows under the gluteus and the thorax, (**c**) inflatable device under the flank

- The further landmarks can now be drawn: the lower margin of the 12th rib and the upper margin of the iliac crest (Fig. 11.7).
- Then the patient is put in a modified lithotomy position, very similar to that used during a semirigid retrograde ureteroscopy, with both glutei on the inferior border of the operating table. The ipsilateral leg is slightly abducted and extended, and the contralateral leg is lifted and partially flexed (Fig. 11.8). Both leg stirrups should be adequately padded, possibly with gelatins as well.
- After positioning maneuvers, check again for possible corrections (especially of the upper and lower limbs) and fix everything with the aid of Peha-haft or similar.

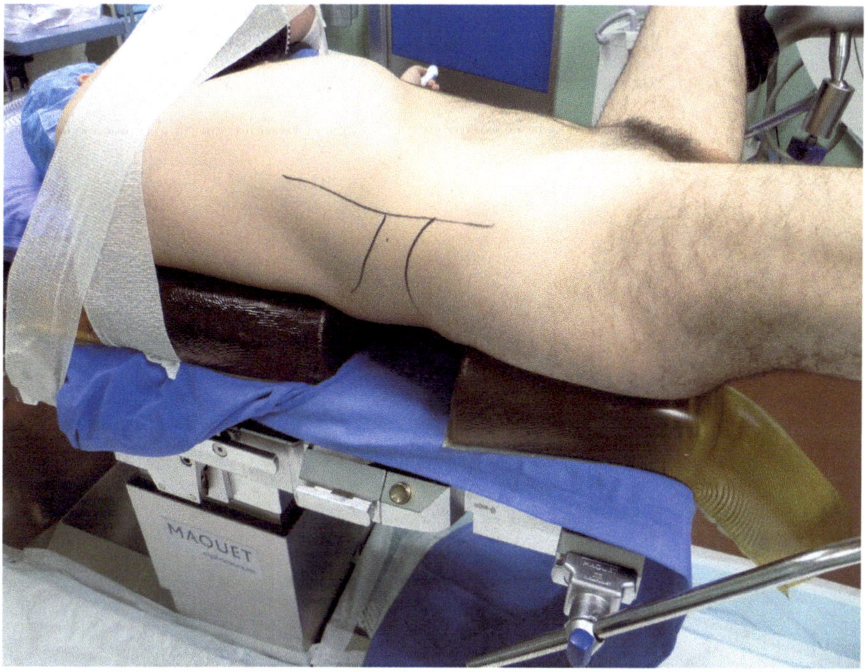

Fig. 11.7 When the patient is in the right position, the remaining reference lines are drawn (12th rib and iliac crest)

11.2 Sterile Draping of the Patient and Preparation of the Surgical Field

- Disinfection of the skin comprises the lumbar region, the anterior abdominal wall, the external genitalia, and the perineum (Fig. 11.9) (see also Chap. 19).
- The sterile draping does not require to be changed intraoperatively. We use a standard cystoscopy set which is not entirely unfolded towards the abdomen and chest, and then the lumbar region is draped with standard abdominal adhesive drapes or with a modified cystoscopy set.
- The irrigation fluid pouring outside the Amplatz sheath needs special handling. A watertight covering of a Mayo table, which is attached to the lateral abdominal drape under the abdominal field near the border of the operative table with two surgical clamps, can be employed. Directing the fluid into the bag is further facilitated by sticking an OPSITE to the operative area. Otherwise, a modified cystoscopy set can be used; in alternative the UroFunnel™ system (Paramount Medical Solutions Ltd.), a malleable metallic mounting frame with a transparent funnel-shaped retrieval bag, is very ergonomic (Fig. 11.10).

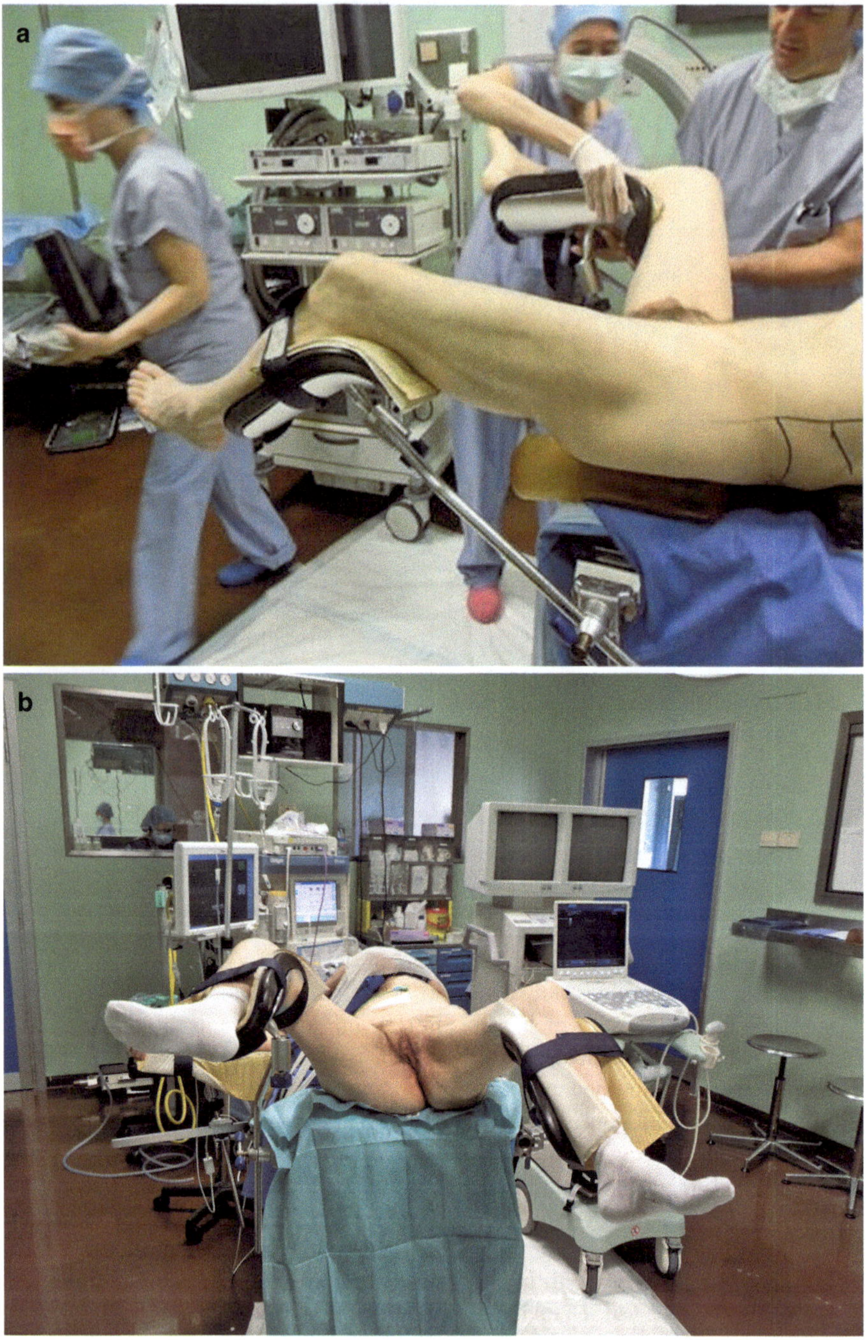

Fig. 11.8 Arrangement of the legs: the ipsilateral one is slightly extended and the contralateral one well abducted. Lateral (**a**) and frontal (**b**) views

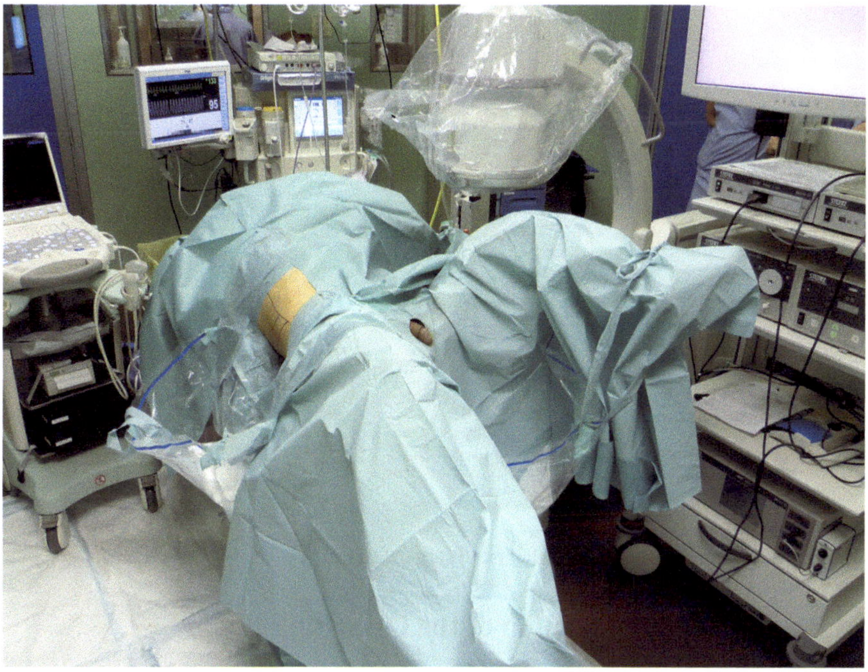

Fig. 11.9 Final sterile draping with the bags for retrieving irrigation fluids

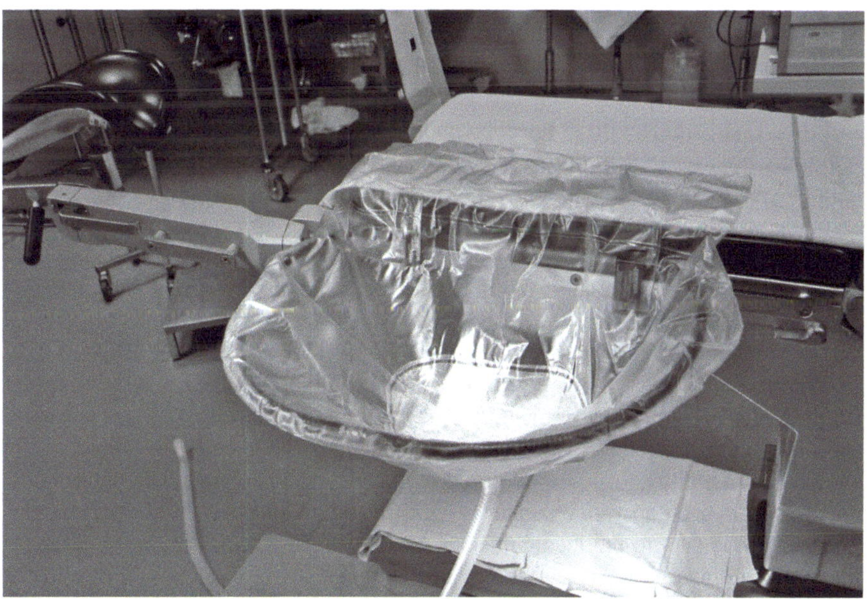

Fig. 11.10 UroFunnel system for retrieving irrigation fluids

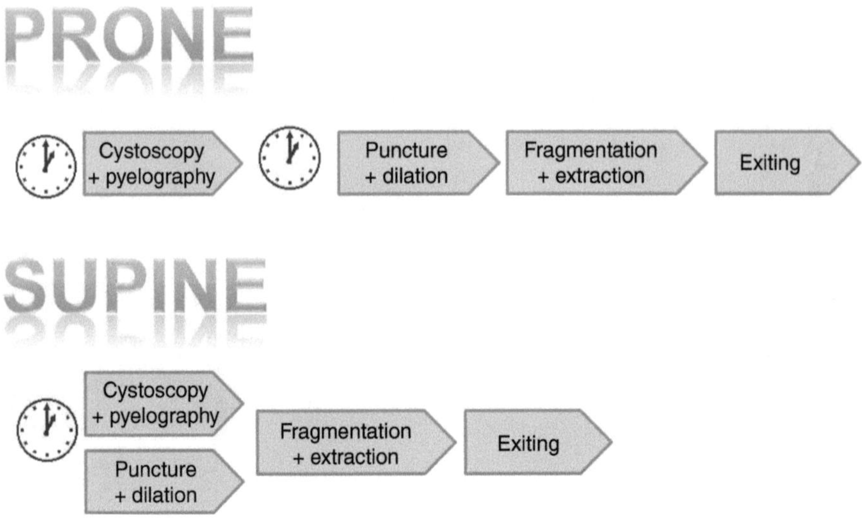

Table 11.1 Timing and duration of the initial surgical steps in prone and supine PNL

11.3 Spatial Organization of the Operating Room

During a supine PNL, and especially during ECIRS in the Galdakao-modified supine Valdivia position, two surgeons work in close cooperation and interaction, optimizing ergonomics of the procedure and improving its time efficiency. Standardized and strategic equipment placement eliminates improvisation, simplifies the training and the work of paramedical staff, and shortens OR occupation time.

Prone PNL begins with cystoscopy and insertion of a ureteric catheter in supine lithotomy position. Then, the ureteric catheter is secured to a Foley catheter. The patient is subsequently repositioned prone for the rest of the procedure (i.e., access creation, stone fragmentation and extraction, drainage). In contrast to prone PNL, during supine PNL it is possible to perform some specific surgical tasks concomitantly rather than sequentially. While one of the surgeons performs the cystoscopy and ureteric catheterization, the second scans the kidney with the ultrasound probe and begins puncturing the collecting system (Table 11.1).

With these considerations in mind, the layout of the OR is extremely important (Fig. 11.11). Each member of the operative team should have an excellent vision on the video screens and the X-ray monitor (Fig. 11.12). The intensity of ambient light should be gradually adjusted as required to improve vision on the different screens.

Obviously, each operative theater is specific and the disposition of different elements should adapt to the local situation. In this chapter, we describe the arrangement we routinely use. Ideally, the operative theater is roomy enough to make it possible to move around all the equipment disposed near the patient. If not, the table can be inclined, leaving more space on the side to be operated. Remember the

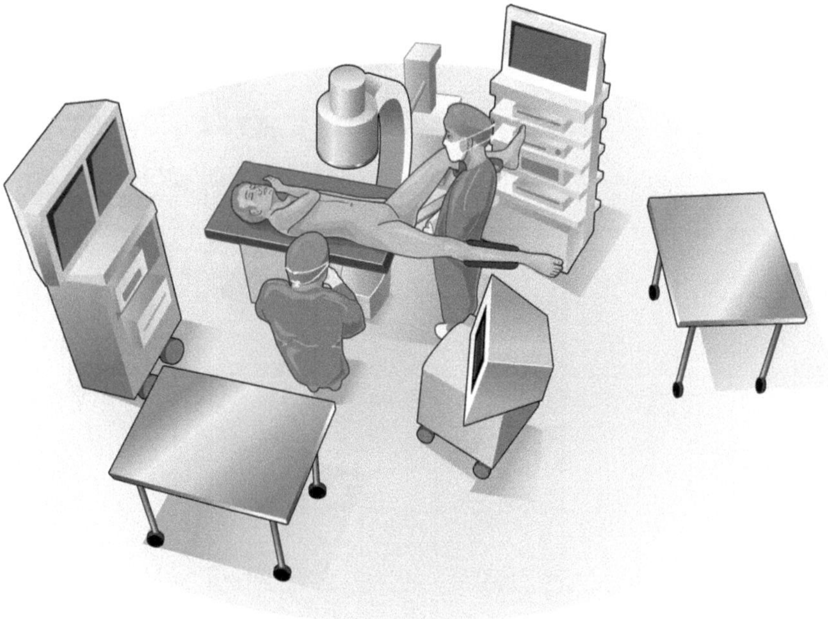

Fig. 11.11 Schematic drawing of OR organization

presence of the anaesthesiologist with all the armamentarium, located at the head of the patient (Fig. 11.5a).

Unfortunately, integrated endourological tables are not optimal for a supine procedure, because usually the X-ray device works only in the anteroposterior plane. Furthermore, the radiological unit is attached to the same side of the operative table, leaving insufficient room at this site to access the kidney. This is probably one of the limiting factors explaining why supine positions are not very popular in some endourological centers (see also Chap. 3).

The X-ray screen is at the level of the head of the patient, on the side of the stone (Fig. 11.12b). The mobile C-arm unit is in front of the surgeon performing the nephroscopy (Fig. 11.9). The X-ray source should be placed under the operative table in order to diminish radiation scattering and exposure of the surgical team. The receptor of the C-arm is draped sterile to facilitate its manipulation by the surgeon. The C-arm should be easily movable by the surgeon himself cephalad and laterally to visualize the kidney and also caudally and medially to see the bladder. Since the patient is tilted 20°, in order to have a nearly anteroposterior view, one should also tilt the C-arm in the same direction and same inclination. Unfortunately, when doing so, the metallic frame of the operative table often interferes with the X-ray picture. To avoid this artifact, we tilt the C-arm only 5°. The foot pedal of the fluoroscopy unit is placed near the foot of the surgeon, so that he can decide the instant and the duration of X-ray monitoring during the procedure without the need of the presence of a person dedicated to this task.

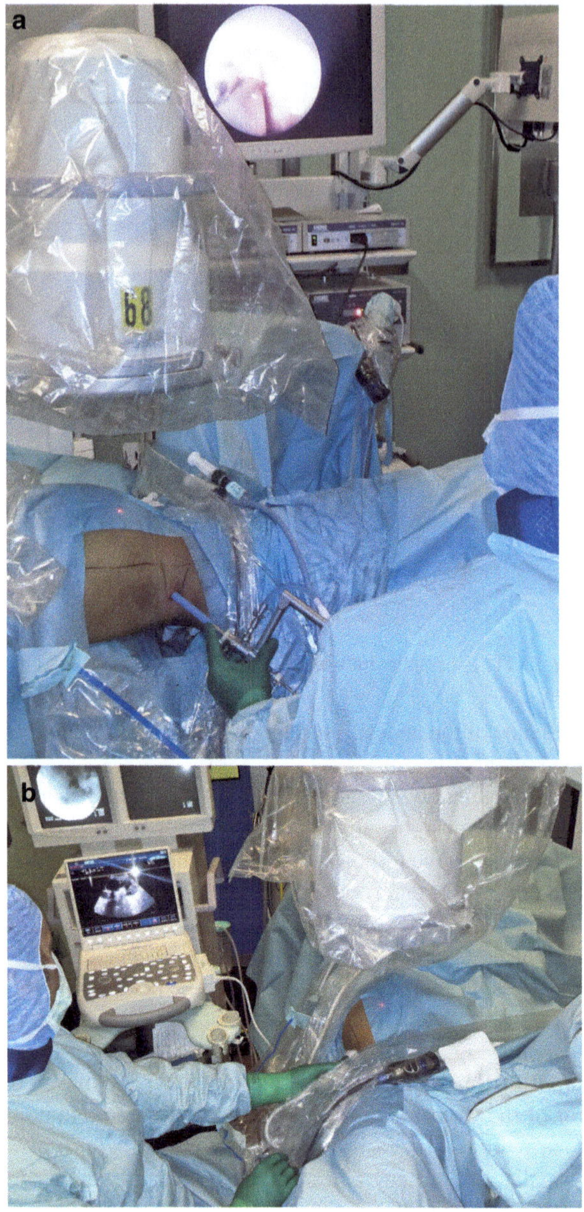

Fig. 11.12 Both video (**a**) and fluoroscopic and ultrasound screens (**b**) should be handy for the surgeons

The ultrasound device is beside the patient, on the side of the stone (Fig. 11.12b). The ultrasound probe is sterilely draped, as well as the keypad and commands, should an adjustment of ultrasound parameters be performed during the procedure.

The video tower (Fig. 11.13) is contralateral to the stone near to the leg of the patient (Fig. 11.12a). This allows each team member to have a vision on the screen.

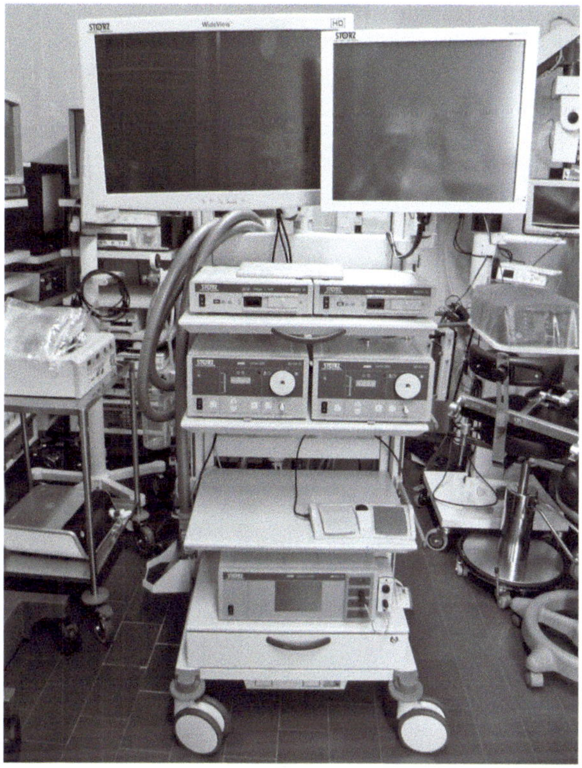

Fig. 11.13 Video tower ready for use

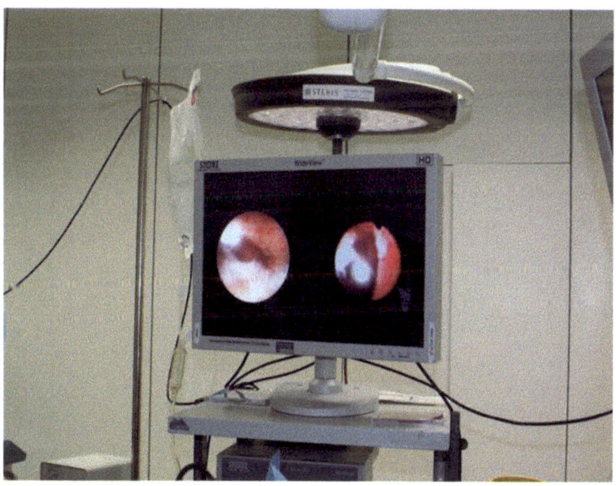

Fig. 11.14 Monitor with the possibility of simultaneous double vision (retrograde and antegrade)

If two endoscopes are used, they are connected to the same wide (16:9) screen using the "picture in picture" function (Fig. 11.14).

The different lithotripters and suction devices (Fig. 11.15) are behind the surgeon who performs nephroscopy. All cables and lines used for the nephroscopy are fixed

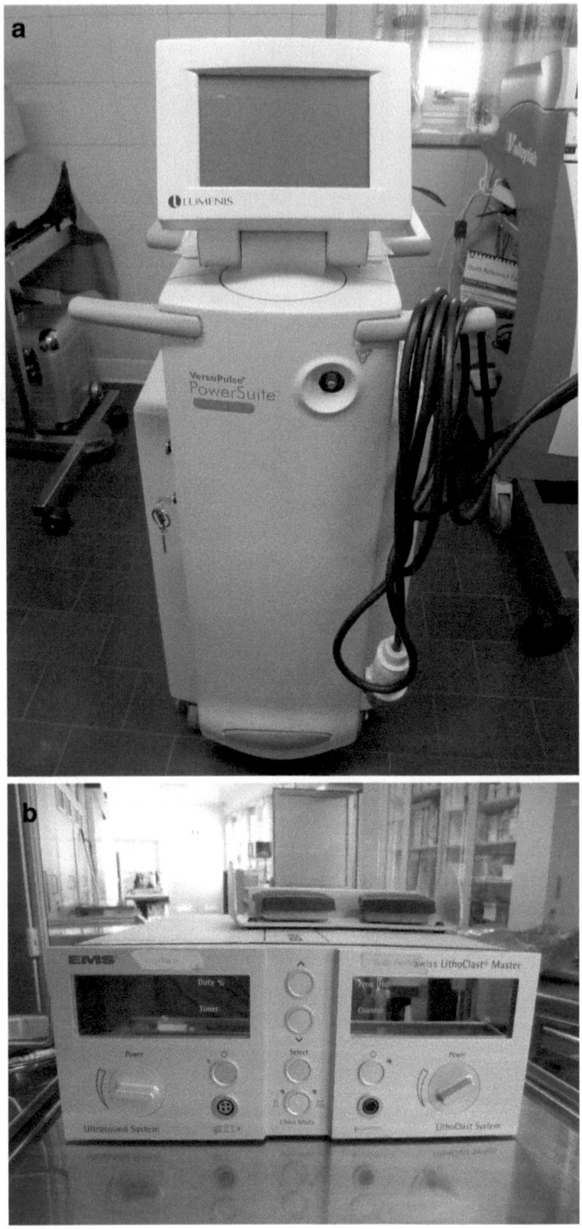

Fig. 11.15 Laser (**a**) and combined ballistic/ultrasound (**b**) devices

near the shoulder of the patient on the side of the stone. The cables required for retrograde endoscopy are connected to the video tower near to the leg opposite to the stone.

A back table is disposed behind each surgeon, one for the surgeon who performs the antegrade approach and another one for the surgeon who deals with retrograde

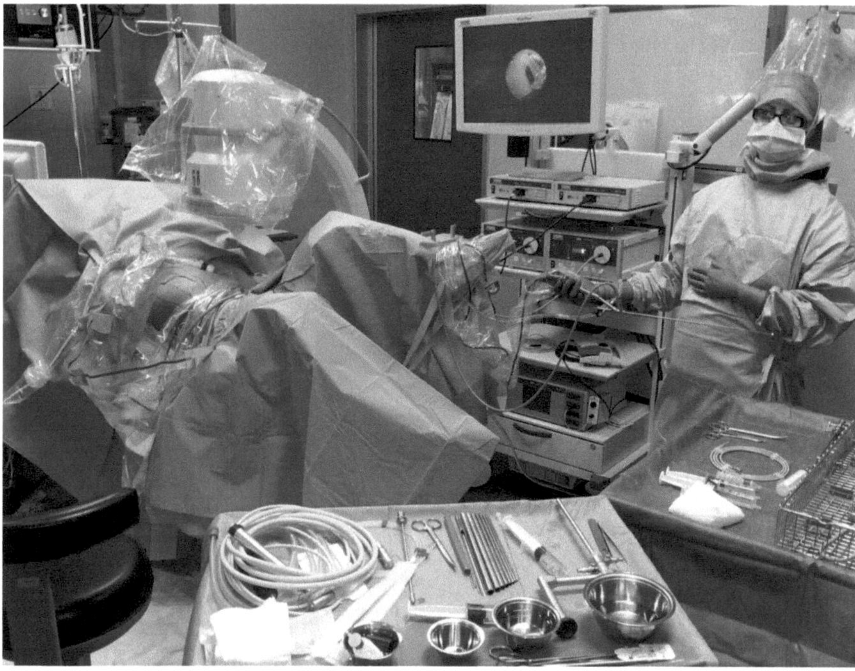

Fig. 11.16 The back tables should be handy for both surgeons, behind them

endoscopy (Fig. 11.16). The setup of these tables should also be standardized and rationalized (see Chap. 19). ECIRS is particularly instrument dependent, and a meticulous organization of the back tables is indispensable especially because of the distribution of different tasks between the two surgeons working in tandem. Rapid and easy accessibility of each instrument is an important factor for optimal time management. On each table the devices are arranged in the order of use.

Because different endoscopes are required at different steps of the procedure and the same scope may be used several times, we found it indispensable to use sterile and watertight camera draping. This avoids desterilizing the endoscopes and the condensation of liquid on the endoscopic camera. If flexible instruments are used, they should be placed in a protected area in order to avoid accidental compression of their delicate and fragile shaft (Fig. 11.17). Any sharp instrument near the flexible instruments is source of risk of instrument sleeve perforation.

A set of small forceps like Kocher or Kelly should also be available. They are used to attach different cables to the draping. Many cables are used during ECIRS including two irrigation fluid lines, two light cables, two camera cables, the ultrasound probe, the LithoClast cable, ultrasound handpiece cable, and another cable for aspiration. All these cables should be arranged without forming loops or knots; an adequate length should also be available to guarantee easy back and forth motions of the nephroscope and fragmentation devices throughout the procedure (Fig. 11.18).

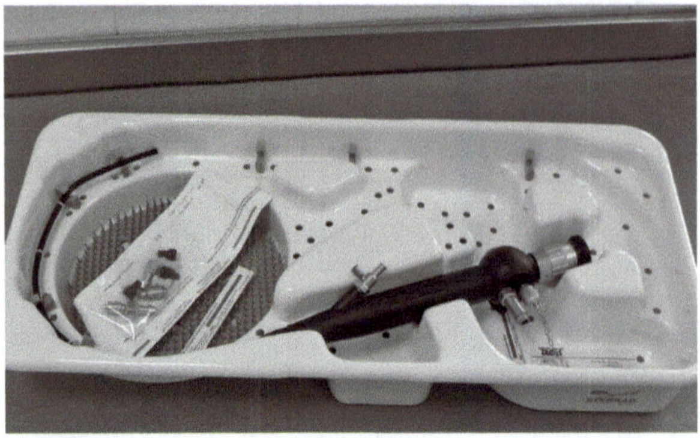

Fig. 11.17 Care should be taken in the correct handling of the delicate flexible ureteroscopes

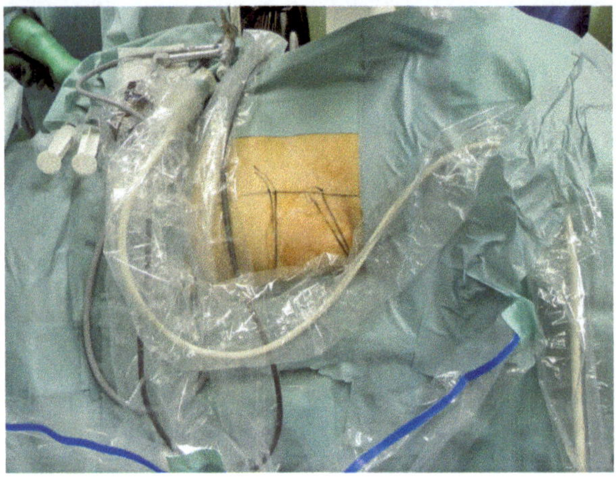

Fig. 11.18 All the cables should be sterile, fixed, and put in a standardized order

References

1. Valdivia Uria JG, Valle Gerhold J, Lopez Lopez JA, Villarroya Rodriguez S, Ambroj Navarro C, Ramirez Fabian M et al (1998) Technique and complications of percutaneous nephroscopy: experience with 557 patients in the supine position. J Urol 160:1975–1978
2. Ibarluzea G, Scoffone CM, Cracco CM, Poggio M, Porpiglia F, Terrone C et al (2007) Supine Valdivia and modified lithotomy position for simultaneous anterograde and retrograde endourological access. BJU Int 100:233–236
3. De Sio M, Autorino R, Quarto G, Calabro F, Damiano R, Giugliano F et al (2008) Modified supine versus prone position in percutaneous nephrolithotomy for renal stones treatable with a single percutaneous access: a prospective randomized trial. Eur Urol 54:196–202
4. Daels F, Gonzalez MS, Freire FG, Jurado A, Damia O (2009) Percutaneous lithotripsy in Valdivia-Galdakao decubitus position: our experience. J Endourol 23:1615–1620
5. Scoffone CM, Cracco CM, Cossu M, Grande S, Poggio M, Scarpa RM (2008) Endoscopic combined intrarenal surgery in Galdakao-modified supine Valdivia position: a new standard for percutaneous nephrolithotomy? Eur Urol 54:1393–1403
6. Cracco CM, Scoffone CM, Scarpa RM (2011) New developments in percutaneous techniques for simple and complex branched renal stones. Curr Opin Urol 21:154–160

7. Miano R, Scoffone C, De Nunzio C, Germani S, Cracco C, Usai P et al (2010) Position: prone or supine is the issue of percutaneous nephrolithotomy. J Endourol 24:931–938
8. Hoznek A, Rode J, Ouzaid I, Faraj B, Kimuli M, de la Taille A et al (2012) Modified supine percutaneous nephrolithotomy for large kidney and ureteral stones: technique and results. Eur Urol 61:164–170

Chapter 12
Instruments and Accessories for ECIRS

Cesare Marco Scoffone, András Hoznek, and Julie Rode

Abstract Since ECIRS offers the possibility of a simultaneous antegrade and retrograde access to the upper urinary tract performed by two distinct urologists, the optimal working environment should comprise a valid video network with adequate settings, a complete imaging equipment, an irrigation system, and a variety of instruments and accessories, which should be well known in terms of features and technological details. In this chapter the authors describe a complete landscape of all the alternatives on the market, with regard to ureteroscopes and nephroscopes, disposable accessories like access needles, guidewires and dilation systems, intracorporeal lithotripsy, and fragments retrieval devices.

12.1 The Video Network

Since ECIRS offers the possibility of a simultaneous antegrade and retrograde access to the upper urinary tract with the contemporary use of two endoscopes, the optimal working environment comprises two digital video cameras, either fixed (Fig. 12.1) or pendulum (Fig. 12.2); two fiber-optic cables of different diameter, from 2.5 to 3.5 mm based upon the diameter of the endoscopes (Fig. 12.3); two adequate Xenon light sources (Fig. 12.4); two control units (Fig. 12.1); and two screens. Alternatively, it is also possible to use a single 16:9 high-resolution screen and to send to the same screen the two video signals with image splitting, with the

C.M. Scoffone, MD (✉)
Department of Urology, Cottolengo Hospital, via Cottolengo 9, 10152 Torino, Italy
e-mail: scoof@libero.it

A. Hoznek, MD • J. Rode
Department of Urology, CHU Henri Mondor, 51. Av. du Ml. de Lattre de Tassigny, 94010 Créteil Cedex, France
e-mail: andras.hoznek@gmail.com; rode.julie@orange.fr

C.M. Scoffone et al. (eds.), *Supine Percutaneous Nephrolithotomy and ECIRS*,
DOI 10.1007/978-2-8178-0459-0_12, © Springer-Verlag France 2014

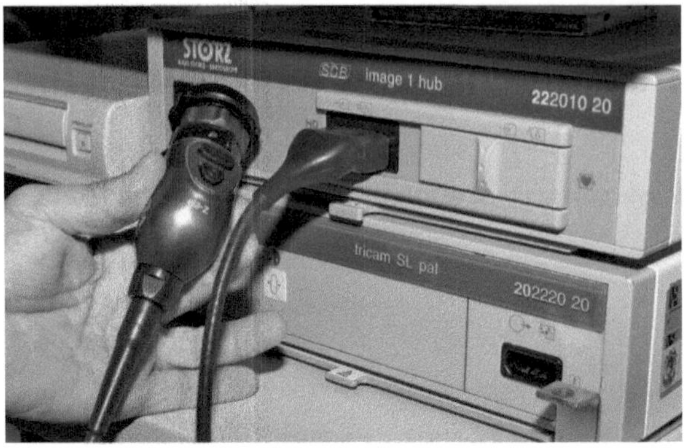

Fig. 12.1 Storz HD fixed video camera with its control unit

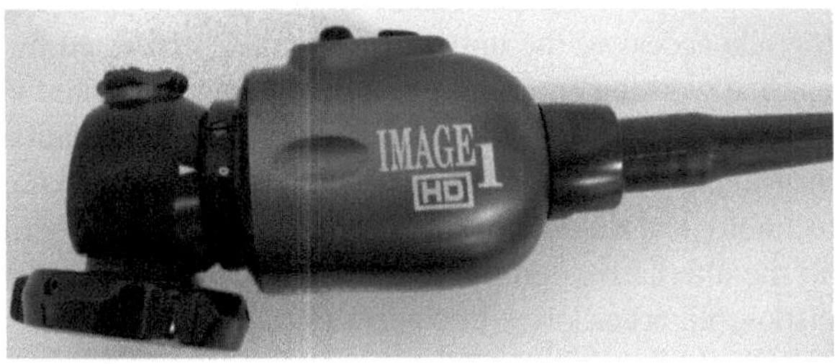

Fig. 12.2 Storz HD pendulum video camera

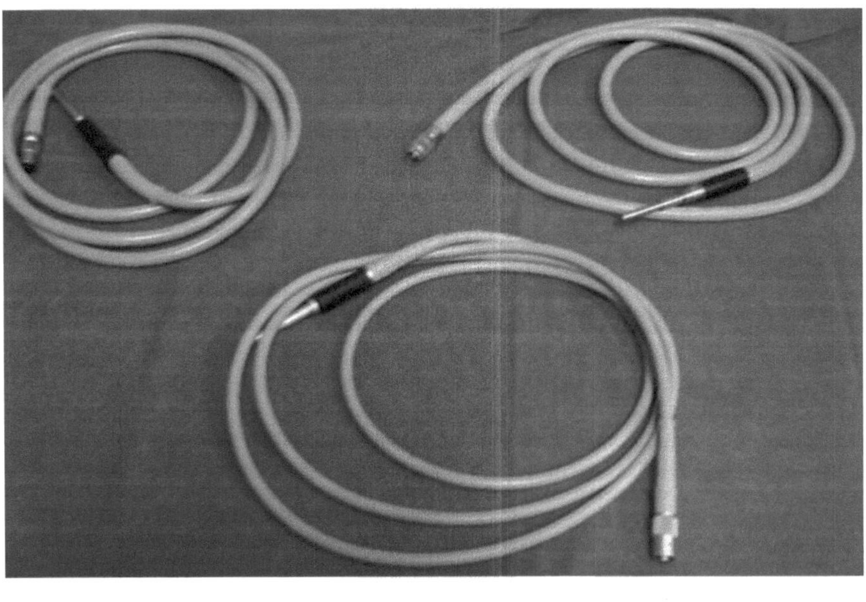

Fig. 12.3 Fiber-optic cables of different diameters

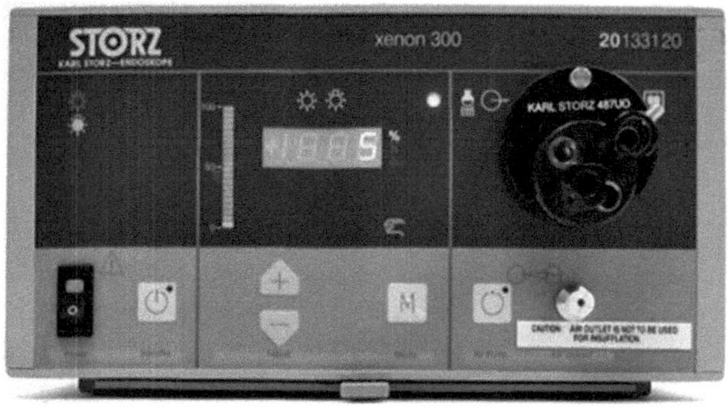

Fig. 12.4 Storz Xenon light source

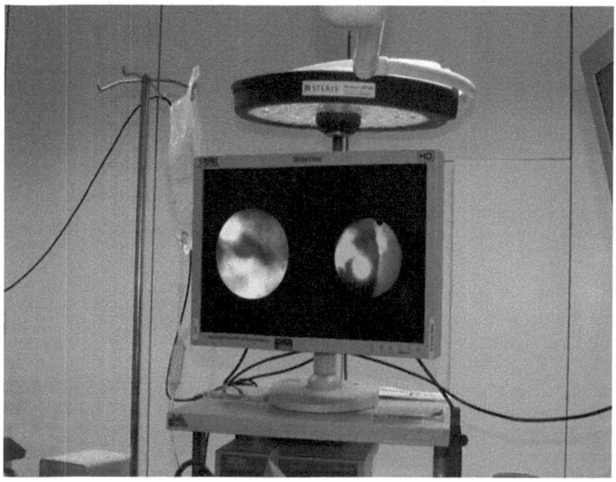

Fig. 12.5 Storz 16:9 HD monitor

additional possibility of the "picture in picture" images (Fig. 12.5). In any case all members of the operative team should have a comfortable view on the screen during the whole procedure. All the video network devices can be expressly housed in a video tower (Fig. 12.6).

The standard-definition (SD) analogic video signal (with the transformation of the endoscopic image into an electromagnetic wave thanks to a chip on the camera head sent to a standard monitor) has been nowadays largely overcome by the digital high-definition (HD) systems (exploiting serial waves of numbers instead of a simple electromagnetic wave). Digital HD systems must be supported by an adequate video network, in order to avoid to lose the advantages of such improved image quality.

12.1.1 Camera Heads and Their Setting

The Storz HD camera heads (H3-Z and the latest pendulum version) (Fig. 12.1, 12.2) have an optimized weight and ergonomic handling, reducing fatigue and improving control during procedures. The integrated 3-chip camera head with the latest CCD (charge-coupled device) sensor technology assures detailed, high-contrast, quasi-3D, and

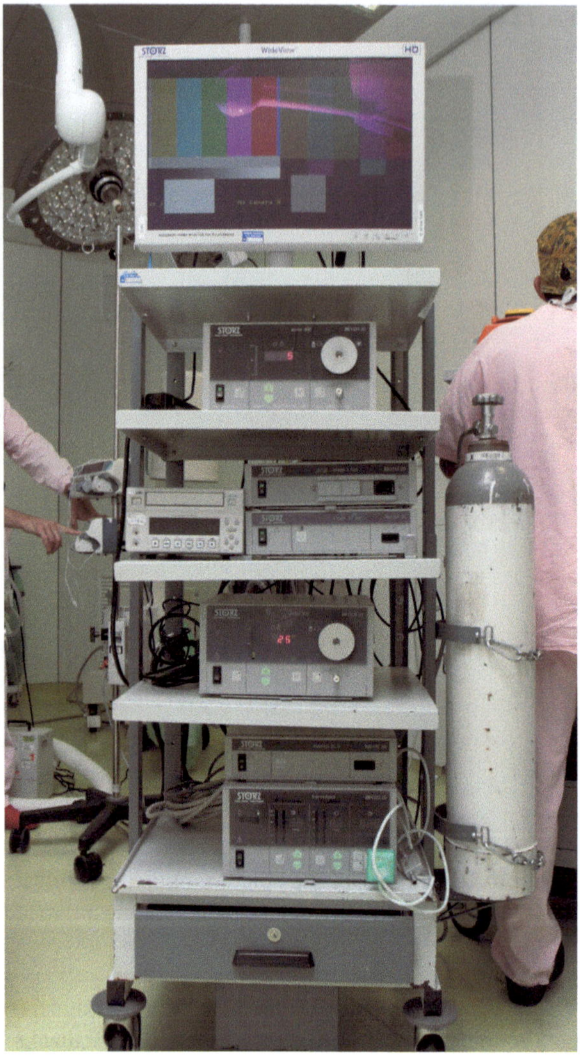

Fig. 12.6 Video tower housing all video network devices

noise-free images, with natural color reproduction across the entire zoom range. Ergonomically located buttons allow to program the camera head features according to the endoscope in use. HD camera heads have a 16:9 aspect ratio versus the 4:3 of the SD camera heads, increasing by more than 35 % the amplitude of the endoscopic field and by five times more the image resolution.

Since these camera heads have been conceived for laparoscopic procedures, thus for vision in wide-body hollows and to be coupled with big optics, the transposition of their use in ureteroscopy and nephroscopy requires a particular setting, in order to obtain an optimal vision.

Rigid, semirigid, and flexible ureteroscopes and nephroscopes require preliminary white balance, with the exception of the digital CMOS flexible nephroscope. Enhancement and brightness are set up according to the instrument to be used and the size/color of the working space (ureter versus renal pelvis and calyces):

- Low enhancement and small endoscope A/low brightness for the rigid nephroscope;
- Filter A enhancement and small endoscope A brightness for the flexible nephroscope;
- Enhancement off and small endoscope B brightness for the semirigid ureteroscope;
- Filter B enhancement and small scope B brightness for the flexible ureteroscope.

12.1.2 Light Source and Optic Cables

Optic cables with different diameters (2.5 mm for all flexible endoscopes and the semirigid ureteroscope, 3.5 mm for the rigid nephroscope) (Fig. 12.3) differ in the amount of light transmitted. The Xenon light source should also be regulated in order to avoid bad vision due to too much light and tissue reflection. In addition, injecting too much light into the cable does not improve luminosity, but light transforms into heat and burns the optical fibers of the endoscope.

The flexible digital CMOS (Complementary Metal-Oxide Semiconductor) nephroscope has a distal chip directly transforming the image into a digital signal on the tip of the instrument and needs no light source nor optic cable or white balance, having an integrated LED (light-emitting diode) technology in the handle (enhancement off, zoom × 2).

12.2 Imaging Equipment

The operating table for RIRS/PNL has to be radiolucent, with the possibility to translate it for housing the C-arm and to avoid radiopaque transverse bars underneath. Furthermore, the patient must have the chance to be put in lithotomic position (see also Chaps. 11 and 19). For a supine PNL, it is better to use an independent C arm rather than an X-ray device integrated to an endourology table, requiring two differ ent tables for the right and left side, or to change the position of the patient upside down (putting the head in the place of the feet) (see also Chap. 3). The individual C-arm (Fig. 12.7) can be placed as required either on the right or on the left side of the patient, leaving all the needed space to the surgeon. If fluoroscopy-only guidance is used, it is also important to be able to tilt the C-arm towards head or legs of the patient. This allows to target the kidney first in the anteroposterior incidence, then with a 30° tilt of the C-arm cephalad, to obtain information about the depth of the needle trajectory (see also Chap. 11) [1]. In order to maximally decrease radiation exposure of both patient and surgical staff and also to improve safety of the puncture, the combined use of ultrasound (Fig. 12.8) is crucial.

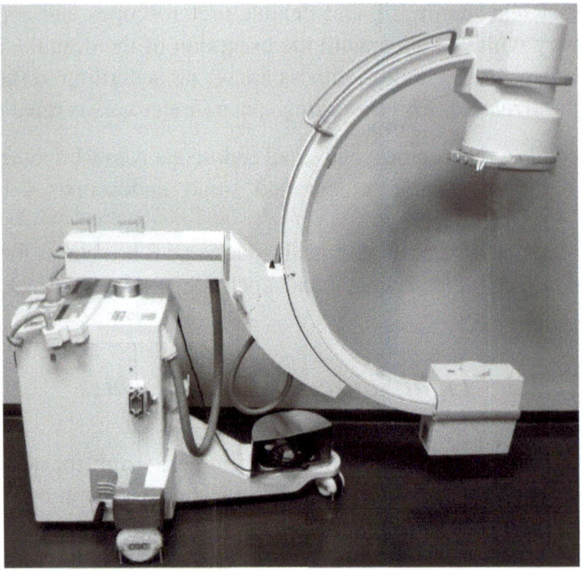

Fig. 12.7 Independent C-arm for fluoroscopy

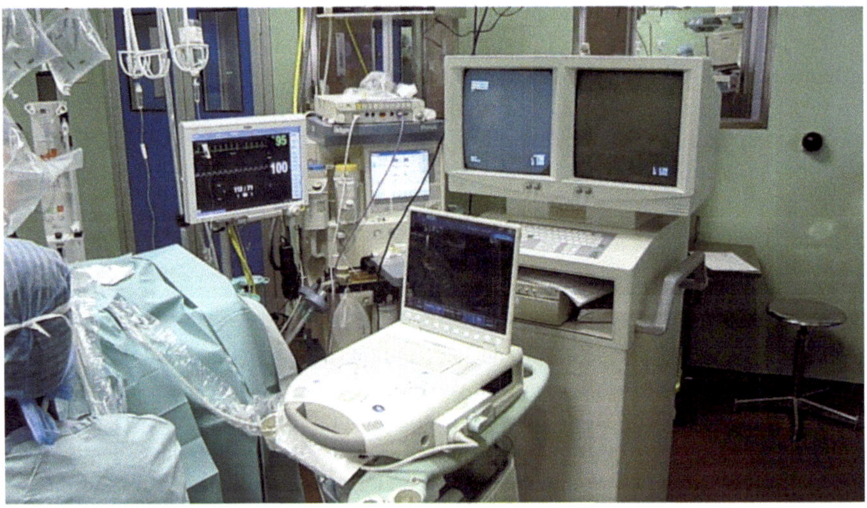

Fig. 12.8 Ultrasound device

12.3 Nephroscopes and Ureteroscopes

The choice of the nephroscope is of utmost importance. Rigid nephroscopes have the advantage of a superior optical quality due to the rod lens system. The optimal nephroscope should have a sufficient working length, a large working channel, a reduced outer diameter, and a watertight entry site for instruments and accessories.

In older nephroscopes the cranked (Fig. 12.9) or 45° offset optics and the light cable were located on opposite sides of the shaft. Therefore, in supine position,

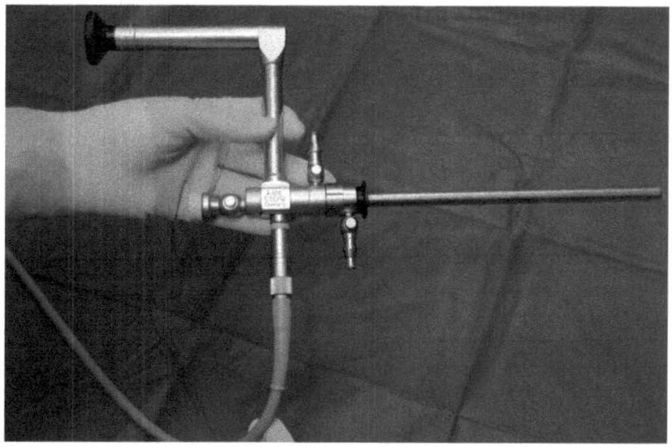

Fig. 12.9 Cranked offset optics with the light cable on the opposite side of the shaft in first-generation nephroscopes

collision with the border of the surgical table of this type of nephroscope could occur, resulting in limited maneuverability. For this reason, when we started with ECIRS years ago, we changed the kind of support under thorax and ankle of the patient, in order to enlarge the space of movement of the instrument.

Presently, all major manufacturers produce models in which the optical and light cables and the irrigation lines are all located on the same side of the shaft (Fig. 12.10a, b). With such nephroscopes, problems due to a conflict with the surgical table are only exceptionally encountered. Most nephroscopes have a continuous flow design, with an inflow and an outflow valve. However, when using a plastic Amplatz sheath, the outer shaft with the outflow valve loses its role; in fact, the irrigation fluid can flow out between nephroscope and Amplatz sheath. Furthermore, the shaft additionally increases the diameter of the scope, and this can be a disadvantage when accessing a calyx with a narrow infundibulum. Therefore, it is preferable to choose a nephroscope that can also be used without the outer shaft.

In the market there are also midi (Fig. 12.11) and mini-nephroscopes (Fig. 12.12a, b, c).

A flexible cystoscope is crucial during a contemporary PNL/ECIRS. It allows to access peripheral calyces that are not reachable with a rigid instrument. This allows to avoid the need for multiple tracts, especially in case of staghorn stones. The limitation of analogic flexible instruments (Fig. 12.13a) is the small diameter of the working channel and their perceived inferior optical quality, because of the "honeycomb" effect produced by the fiber-optic bundles. Actually this can be adequately corrected by the right set up of the filters. Digital nephroscopes (Fig. 12.13b) have a very high quality of imaging. Usually the lithotripsy energy source for any flexible instrument is the laser, because of the reduced diameter and significant flexibility of the fibers employed.

One of the major advantages of the supine position is its ability to use two endoscopes simultaneously, one through the Amplatz sheath and the other transurethrally. In case of simultaneous renal and ureteral stone, the latter can be treated with a rigid ureteroscope (Fig. 12.14a, b, c) and holmium laser. The use of a ureteroscope has also the advantage of preventing the migration of small fragments into the ureter during fragmentation. In addition, through the ureteroscope it is possible to

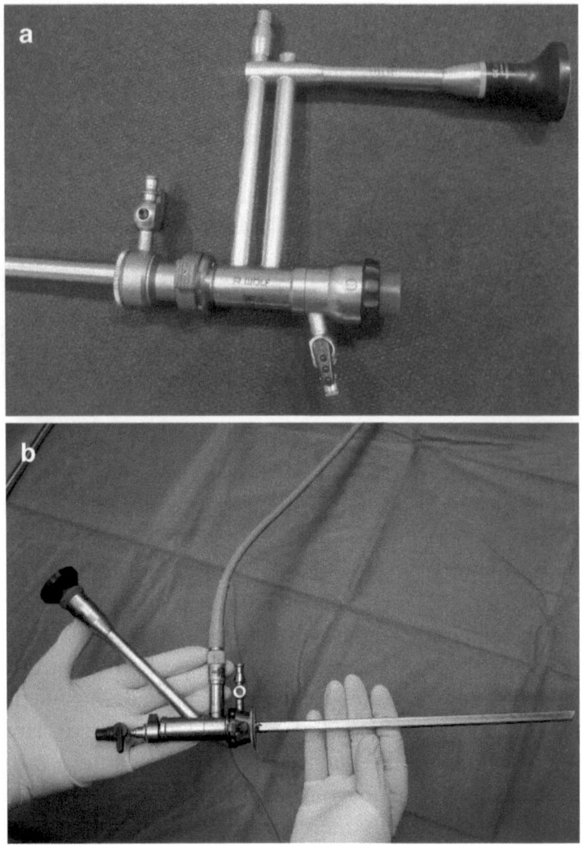

Fig. 12.10 Wolf (**a**) and Olympus (**b**) nephroscopes

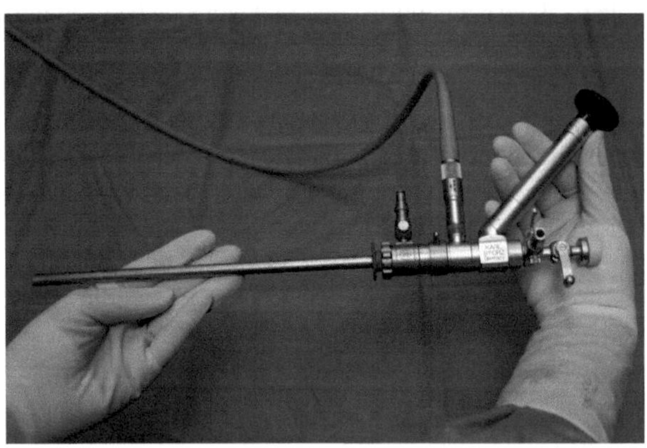

Fig. 12.11 Storz 17 Ch with outer shaft of 22 Ch rigid nephroscope

maintain a continuous and abundant irrigation which helps washing out small fragments through the Amplatz throughout the fragmentation process.

The use of flexible ureterorenoscope (Fig. 12.15) retrogradely together with a rigid or flexible nephroscope anterogradely allows to reach any district of the renal cavities. For this reason among the instruments semirigid and flexible ureteroscopes must be at disposition.

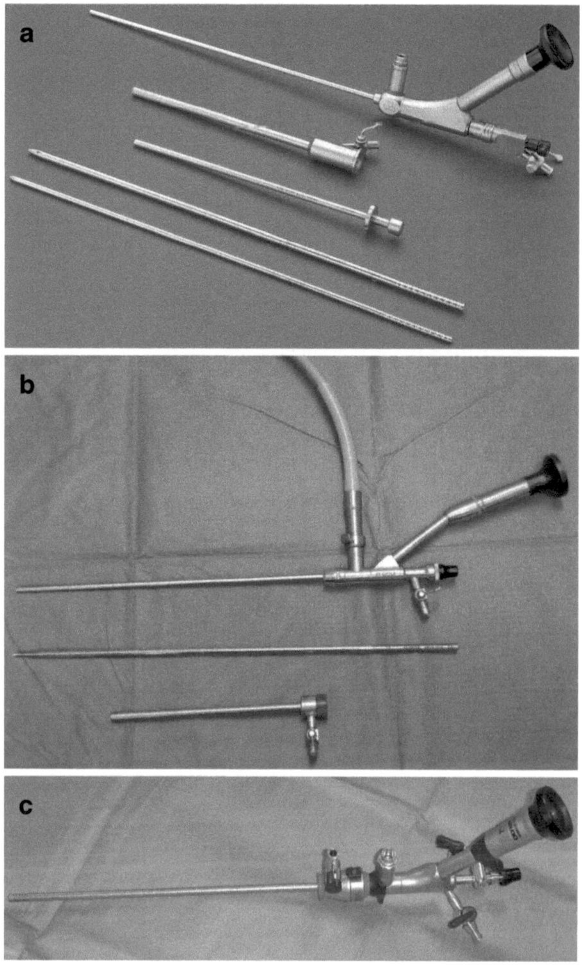

Fig. 12.12 Mini-PNL set with Storz (**a**) Wolf (**b**) Olympus (**c**)

In summary, in order to achieve maximal efficiency during ECIRS, the optimal set of endoscopes includes rigid and flexible nephroscopes and rigid and flexible ureteroscopes.

12.4 Irrigation Systems

12.4.1 Facing the Issue of Hypothermia

During percutaneous surgery, continuous irrigation with saline is required. Because of the amount and duration of such irrigation at room temperature, hypothermia is a concrete risk for the operated patient. Thus, heating to 38 °C of the irrigant fluids is fundamental. There are specific urologic systems that deliver large volumes of irrigation at body temperature, with optimal flow rates and offering a bubble-free field

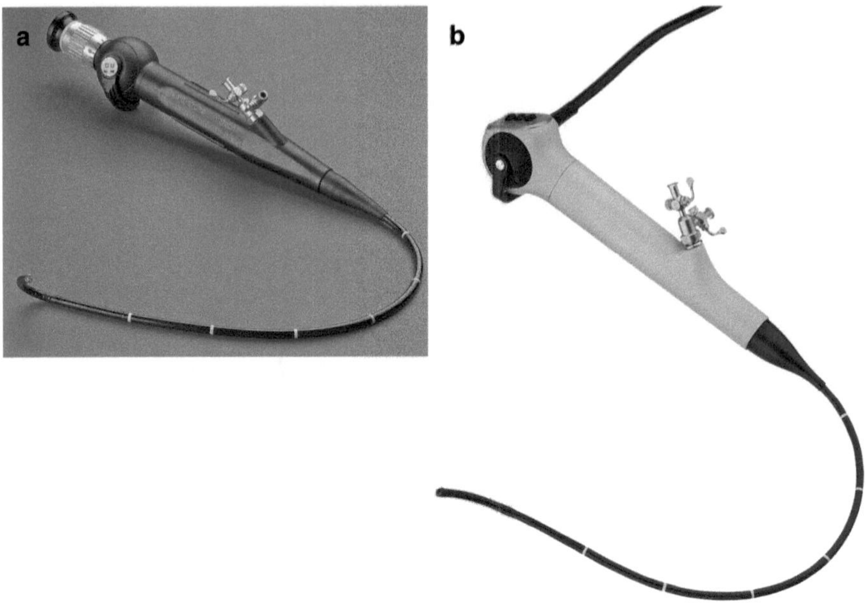

Fig. 12.13 Analogic (**a**) and digital (**b**) flexible Storz nephroscopes

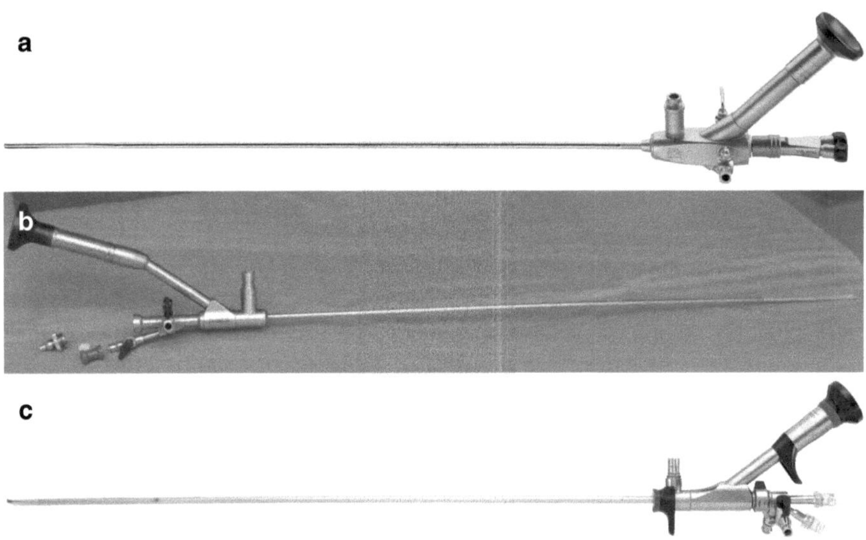

Fig. 12.14 Storz (**a**) Wolf 6–7.5 Ch (**b**) and Olympus (**c**) semirigid ureteroscopes

of vision (Fig. 12.16). If such a device is not available, an alternative is the use of a microwave oven. The only thing to remember is to switch off the heating during ultrasound lithotripsy, in order to avoid overheating. This precaution is not necessary when using laser and ballistic lithotripsy.

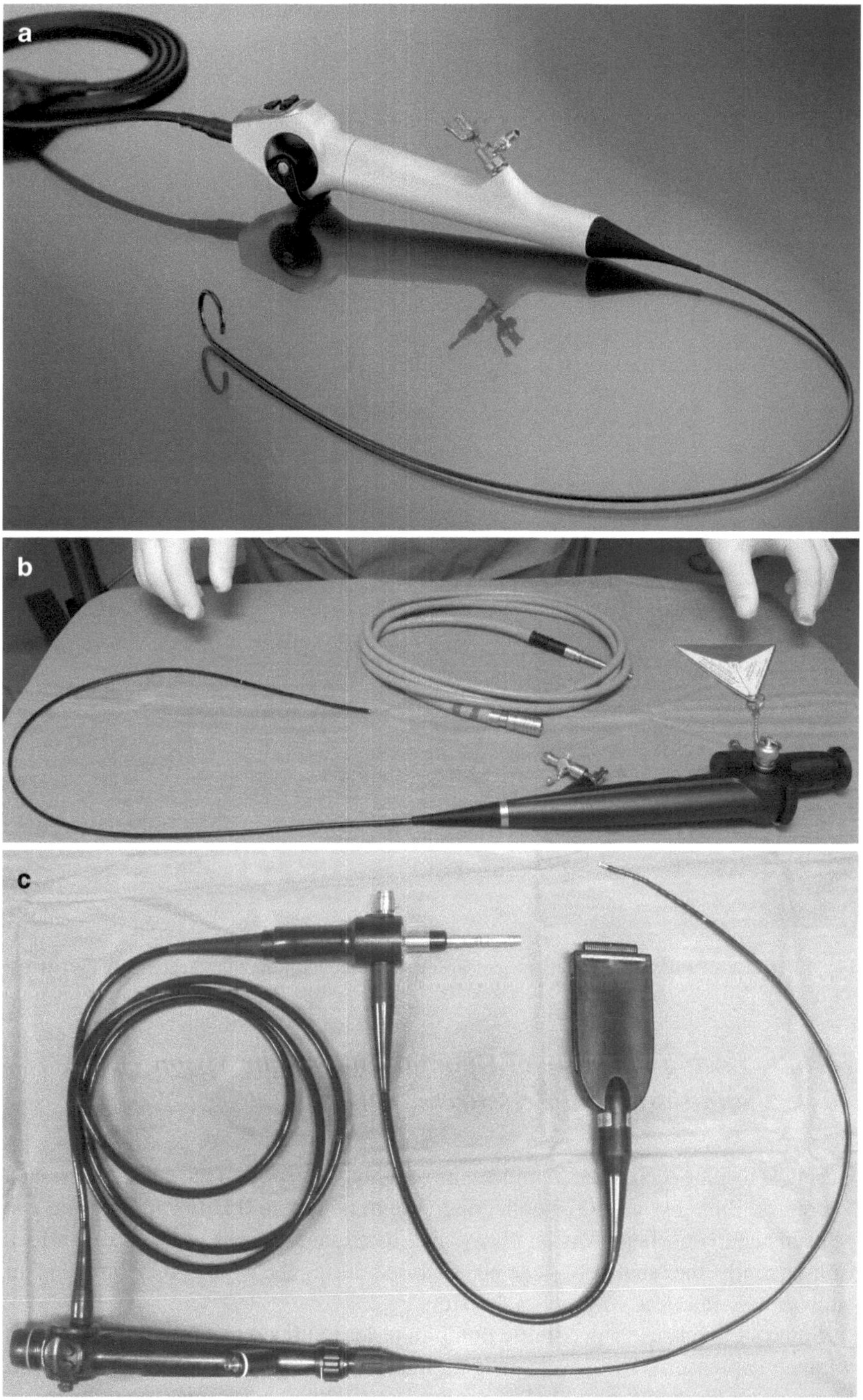

Fig. 12.15 Storz flexible video-ureterorenoscope Flex-XC (**a**) Wolf fiber-optic analogic Viper (**b**) and digital Olympus (**c**) flexible ureteroscopes

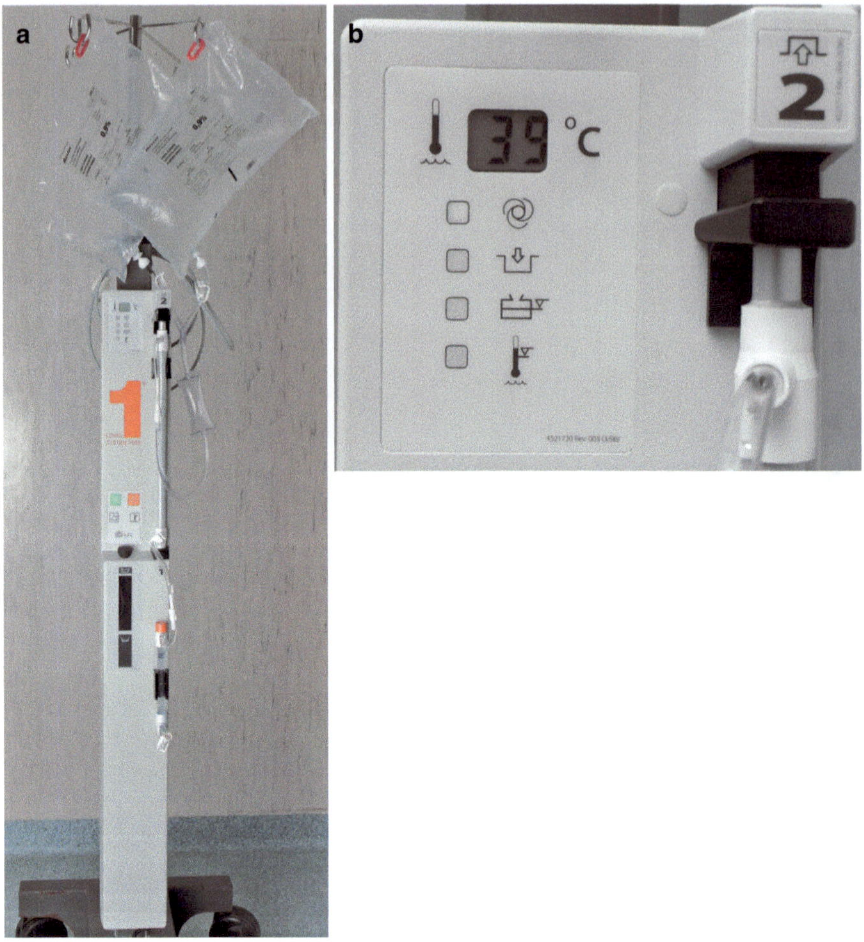

Fig. 12.16 Level 1 device by Smiths Medical for sustaining/elevating the irrigation bags (**a**) and for heating (**b**)

12.4.2 Facing the Issue of Optimal Endoscopic Vision and Intrarenal Pressures

During a supine PNL, the Amplatz is roughly horizontal (see also Chap. 13). Therefore, the pressure in the collecting system is near to 0 H_2O cm. Pressure can be even negative, when using an ultrasonic lithotripter, because of its suction effect. Consequently, the renal pelvis can be collapsed during the whole procedure, and air bubbles may interfere with optimal vision.

Some surgeons use a peristaltic pump in order to obtain increased flow rate and intrapelvic pressure. The Level 1 irrigation and heating column produced by Smiths Medical can be used for all kind of nephroscopes and ureteroscopes (and for resectoscopes as well), combining the advantage of heating the irrigation fluid flowing without air bubbles with the possibility to vary the height of the column (see also

Chap. 14), thus varying the gravity pressure of the flow of one or two simultaneous fluid bags (Fig. 12.16).

If a retrograde ureteroscopy is performed at the same time of PNL, the ureteroscope should have its own irrigation line. The role of a port seal is essential to avoid to lose fluid from the endoscope (see also Chap. 19). Because of the presence of the Amplatz sheath, higher pressures can be used than during a standard ureteroscopy, without the risk of overdistension of the renal cavities. This has also the advantage of washing out the small stone fragments created by the ureteroscope through the Amplatz.

Several irrigation devices are disponible for ureteroscopic irrigation, especially when using flexible instruments. In fact, deflection and full working channels decrease irrigation, worsen endoscopic vision, and increase renal pelvic pressures. Gravity irrigation can be increased with occasional manual pressure; there are also manual (hand- or foot-assisted) devices (Fig. 12.17), pneumatic cuffs for pressurized flow, and automated devices. Care should be taken to choose a pump that is validated for urologic use, in order to avoid medicolegal consequences in case of accidents. In any case, the main issue should be to be aware of the importance of avoiding prolonged high intrarenal pressures, predisposing to pyelorenal reflux and infectious complications (see also Chap. 19).

12.5 Disposable Accessories

12.5.1 Access Needle

Accurate puncture of the collecting system is the fundamental initial step of percutaneous surgery. The needle should be only slightly flexible and enable soft tissue penetration, reaching deep targets without excessive deviations (Fig. 12.18). Enhanced visualization of the needle tip when used with ultrasonic imaging is essential. The 18 gauge Chiba needle is composed of a 22 gauge cannula and fitted stylet. Some urologists use a small trocar instead.

12.5.2 Guidewires

Guidewires play an important role throughout the whole procedure, thus their correct selection is essential. They are available in variable diameters, lengths, stiffness, tip configuration, and coatings. The knowledge of all the features and behavior of a given wire is crucial for choosing the optimal one, depending upon its role during surgery.

Hydrophilic wires are made of a nickel titanium core and a polyurethane shell coated with a hydrophilic polymer. There are many hydrophilic guidewires on the market, like the Glidewire (Terumo), the HiWire (Cook), and the ZipWire (Boston Scientific), conceived to decrease friction when wet. They are optimal during bypassing impacted stones and negotiating difficult ureters. Their inconvenient is their tendency to slip out of the collecting system during the procedure. If a hydrophilic guidewire (0.038″, 150 cm) is passed down the ureter and outside the meatus (easy

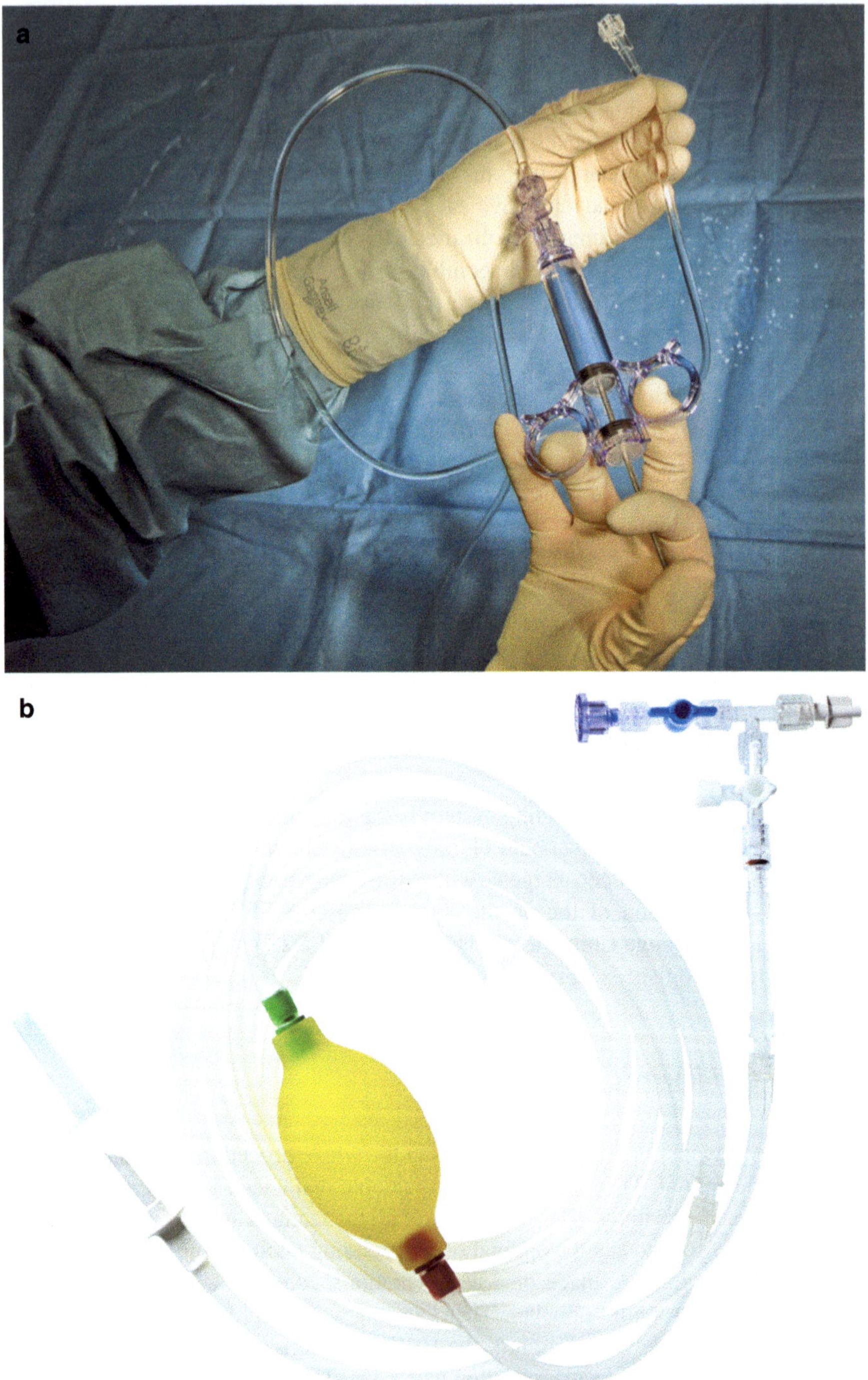

Fig. 12.17 Boston Scientific manual pump device (**a**) and Coloplast Porgés HiLine irrigation device (**b**)

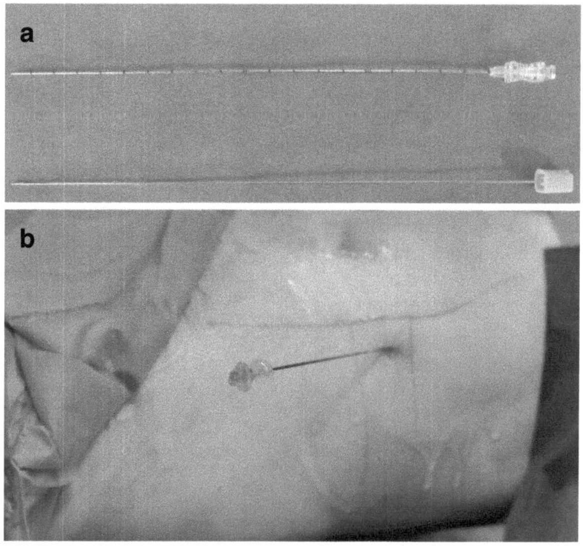

Fig. 12.18 A 18 G Chiba needle (**a**) and the same needle after renal puncture and removal of the stylet (**b**)

maneuver in the supine position), this functions both as safety and working wire. If this kind of through-and-through passage of the working wire is not possible, it is always advisable to place a second 035″ J-Tip PTFE-coated guidewire as a safety wire.

As a safety wire, it is better to use high-friction guidewires. They are made of a central mandrel covered by a tightly coiled steel wire coated with polytetrafluoroethylene (PTFE, Teflon).

During tract dilatation, a super-stiff or an extra-stiff, unkinkable Amplatz wire is recommended. The stiffness is proportional to the diameter of the central mandrel. This is an important characteristic during the dilatation process, in order to avoid kinking during passage of serial dilators at the level of the fascia and the renal capsule. Depending on the method used for dilatation, the coating of the wire may be different. When using metallic dilatators a more resistant PTFE-coated wire is preferable. With the balloon, hydrophilic wires are also suitable.

The Roadrunner (Cook) and Sensor (Boston Scientific) guidewires combine the advantages of both glidewires and super-stiff Amplatz wires. The Roadrunner guidewire is covered by a microthin layer of hydrophilic polymer allowing smooth passage around the stone and the ureteropelvic junction and has a platinum tip for fluoroscopic visualization and a stiff Nitinol core. The Sensor guidewire has a hydrophilic floppy tip for negotiating tortuous anatomy, a tungsten-filled radiopaque tip, a PTFE coating, and a Nitinol core.

After puncture, a sufficient length of guidewire should be inserted into the collecting system. Optimally, the guidewire is directed into the ureter. This is usually quite straightforward if an upper or a mid-calyx is punctured. However, in an effort to diminish the risk of hemorrhagic complications or thoracic injuries, many urologists prefer to puncture the posterior lower calyx. This is considered by many as the safest area regarding the distribution of renal vessels (see also Chaps. 6 and 13). There are several possibilities to bring down the guidewire to the ureter after a lower pole puncture. If a retrograde ureteroscopy is performed (Endovision puncture), the tip of the guide can be grasped with forceps or a basket and simply pulled

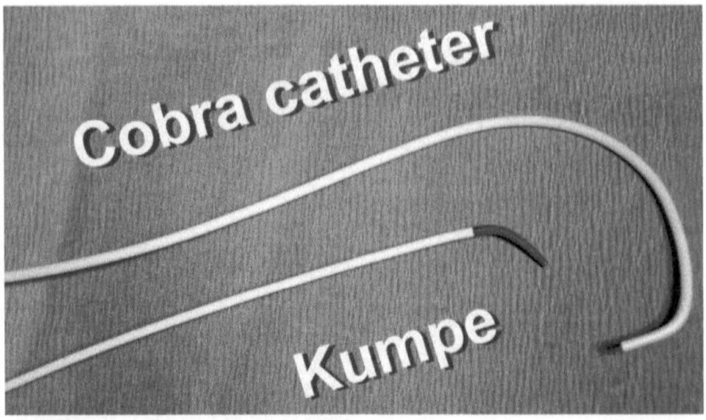

Fig. 12.19 The Cobra catheter is used to direct a 0.038″ guidewire to a specific renal area. It is made up by a material imparting torque control to the catheter shaft. The Kumpe catheter is used in combination with flexible-tipped guidewires to gain difficult ureteral access beyond a redundant or tortuous ureteral segment

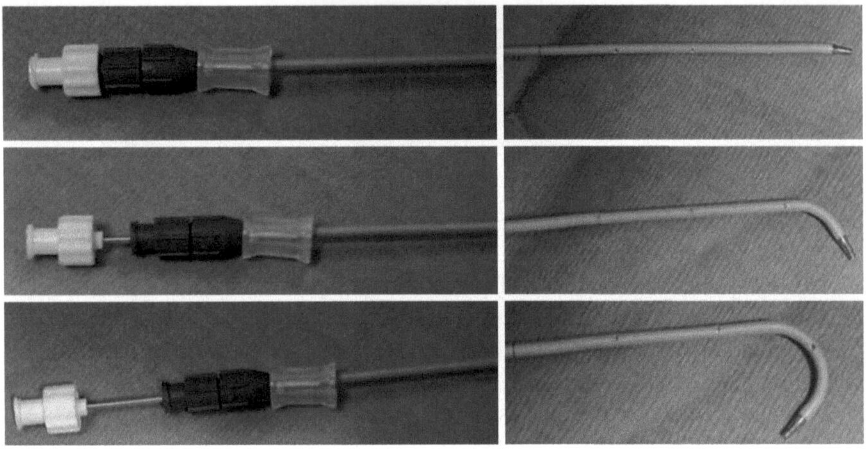

Fig. 12.20 Modification of the angulation of the tip of a Coloplast Colibri nephrostomy by progressively pulling the hollow metallic stylet allows directing the guidewire down the ureter

downwards. Alternatively, curved catheters like the Cobra or Kumpe (Fig. 12.19) catheter can be used. Another alternative is to use a pigtail nephrostomy with a hollow metallic stylet that allows modifying the curvature of the tip of the nephrostomy (Fig. 12.20). If the ureteropelvic junction or the ureter is difficult to negotiate, a guidewire with a prefashioned Coude tip on the floppy end can be of help. This kind of guidewire has a good combination of floppy, lubricious tip and a stiffer core. However, a guidewire should not be used as a safety wire, because it has only limited friction, and therefore it can be easily dislodged during the case.

12.5.3 *Fascial Dilators*

After having introduced the working guidewire, the tract is dilated to approximately 10 Ch. For this purpose, different fascial dilators are disponible. In our hands, the dilator of any 8 or 10 Ch nephrostomy set works well; at the end of the procedure, this nephrostomy can be used for drainage of the collecting system.

12.5.4 Alken Dilators

Historically, during the very first PNL, percutaneous tract creation was a 2-week procedure accomplished during several sessions [2]. It consisted in the sequential insertion of several nephrostomies, progressively upsized every other day until reaching a 20–24 Ch mature channel. However, this method considerably prolonged hospital stay and comprised difficulties such as kinking of the guidewire, bleeding, infection, and false passages.

To overcome these difficulties Alken developed a metallic telescopic dilatator set (Fig. 12.21), allowing a one-step nephrolithotomy [3]. The purpose was to maintain the initial straight puncture path during the dilation procedure, establishing a large percutaneous tract in one session with minimal bleeding. The last step of the dilation process was the insertion of the external shaft of the continuous flow nephroscope over the last and largest metallic dilator.

The Alken dilators have many advantages. First, they are reusable, therefore less expensive than other dilator systems. Furthermore, because of their rigidity, they are particularly fit for patients with previous surgery, presenting perirenal fibrous tissue. Lastly, during the dilation process, the shape of the terminal tract remains squared rather than conical. In case of complete staghorn calculus or a calyceal stone entirely filling the targeted calyx, the use of a tapered dilation system may be responsible for significant tract bleeding in case of insufficient intrarenal introduction. The only inconvenient of the Alken dilators is that in inexperienced hands they can be harmful and even cause renal pelvis perforation.

12.5.5 Semirigid Serial Amplatz Dilators

Kurt Amplatz has conceived a different dilation system, which consists of an 8 Ch flexible polyurethane dilator sliding over the working guidewire and whenever it is possible descending into the ureter [4].

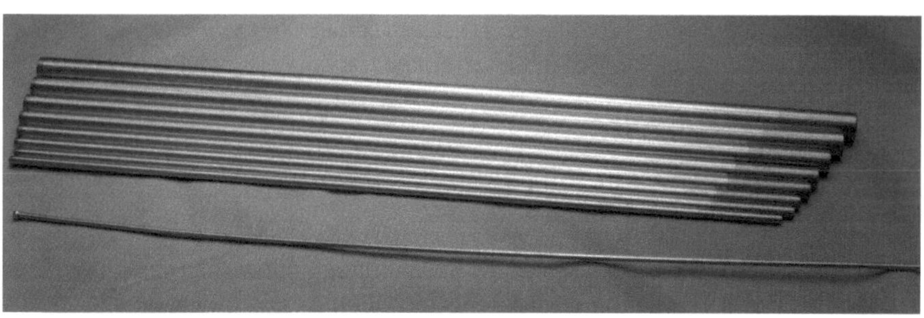

Fig. 12.21 Metallic telescopic Alken dilators

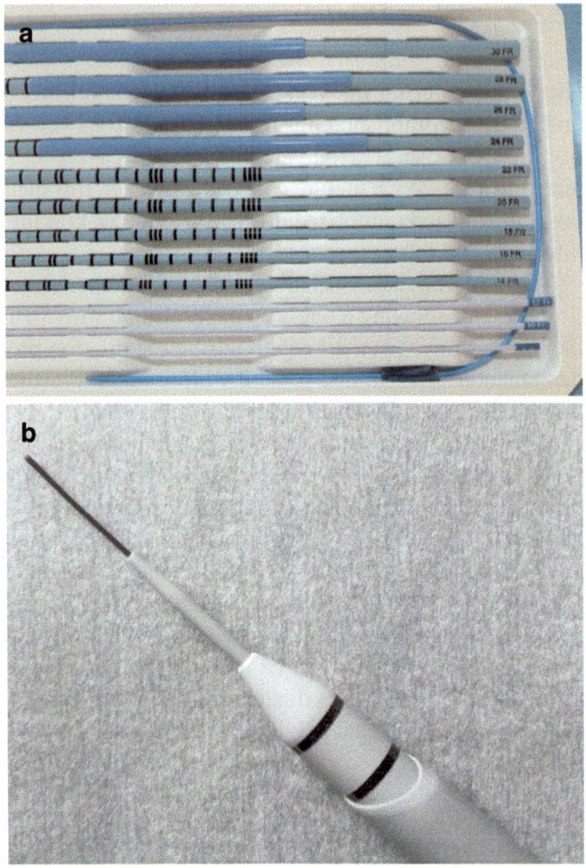

Fig. 12.22 Semirigid serial Amplatz dilators (**a**) and one-shot dilation (**b**)

The polyurethane dilator protects the guidewire and prevents kinking during progressive dilation. The nephrostomy tract is dilated in a stepwise fashion with the full set until the desired caliber (Fig. 12.22a). Single Amplatz dilators of different calibers are also in the market. Then a beveled-tip stiff and thin-walled Teflon sleeve is inserted over the last dilator. Originally, the purpose of this dilation method was to achieve the largest possible nephrostomy tract, up to 30–32 Ch, in order to remove large stones without the necessity of fragmentation. Nowadays, the one-shot technique is also used (Fig. 12.22b).

The inconvenient of serial dilators is that each dilator has to be removed before the larger one is inserted, and, in the interval, the tract may somewhat bleed.

12.5.6 Balloon Dilator

Due to the fact that the balloons produce radial dilation rather than shearing forces like the two previous dilation devices, this technique is less traumatic and causes less hemorrhage. Furthermore, the balloon dilation is quicker and requires less X-ray monitoring during the dilation process. However, it is more expensive than the two other systems.

This dilation system consists of a balloon which can be loaded until the renal parenchyma over the working guidewire. There are two main devices on the market, the Boston Scientific Nephromax (Fig. 12.23a) and the Cook UltraXX (Fig. 12.23b). Usually, a metallic ring at the extremity of the balloon serves as a radiopaque marker to adequately place the device at the limit of the calyx and papilla. Then the balloon is inflated up to 16–20 (and even 30) atmospheres (Fig. 12.23c) with a syringe equipped with a screw-operated inflation system. Care should be taken not to forget to load the Amplatz sheath behind the balloon before its placement into the nephrostomy tract (see also Chap. 19) (Fig. 12.23d). In case of perirenal scarring, an

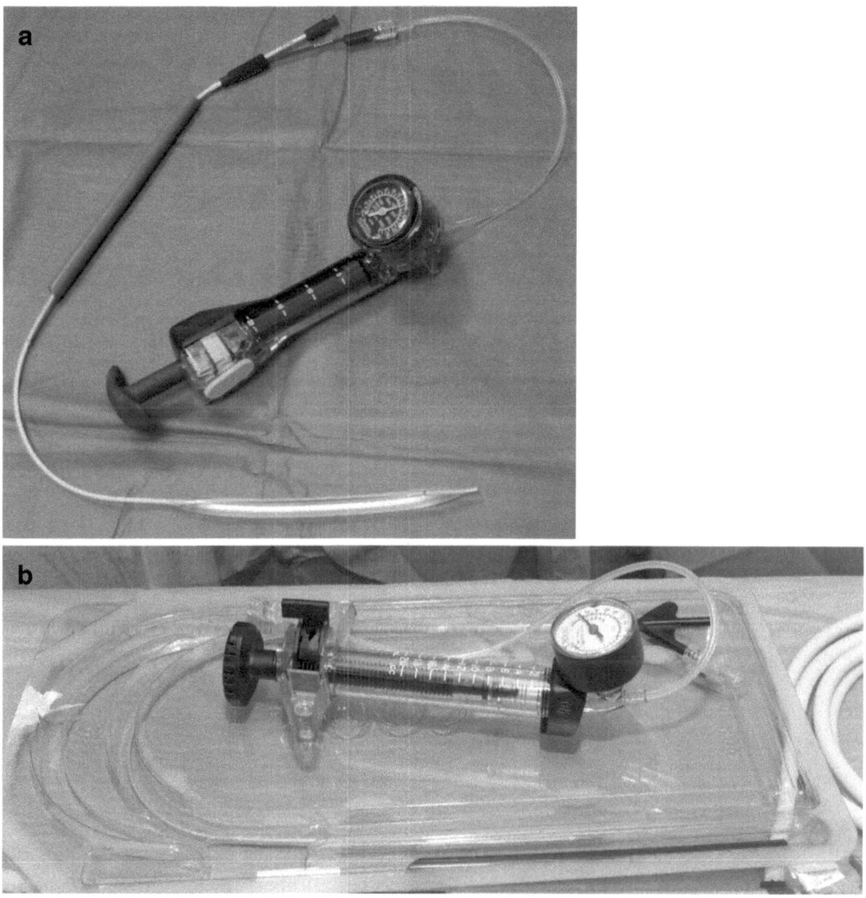

Fig. 12.23 Balloon dilators by Boston Scientific (**a**) and Cook (**b**) to be inflated up to 16–20 atm (**c**) without forgetting to load the Amplatz sheath before (**d**). The Bard balloon can be inflated up to 30 atm, useful in case of perirenal scar (**e**)

Fig. 12.23 (continued)

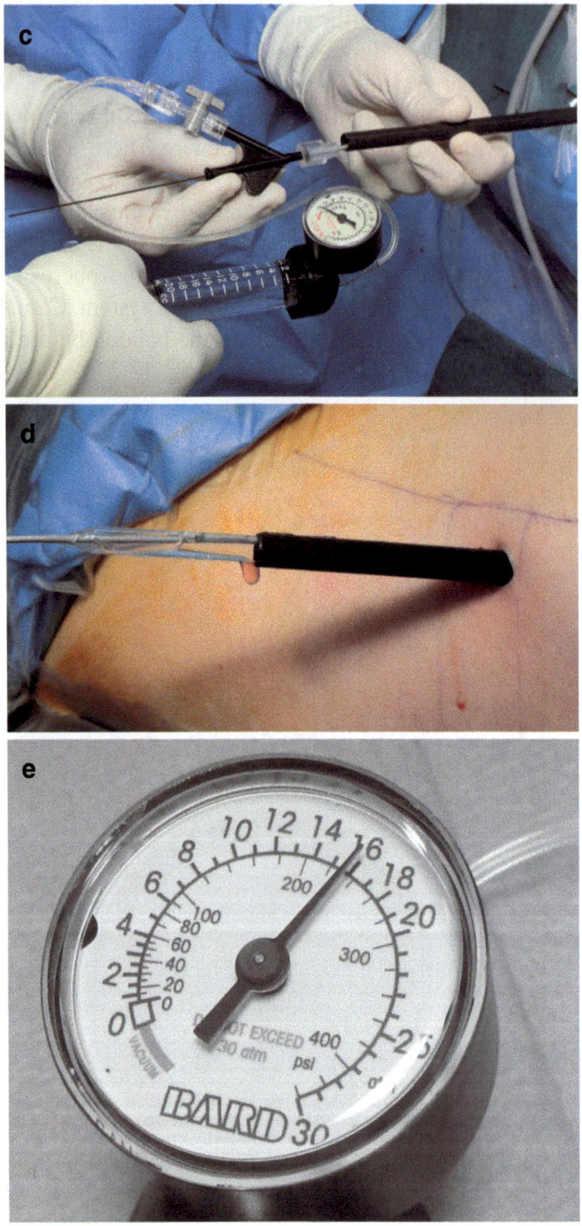

inflation pressure of 20 atm may not be sufficient. The Bard balloon was conceived to reach higher pressures up to 30 atm for such situations (Fig. 12.23e).

The balloon dilation is not always suitable (see also Chap. 13). In case of stones entirely filling the target calyx such as complete staghorn calculi, there is not enough space for balloon application. If the balloon is advanced too far to the calyx besides the stone, dilation may provoke massive bleeding. On the other hand, if the tip of the balloon does not reach the calyx, the tract through the parenchyma has a conical shape, and a troublesome bleeding is encountered during initial insertion of the nephroscope. Sometimes balloons also fail to dilate dense scar tissue, such as a perirenal fibrosis after previous surgery. Another problem is the limited choice in the size of balloons (18, 24, and 30 Ch).

12.5.7 Amplatz Sheath

There are different sizes of Amplatz sheaths, the choice depending upon several factors (see Chap. 13). In the past the continuous flow nephroscope with its sheath was used without the Amplatz sheath. Now its use makes the procedure safer and less traumatic. Large, 30 Ch sheaths allow to remove stones up to 1 cm in diameter. However, their use is not recommended on non-dilated systems especially if the target calyx has a narrow infundibulum. In such circumstances, the advancement of the sheath would provoke troublesome bleeding. The other drawback with the use of large nephrostomy tract is the increased occurrence of urinary fistula. Recently, the trend is to use smaller caliber Amplatz sheaths, to perform a "midi" or "mini" PNL. A 24 Ch Amplatz sheath is usually compatible with standard 22 Ch nephroscopes.

Some authors even recommend 15–16.5 Ch Amplatz sheaths (mini-PNL). However, some urologists argue that diminishing the diameter of the Amplatz sheath makes it more difficult to remove stone fragments, and in this case, the advantage of a PNL compared to a retrograde flexible ureteroscopy with a 14 Ch ureteral access sheaths is debatable.

There are also different lengths available. For morbidly obese patients, extra-long, 20 cm Amplatz sheaths can be of help. Obviously, a long nephroscope is also required. A potential problem in obese patients is the possibility of inward migration of the Amplatz sheath. If the sheath is inadvertently pushed under the skin, this can be quite bothersome and removal of the sheath somehow difficult. The solution is to place a suture at the outer extremity of the Amplatz sheath which prevents its inward migration.

The choice of the transparency of the sheath depends on the individual preference of the surgeon. Transparent sheaths with a longitudinal marker line have been proposed to visualize small stones located laterally to the tract. However, in case of bleeding during the procedure, it is more difficult to identify the extremity of the sheath, and the longitudinal marker line may be confounded with the guidewire. Some sheaths also have a small incision at their outer extremity, helping to stabilize the guidewire.

12.5.8 Other Disposable Accessories

Rarely, a ureteral access sheath (UAS) might be useful, in case of combined active retrograde ureteroscopy and laser lithotripsy conducted simultaneously to the percutaneous procedure. In this case, the UAS is not useful in order to protect the collecting system from high intrarenal pressures, because the large Amplatz sheath

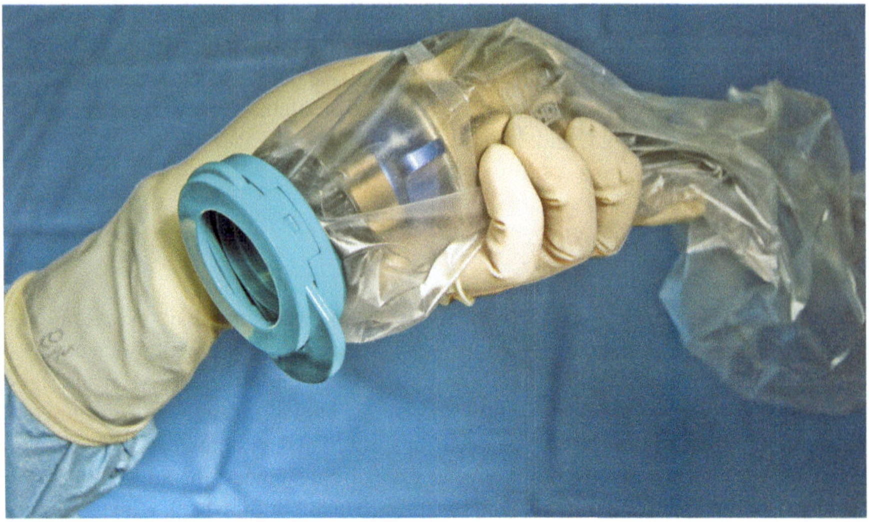

Fig. 12.24 Camera head sterile watertight covering

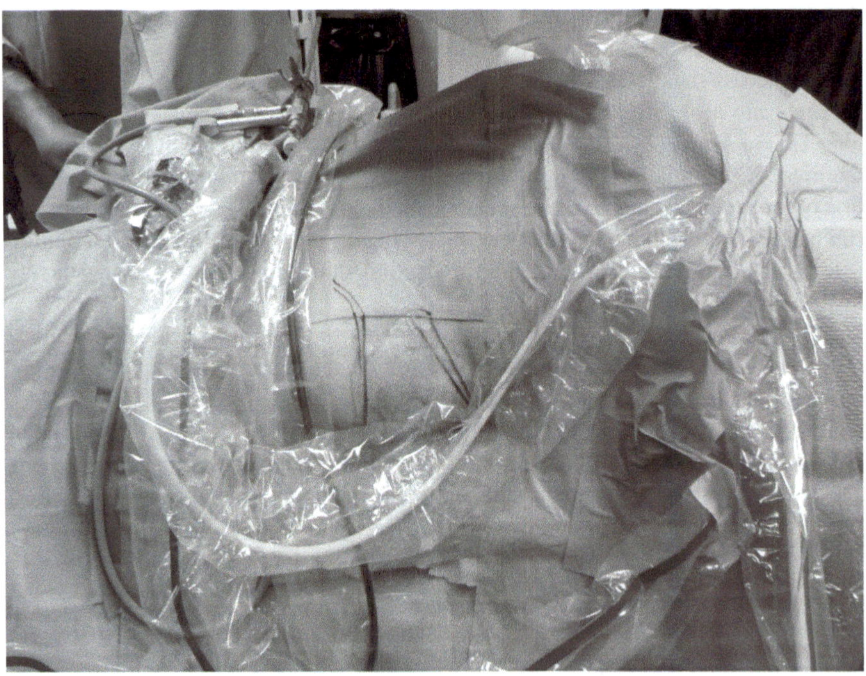

Fig. 12.25 Sterile coverings for all the cables, which are somehow fixed to maintain the surgical field in order

already works in that direction; all the same a UAS may protect the ureter during the multiple passages of the endoscope and facilitate the procedure.

Sterile coverings for the video cameras (Fig. 12.24), the ultrasound probe (Fig. 12.25), the C-arm head, and eventually the surgeon's seat may be needed.

12.6 Intracorporeal Lithotripsy

Several fragmentation devices are available for clinical use.

In 1950, Yutkin patented the principle of electrohydraulic lithotripsy (EHL), based on the effect of a high-voltage electrical discharge in a water environment. Water suddenly vaporizes, leading to the creation of an explosively expanding steam bubble that produces a shockwave. In 1957, the original prototype was used in Riga (Latvia) by Victor Goldberg. The first EHL device, the Urat-1, was clinically applied to bladder stones. Its use for PNL was rapidly abandoned because it produced too high pressure peaks, responsible for excessive bleeding within the collecting system.

Contemporary intracorporeal lithotripsy devices include ultrasound, ballistic and laser lithotripters, or the combination of these energies.

12.6.1 Ultrasound Lithotripsy

In 1952, in an experimental model, Mulvaney used a metal probe attached to a piezoelectric element with the purpose of stone disintegration [5]. In 1971, Gasteyer described the use of a prototype device for fragmenting bladder calculi, but the probe design did not permit evacuation of fragments [6]. The main problem of these first-generation ultrasound devices was the accumulation of heat.

The solution was found by Hautmann and colleagues, who developed in collaboration with Karl Storz company (Tuttlingen, Germany) the "Aachen model." They combined irrigation with suction through a hollow metallic probe, preventing overheating.

12.6.1.1 Pure Ultrasound Lithotripters

Contemporary ultrasonic lithotripters (Fig. 12.26) consist of a handpiece containing a piezoelectric crystal, stimulated by electric energy. The lithotripter is activated by a pedal switch. The expansion and contraction of the crystal results in high-frequency vibration (23.000–27.000 Hz). The longitudinal vibration is transmitted to the stone with the help of a hollow probe. The handpiece has also a central channel on the same axis of the probe, allowing suction of the irrigation fluid and stone debris during all the fragmentation

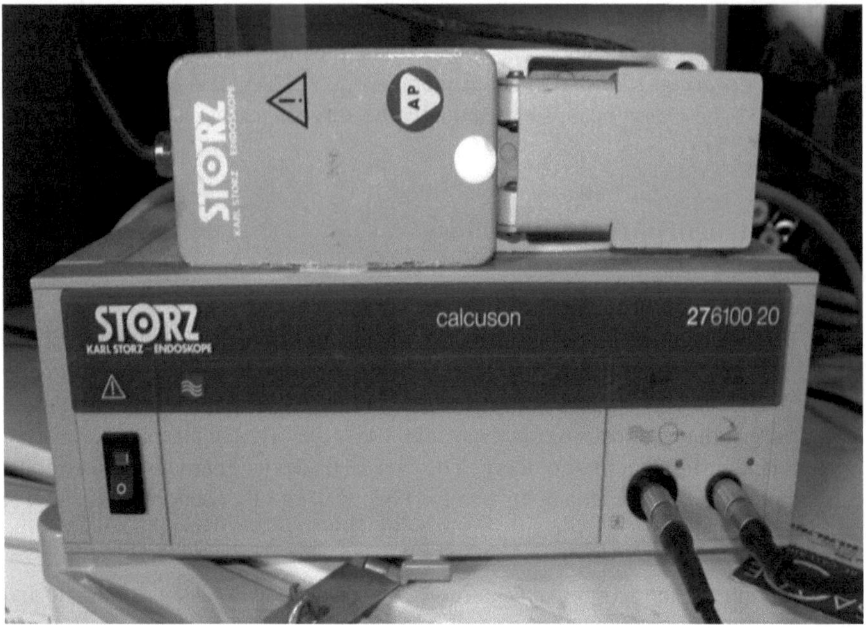

Fig. 12.26 Storz Calcuson ultrasound lithotripter

process. This also helps to cool both probe and handpiece. For PNL, 10 Ch probes are used. The advantage of this method is its ability to remove sand during fragmentation in an atraumatic way; however, a complete efficacy is often lacking on hard stones. Furthermore, the probe gets occasionally obstructed with sand.

Not all nephroscopes are suitable for the ultrasonic lithotripter, because of the 10 Ch diameter of the probe. If the nephroscope is used without the shaft, the working channel should be significantly larger than 10 Ch, otherwise there is not enough irrigation. When using a nephroscope with a 10 Ch working channel, the shaft should be mounted and the irrigation connected to the "outflow" valve of the shaft (Storz model).

12.6.1.2 CyberWand

The CyberWand (Olympus/Gyrus ACMI) (Fig. 12.27) consists of two coaxial ultrasonic probes with an 8 Ch outer diameter inner probe and an 11 Ch outer diameter outer probe. The inner probe, fixed to the handpiece, vibrates at 21 KHz and works as a conventional ultrasonic lithotripter. The outer probe glides over the fixed inner probe and vibrates at 1 KHz producing a "jackhammer" effect. The outer probe never passes the tip of the inner probe since it is 1 mm shorter than the inner probe and its maximal excursion is 1 mm.

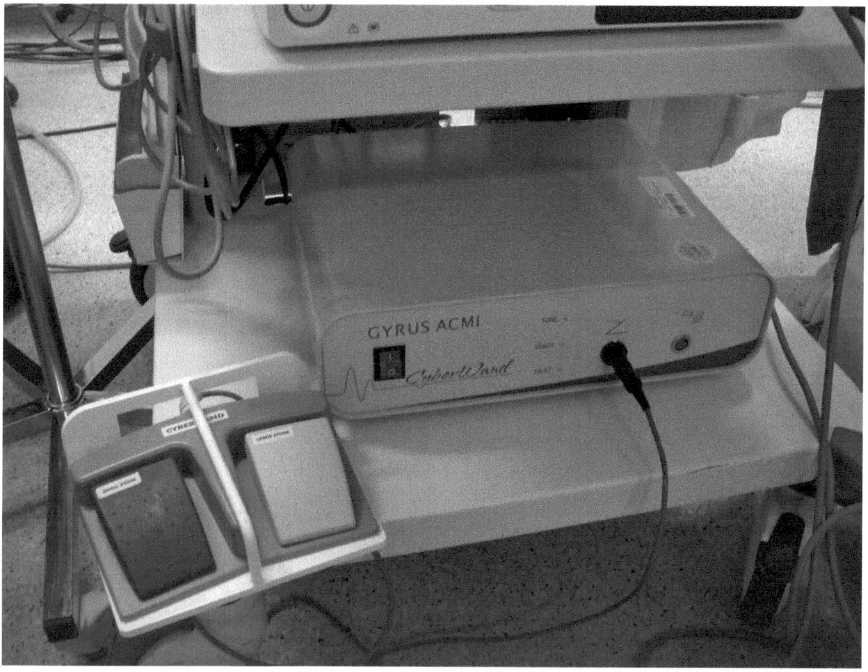

Fig. 12.27 Dual ultrasound lithotripter CyberWand (Olympus/Gyrus ACMI)

12.6.2 Pneumatic Lithotripsy

12.6.2.1 LithoClast

Pneumatic or ballistic lithotripsy was developed in a collaborative work between the Departments of Urology and Medical Electronics of the University Medical School and Electro Medical System, in Lausanne, Switzerland, and introduced in the early 1990s. The LithoClast device by EMS (Fig. 12.28) works similarly to a pneumatic jackhammer. It is powered by compressed air available in the operative room, which necessitates attachment to a central unit; there is a metallic projectile in the handpiece propelled by measured bursts of compressed air against the head of the metal probe at a frequency up to 12 cycles per second. Shots are triggered with the help of a foot pedal. LithoClast can be used with single- or multiple-shot setting. Some urologists prefer the single-pulse mode, because it is associated with controlled fragmentation of the stone, formation of larger fragments, less stone scatter, and less residual fragments [7], being larger fragments easier to pick up and remove.

12.6.2.2 StoneBreaker

The StoneBreaker (Laryngeal Mask Airway [LMA] Company, Switzerland, distributed by Cook Medical) is a compact, autonomous, and cordless handheld lithotripter without

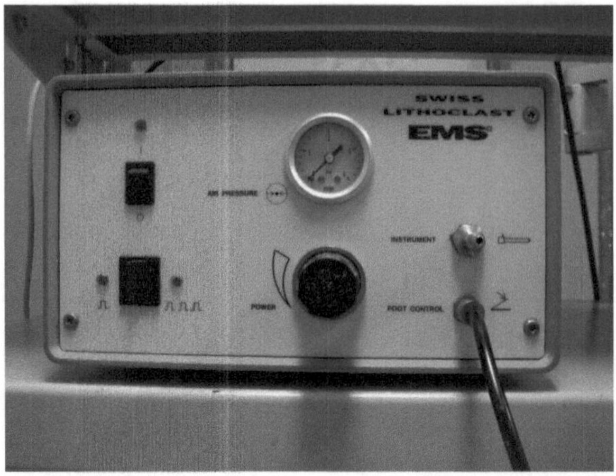

Fig. 12.28 Pneumatic LithoClast by EMS

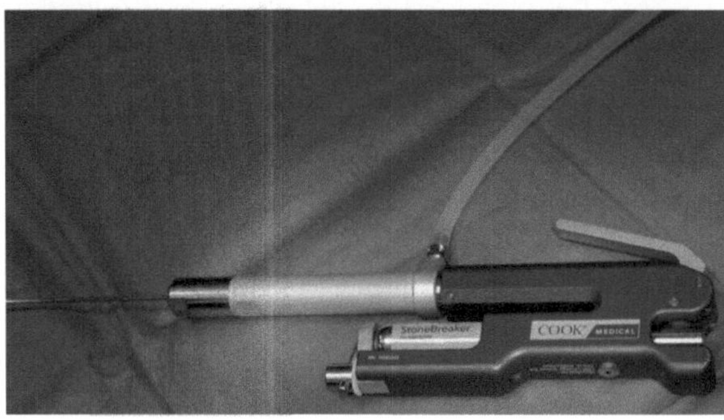

Fig. 12.29 StoneBreaker device by LMA/Cook

the need of an external energy source (Fig. 12.29). The shut is initiated by a hand-activated trigger rather than a foot pedal, which also eliminates cords near the operative field. The StoneBreaker is powered by a disposable, detachable compressed carbon dioxide (CO_2) cartridge. When the CO_2 abruptly expands, its pressure projects the hammer against the firing pin that transmits the kinetic energy to a metallic probe held in contact with the stone. One foremost advantage of this device is the minimal displacement at the tip of the probe, despite the high energy of the mechanical shock. The amount pressure transmitted to the stone is 31 bars, compared with the 3 bars of standard pneumatic lithotripters. Large fragments are easily generated and can be quickly extracted. Because of progressive drop of the gas pressure inside the cartridge, the energy of the impulses simultaneously decreases. One cartridge provides approximately 70 shocks.

12.6.2.3 Swiss LithoBreaker

The Swiss LithoBreaker (EMS) (Fig. 12.30) is a cordless, mobile lithotripsy device, incorporating a battery-driven electromechanical impulse generator (single or continuous at 3 Hz).

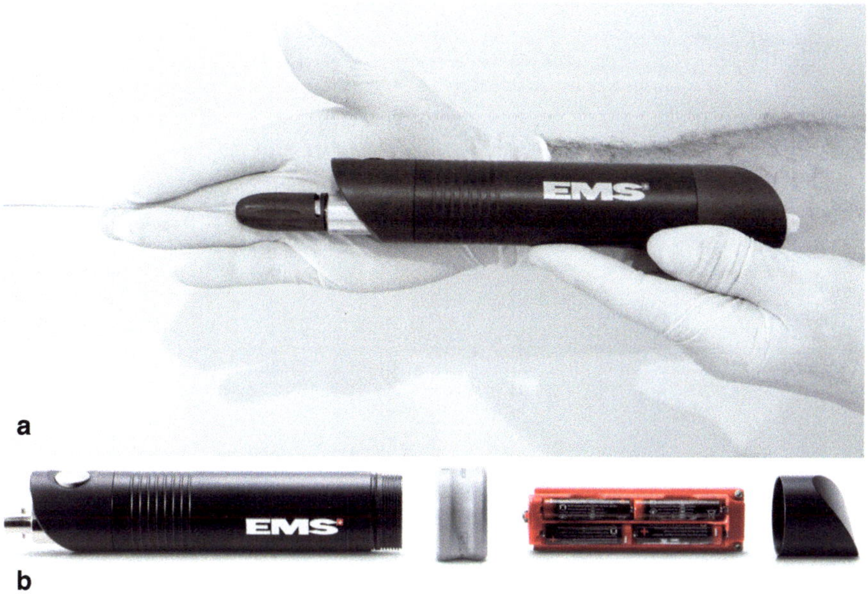

Fig. 12.30 Swiss LithoBreaker by EMS (© EMS Electro Medical Systems) assembled probe (**a**) single elements of the probe (**b**)

12.6.3 Combined Lithotripsy

12.6.3.1 LithoClast Master

The LithoClast Master consists of a dual-energy generator delivering simultaneously pneumatic ad ultrasonic energy (Fig. 12.31a). The two kinds of energy are transmitted to a handpiece (Fig. 12.31b) and triggered with a dual foot switch (Fig. 12.31c). The 1.0 mm LithoClast probe is advanced through the hollow 10 Ch ultrasonic probe without protruding (see also Chap. 19). The ballistic shockwave produces gross fragmentation. The ultrasound completes the fragmentation and allows sand aspirating. The LithoClast probe prevents the ultrasonic probe to get obstructed by sand. The suction tube is attached to a stone-catcher device. Suction is synchronized with ultrasound fragmentation. When the foot pedal is activated, a pinch valve releases the outlet suction tube of the stone catcher.

Care should be taken to use the optimal settings. The LithoClast is set to a frequency of approximately 5 Hz. It is not recommended to use higher frequencies, because the power of the individual shockwaves will diminish. The ultrasound is set to 60 % of its full power. Otherwise there is the concrete risk of overheating. However, the full energy can be used for short periods.

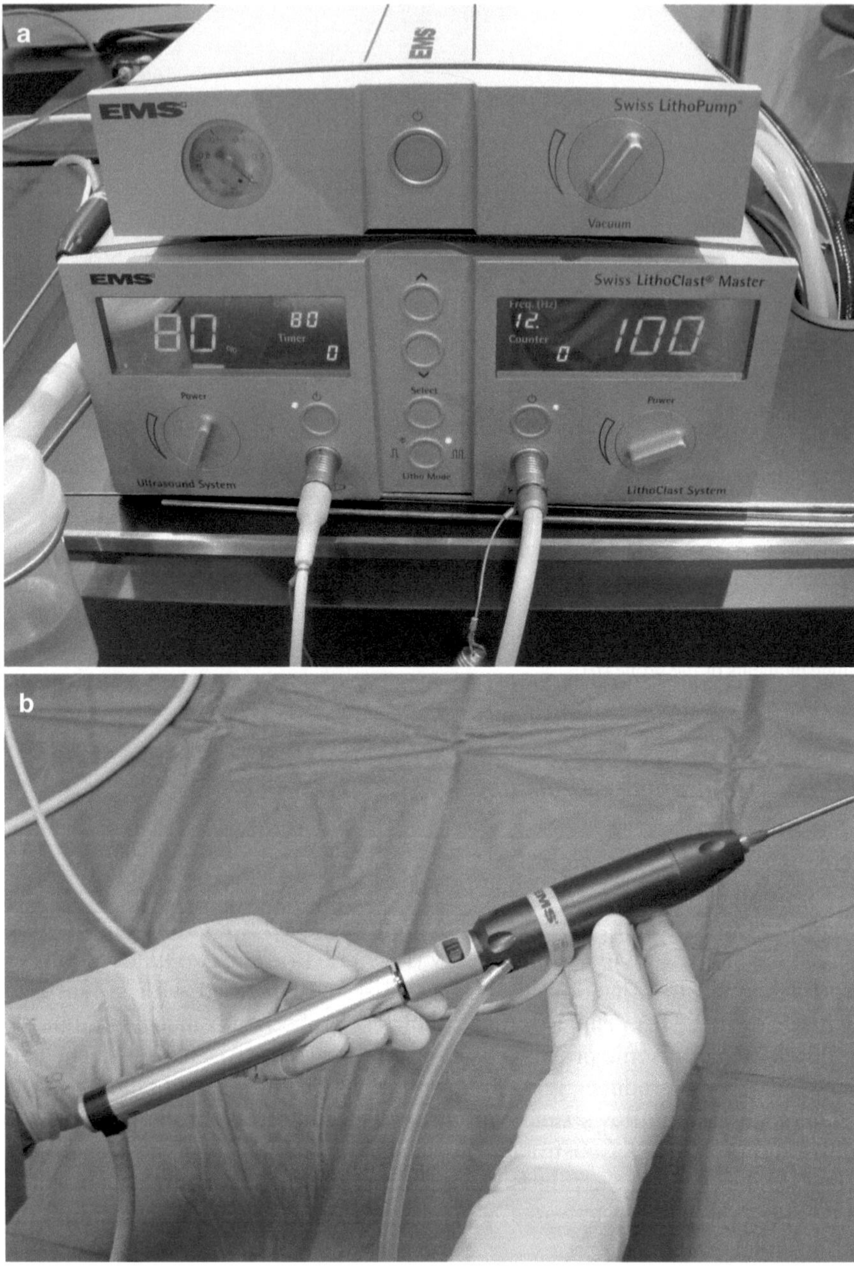

Fig. 12.31 LithoClast Master by EMS (**a**) with handpiece (**b**) foot switch (**c**) and pitch valve on aspiration tube (**d**) for single and combined lithotripsy

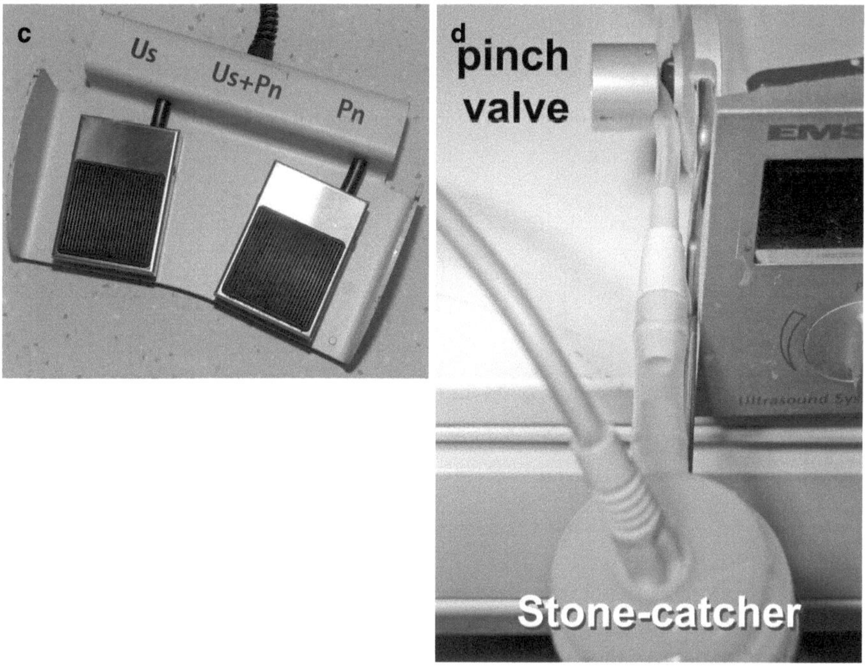

Fig. 12.31 (continued)

12.6.4 Laser

During the few last decades lasers gained increasing popularity in the treatment of stone disease. Basically, the laser is a special form of light energy which is unidirectional, coherent, and monochromatic. As any other forms of light, the laser energy transforms into heat as soon as it is absorbed.

During laser treatment, the stones are surrounded by urine and irrigation fluid. The principle of the laser fragmentation of the stones consists of the localized explosive boiling of water near the stone, resulting in a shockwave. In other words, the target of the laser during stone disintegration is water. The optimal laser should have a wavelength which is highly absorbed by water. This high absorption prevents penetration of the energy in the surrounding tissues and allows vaporization confined to a small area. These criteria are fulfilled by lasers having a wavelength belonging to the infrared spectrum, such as erbium:YAG, holmium:YAG, or CO_2. Additionally, lasers used for stone treatment should also be characterized by a wavelength allowing its transmission via optical fibers. This explains why CO_2 laser is not suitable, and most lasers for stone surgery use holmium:YAG technology.

The holmium:YAG laser is characterized with a high absorption by water and a penetration that does not exceed 0.4 mm. Safety issues (especially the issue of ocular risk) should be known and respected by the urologist. Because the penetration of

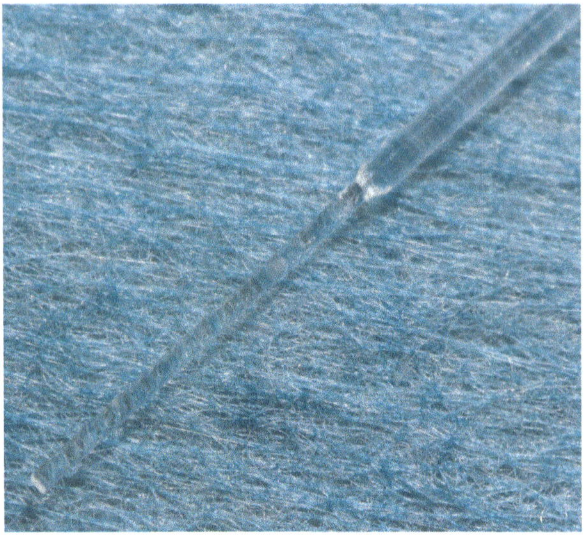

Fig. 12.32 Laser fiber (365 μm in diameter)

the wavelength of holmium laser is weak in human tissues, the beam is absorbed by the transparent parts of the eye before it reaches the retina. Therefore, the main risk consists of corneal burning, but not retinal injury. Each wavelength is characterized by its Maximal Permissible Exposure (MPE), which is the highest power of the laser source considered safe on the cornea. The Nominal Ocular Hazard Distance (NOHD) is the distance from the source at which the energy per surface unit becomes lower than the Maximum Permissible Exposure. In case of holmium:YAG laser, the NOHD is 102 cm. Although the tip of the fiber is inside the urinary tract of the patient during use of the laser, accidental breaking of the fiber may occur during the shot, leading to laser injury. Laser manufacturers recommend that all the staff working in proximity of the laser or the fiber should wear protective glasses.

Although holmium laser is the first-line method during ureteroscopic lithotripsy, the presently available devices are not commonly used for standard PNL. Its use is reserved to smaller stones or during endoscopic combined intrarenal surgery through rigid ureteroscope or flexible nephroscope or ureteroscope. Laser vaporization is also extensively used during mini- or micro-PNL.

There are three parameters that should be specified: pulse duration, energy, and frequency. For stones, pulse duration varies from 150 to 1,000 μs. For hard stones containing small amounts of water, a shorter pulse duration is optimal, while soft stones rich in water require longer pulse durations. The energy depends on the effect the urologist wants to obtain (see also Chap. 14). Higher energy levels up to 2.5 J allow obtaining big fragments, while lower energy, less than 1 J results in vaporization. However, whatever the energy setting, laser fragmentation tends to produce smaller fragments than the pneumatic lithotripter [8].

Another important issue is the quality of laser fibers (Fig. 12.32). They are made of silicium. For endoscopic stone surgery, the size of the fiber depends on the caliber of the working channel of the endoscope. Obviously, more energy can be transmitted with larger fibers. When using a rigid nephroscope, 550 μm fibers may be used.

In the flexible cystoscope and ureterorenoscope, smaller fibers are used for two reasons. First, the smaller the fiber, the better it bends during flexion or deflexion of the instrument. Secondly, because of the narrow working channel, enough space is required around the fiber to allow irrigation. However, because a percutaneous tract with an Amplatz sheath is established and irrigation is also provided with the rigid nephroscope, during a combined antegrade and retrograde procedure, the flow rate through the ureteroscope has only limited importance. The 365 μm fibers are robust, and higher amounts of energy can be transmitted to the stone. If maximal deflection of the ureterorenoscope is indispensable, for example, when dealing with lower calyceal stones retrogradely, a 265 μm fiber is preferable. In our experience 200 μm fibers are too fragile, and their rupture during fragmentation inevitably leads to firing into the working channel of the instrument, destroying optical fibers and water tightness.

12.7 Stone Fragment Retrieval

12.7.1 Graspers

Different graspers with active or passive grasping mechanism are available for percutaneous surgery. The active graspers are similar to surgical forceps with a handle allowing to open and close the jaws of the grasper (Fig. 12.33a). The advantage of this instrument is that they can be used for stone removal and also “dissection” of the nephrostomy tract along the guidewire, in case of inadequate placement of the Amplatz at the beginning of the procedure (Fig 12.33b). Passive graspers are operated with U-spring handle (Fig 12.33c). The jaws can be fenestrated or triple serrated (Fig. 12.33d).

12.7.2 Baskets

The preferred baskets for semirigid and flexible ureteroscopy should be ready for use, to help from the retrograde access. Through the percutaneous access and via the rigid nephroscope, the Perc NCircle tipless basket by Cook (Fig. 12.34a, b) is very useful for the extraction of large fragments. Its advantage is the small caliber of the wires compared to the jaws of a metallic grasper. This allows removing larger fragments through the Amplatz sheath [9]. Via the flexible nephroscope the 2.4 Ch NCircle Delta Wire Tipless Stone Extractor, always by Cook, has the same essential function.

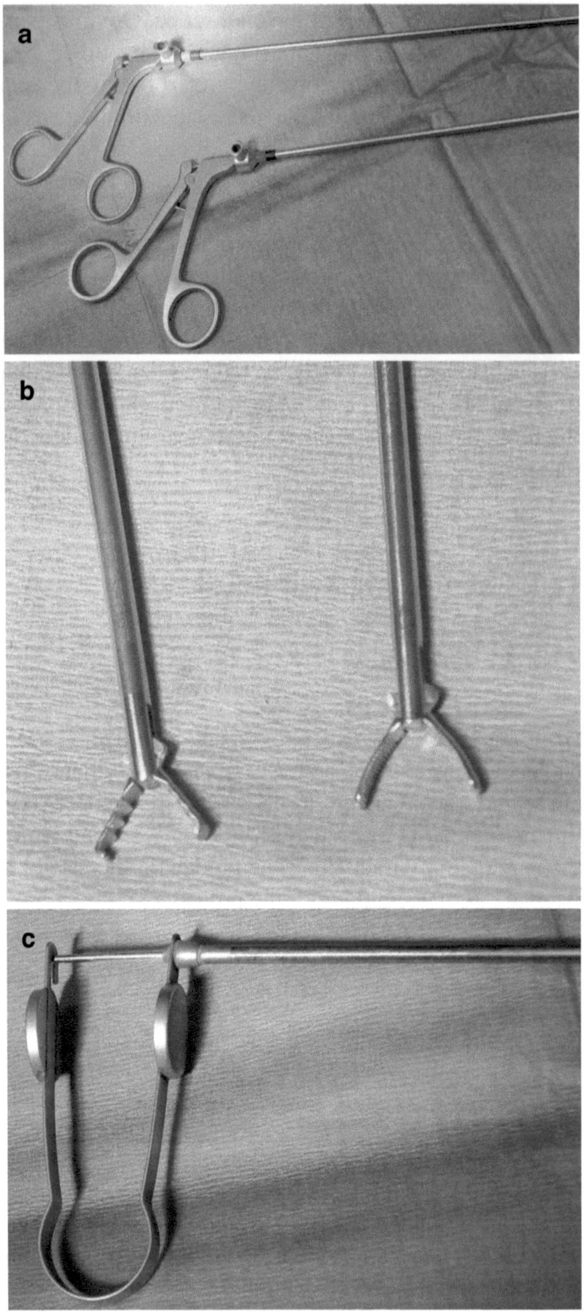

Fig. 12.33 Graspers for PNL: handle (**a**) and jaws (**b**) of an active grasper, handle (**c**) and jaws (**d**) of a passive tripod grasper

Fig. 12.33 (continued)

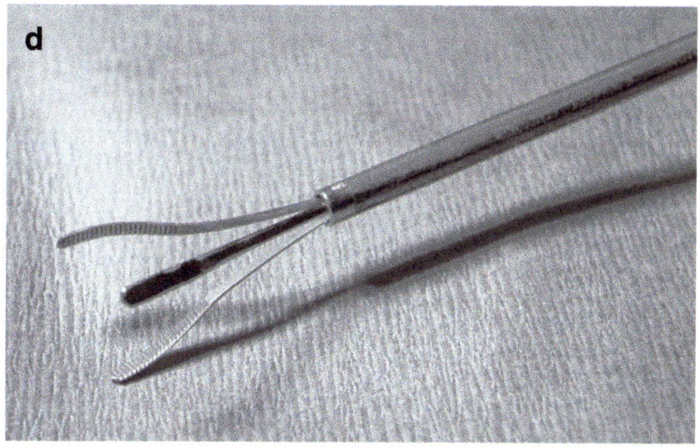

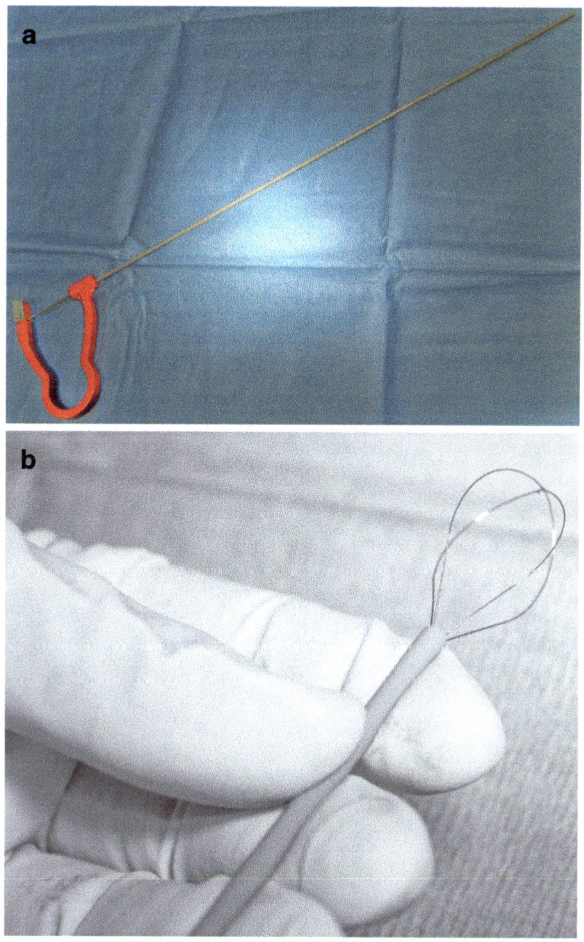

Fig. 12.34 Perc NCircle basket by Cook: handle (**a**) and basket (**b**)

References

1. Hoznek A, Ouzaid I, Gettman M et al (2011) Fluoroscopy-guided renal access in supine percutaneous nephrolithotomy. Urology 78:221–224
2. Fernstrom I, Johansson B (1976) Percutaneous pyelolithotomy. A new extraction technique. Scand J Urol Nephrol 10:257–259
3. Alken P (1981) Telescopbougierset zur perkutanen Nephrostomie. Aktuel Urol 12:216–219
4. Rusnak B, Castaneda-Zuniga W, Kotula F, Herrera M, Amplatz K (1982) An improved dilator system for percutaneous nephrostomies. Radiology 144:174
5. Mulvaney WP (1953) Attempted disintegration of calculi by ultrasonic vibrations. J Urol 70:704–707
6. Gasteyer KH (1971) Eine neue Methode der Blasensteinzertrummerung: Die Ultraschall-Lithotripsie. Urologe 10:30–32
7. Hemal AK, Goel A, Aron M et al (2003) Evaluation of fragmentation with single or multiple pulse setting of Lithoclast for renal calculi during percutaneous nephrolithotripsy and its impact on clearance. Urol Int 70:265–268
8. Teichman JM, Vassar GJ, Bishoff JT, Bellman GC (1998) Holmium:YAG lithotripsy yields smaller fragments than lithoclast, pulsed dye laser or electrohydraulic lithotripsy. J Urol 159:17–23
9. Hoffman N, Lukasewycz SJ, Canales B et al (2004) Percutaneous renal stone extraction: in vitro study of retrieval devices. J Urol 172:559–561

Chapter 13
ECIRS: Access Creation

Cesare Marco Scoffone, András Hoznek, and Cecilia Maria Cracco

Abstract A suitable percutaneous access is the key point of the success of any PNL, maximizing the effectiveness of the procedure in terms of stone-free status and minimizing the risk of complications. The selection of the best calyx of entry should be preoperatively planned, to define the better strategy for a definite patient with a given urolithiasis. The first operative step of ECIRS (preliminary flexible ureteroscopy) has a fundamental diagnostic importance for defining stone and collecting system features impossible to define by means of any preoperative investigation. Renal puncture and tract dilation modalities are discussed. Fluoroscopy and ultrasound guidance, and Endovision control of the supine renal puncture are described and other guidance methods considered (retrograde nephrostomy application, all-seeing needle, image-fusion and iPad guidance, electromagnetic tracking system, navigation systems, and telerobotic arms). Guidewire application and management and tract dilation-related problems are afforded, according to the authors' expertise.

C.M. Scoffone, MD (✉) • C.M. Cracco, MD, PhD
Department of Urology, Cottolengo Hospital, via Cottolengo 9, 10152 Torino, Italy
e-mail: scoof@libero.it; cecilia.cracco@libero.it

A. Hoznek, MD
Department of Urology, CHU Henri Mondor, 51. Av. du Ml. de Lattre de Tassigny, 94010 Créteil Cedex, France
e-mail: andras.hoznek@gmail.com

C.M. Scoffone et al. (eds.), *Supine Percutaneous Nephrolithotomy and ECIRS*,
DOI 10.1007/978-2-8178-0459-0_13, © Springer-Verlag France 2014

13.1 Introduction

Theoretically, PNL can be performed as a single-stage or as a two-staged procedure, with the puncture in a first step and tract dilation with stone extraction in a second step. The latter solution was mainly applied in the past, in patients with increased anaesthesiological risk factors to reduce the surgical stress [1] or for organizational reasons in centers where the puncture was performed by the radiologist rather than by the urologist [2]. According to recently published data, most urologists (about 90 %) now puncture the collecting system themselves [3], while earlier published data in the United States showed that only 11–27 % of the urologists gained the renal access on their own [2, 4]. In fact, access-related complications are less, and stone-free rates improved when the percutaneous access is gained by the urologist rather than by the radiologist. Moreover, access obtained by radiologists for decompression of infected or obstructed systems may not be adequate for PNL [5, 6]. Therefore, PNL presently consists in a single-stage procedure, with the access usually gained by the urologist at the time of surgery.

13.2 Site and Path of the Renal Puncture

A suitable percutaneous access is the key point of the success of any PNL. The selection of the best calyx of entry should be preoperatively planned on the base of CT and other imaging studies (see Chap. 7), able to define the better strategy for a definite patient with a given urolithiasis according to the modern principles of tailored therapies and personalized medicine. The ideal puncture should maximize the effectiveness of the procedure in terms of stone-free status and minimize the risk of complications, particularly bleeding and visceral damage.

The first operative step of ECIRS consists in a preliminary flexible ureteroscopy, having a fundamental diagnostic importance for the definition of some features of the urolithiasis (such as stone mobility and hardness) and of the collecting system (such as calyceal and pyelic elasticity, infundibular size and compliance, mucosal inflammation) impossible to determine by means of any preoperative investigation. Therefore, based upon our experience, preliminary flexible ureteroscopy should become a standardized diagnostic tool, essential for the optimal planning of any endourological stone treatment, as the deriving information effectively integrate the data deduced from preoperative imaging studies and may also change at the beginning of surgery a prearranged indication from RIRS to PNL and vice versa.

Taking into consideration the retroperitoneal position of the kidney, its anatomical relationships with the neighboring organs (which may vary according the patient's decubitus), and its particular vascular and calyceal distribution (see Chap. 6), it is accepted that most of the times the safest access from the skin to the urinary tract passes through the longer axis of a lower renal calyx papilla, generally a posterior one, allowing to develop a path running parallel to the axis of the infundibulum [3].

This is the least traumatic access, reducing the risk of bleeding because the needle passes along the Brodel's bloodless line, i.e., the avascular field between anterior and posterior divisions of the main renal artery, avoiding contact with large vessels.

Most accesses are subcostal (63–83 %) but may also be intercostal or supracostal [3, 6]. The important thing is not to be too close to the rib, with the risk of injurying intercostal nerves and vessels and provoking postoperative pain. The risks of visceral lesions (colon, liver, and spleen) are discussed in detail in Chaps. 6 and 20.

Upper pole punctures have an increased risk of hydrothorax. With a supracostal 11th rib approach, the risk is 14 % on the left side and 29 % on the right side in prone position and 16 % on the left and 8 % on the right side in the supine position. A 10th rib supracostal approach is prohibitive, with more than 50 % risk of puncturing the lung [7]. However, it should be observed that an upper pole puncture in the supine position allowing ECIRS is often unnecessary because of the possibility of using flexible antegradely and retrogradely inserted endoscopes.

The resulting renal access in the supine and supine-modified positions through the lumbar area is horizontal or slightly inclined downwards, thus lowering the pressure within the collecting system, favoring the spontaneous evacuation of stone fragments and minimizing the possibility of stone migration into the ureter during fragmentation.

The step of the renal access is divided into three main parts:

1. Puncture of the collecting system.
2. Dilation of the percutaneous tract.
3. Application of the Amplatz sheath.

13.3 Renal Puncture

The puncture of the collecting system is usually performed from the skin to the collecting system, exploiting different guidance methods. None of them can be considered the best one alone, but their combined use exploiting the respective advantages may supply a valid support. Presently the optimal guidance for renal puncture is still to be sought out.

13.3.1 Fluoroscopy Guidance

Biplanar fluoroscopy with the use of the C-arm is an essential intraoperative tool for renal puncture, used in more than 60 % of cases alone [1, 8, 9]. There is also the possibility of using digital 3D reconstruction systems. In prone position fluoroscopic-only percutaneous access requires the retrograde contrast filling of the renal collecting system. Therefore, traditionally, contrast medium is instilled via a cystoscopically placed ureteral catheter, with the patient in a dorsal lithotomy position; then, the patient is turned prone for PNL. Always in the prone position, the bull's eye and the triangulation technique may be employed.

As to the fluoroscopy-guided renal puncture in the supine and supine-modified positions (Fig. 13.1a), the technique has been adapted and described in detail [10]. The first part of the procedure (i.e., the retrograde pyelography via a ureteral catheter or the retrogradely applied flexible ureteroscope) is easier with the patient in the Valdivia supine or Galdakao-modified supine Valdivia position, with no need of changing the decubitus intraoperatively. Biplanar fluoroscopy identifies the x/y reference point of entry of the needle (Fig. 13.1b), using a reference clamp placed in the vertical projection of the target calyx (Fig. 13.1c). As to the third dimension of the puncture, the 30° cephalad tilting of the C-arm is employed (Fig. 13.1d), with the needle moving in the same direction of the reference clamp if located above the

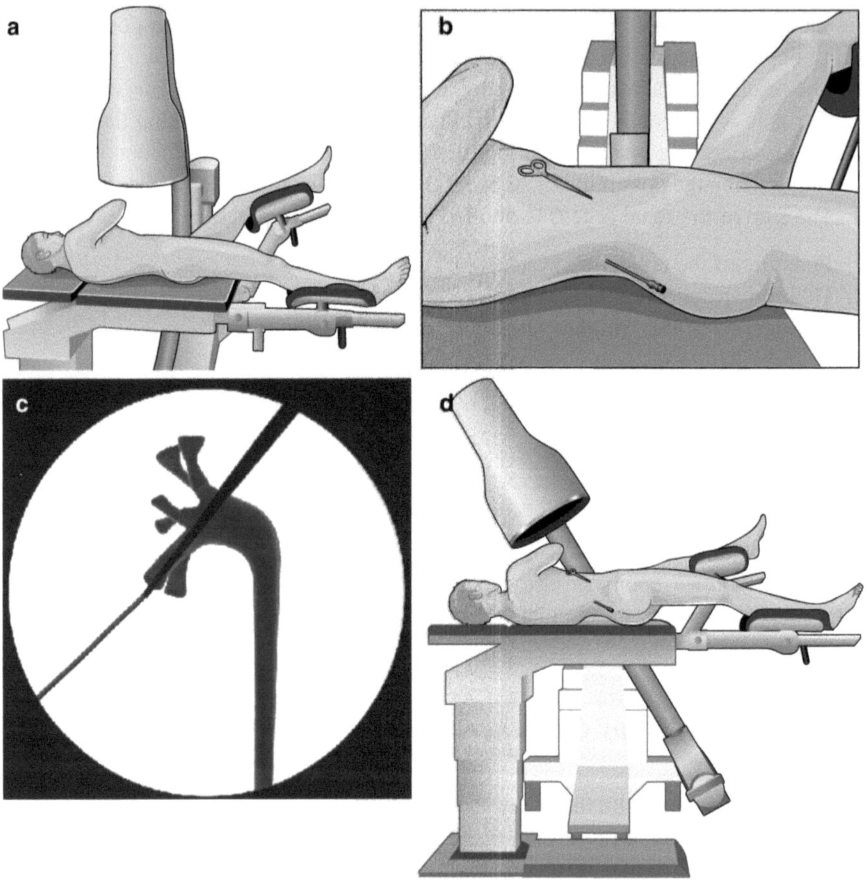

Fig. 13.1 Cephalad 30° tilting of the C-arm to puncture the kidney under fluoroscopic guidance (© Carole Fumat): Initial position (**a**) Placing a reference clamp on the abdominal wall (**b**) The clamp is placed in the vertical projection of the target calyx, and the needle is advanced towards the calyx (**c**) If no urine appears at the extremity of the needle, the C-arm is tilted cranially (**d**) In this example, the needle moves opposite to the displacement of the clamp on the fluoroscopy screen, meaning that the needle is behind the calyx (**e, f**) The needle is repositioned accordingly (**g, h**)

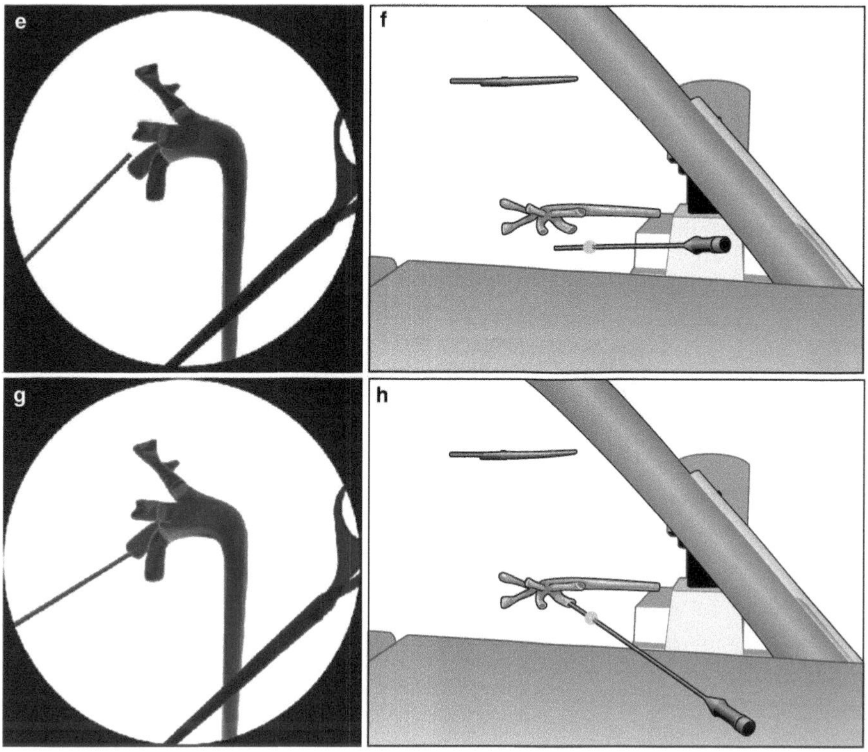

Fig. 13.1 (continued)

calyx, in the opposite direction if its tip is below the calyx (Fig. 13.1e, f). Accordingly, the needle can be slightly withdrawn and repositioned (Fig. 13.1g, h), modifying its inclination upwards or downwards. With this technique most punctures have been reported to be successful in less than one-minute radioscopy time, but its limit is that you verify and correct the position of the needle after having inserted it, without knowing in advance its exact target, thus puncturing the kidney more than once.

13.3.2 Ultrasound Guidance

Ultrasound guidance alone is possible but rarely employed as unique method (about 10 % of the procedures), exclusively in experienced centers and, namely, in children and young women [3, 11]. Totally ultrasound percutaneous procedures in supine position have also been successfully performed [12]. The advantages of ultrasound guidance include avoidance of radiation exposure and monitoring of adjacent viscera that could be injured (although the occurrence of retrorenal colon, <2 % in the supine position, is fundamentally foreseen with the preoperative CT scan) [13, 14].

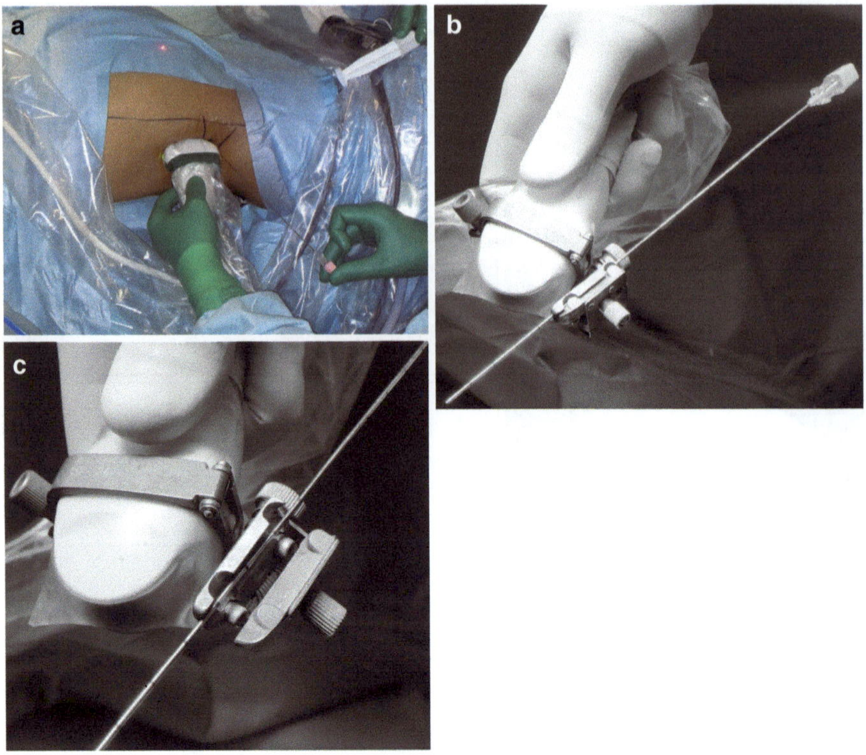

Fig. 13.2 Freehand ultrasound-guided renal puncture (**a**) needle guidance for the same ultrasound-guided puncture (**b**) and release mechanism of the needle (**c**)

The real-time contribution of 3D, 4D, and contrast-enhanced US (CEUS) has also been evaluated [15, 16].

Ultrasound-guided puncture can be performed freehand (Fig. 13.2a) or using a puncture attachment with a needle guide (Fig. 13.2b). The advantage of freehand puncturing is that the axis of the probe can be adjusted without modifying the axis of the needle; however, it requires specific skill and experience. Puncturing with the help of the needle guide may be preferred by some surgeons, because the axis of the needle relative to the probe is constant and the trajectory of the puncture is displayed with a dotted line on the ultrasound screen. Care should be taken to choose the optimal ultrasound probe for renal puncture. One important issue is the releasing mechanism of the needle guide, once the needle is in place in the target calyx, which can cause its accidental displacement. We prefer a re-sterilizable needle guide, releasing the needle with the help of a spring mechanism (Fig. 13.2c). Another relevant feature of the probe is its size. With large probes, occasionally the needle path may be obstructed by the iliac crest because of the peripheral position of the needle. Therefore, we prefer narrower probes, easier to manipulate between the lower edge of the ribs and the iliac crest.

13.3.3 Renal Puncture Under Ultrasound-Assisted Fluoroscopic Guidance

Fluoroscopy and ultrasound guidance can be usefully combined for performing a good renal puncture, although this approach is not very commonly applied (less than 15 % in the CROES series) [3].

According to our standardized experience, we start the procedure performing a thorough ultrasound evaluation of kidney, stone disease, and adjacent organs (Fig. 13.3a). Then, we identify the exact target of our puncture (the calyx or the

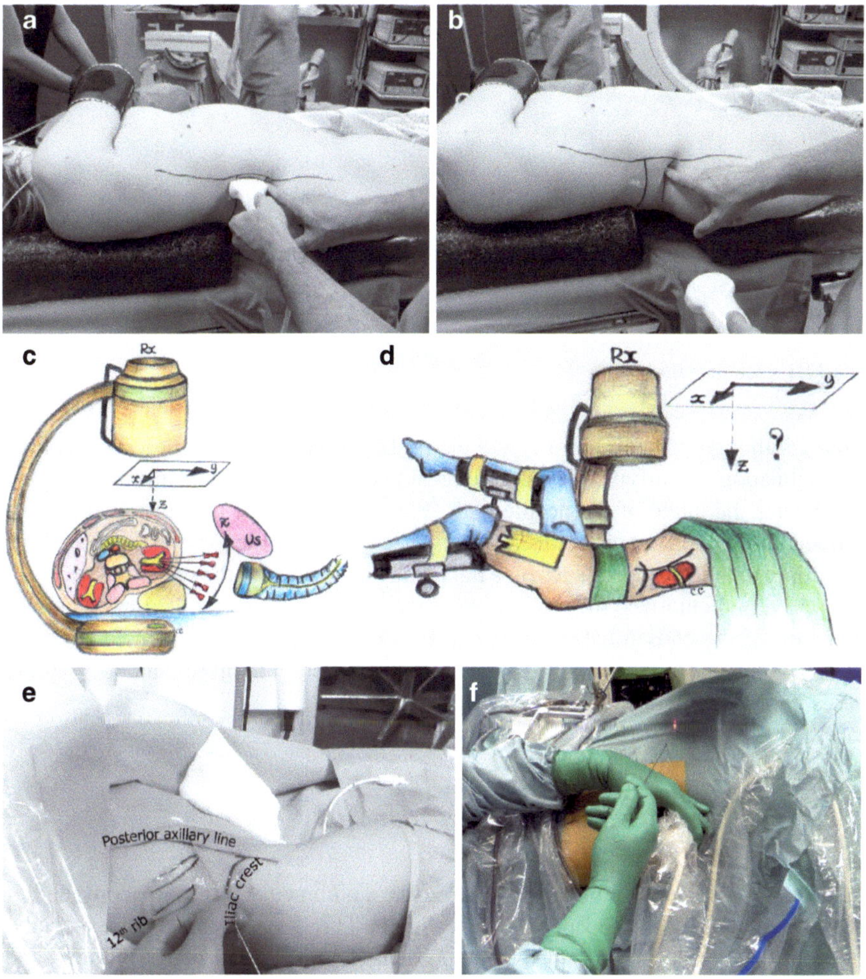

Fig. 13.3 Preliminary ultrasound examination (**a**) followed by the identification of the inclination of the needle on the third plane (**b**, **c**). Subsequent biplanar fluoroscopic-guided renal puncture identifying the other two dimensions (**d**, **e**) maintaining the inclination of the needle indicated by the previous ultrasound (**f**, **g**, **h**, **i**)

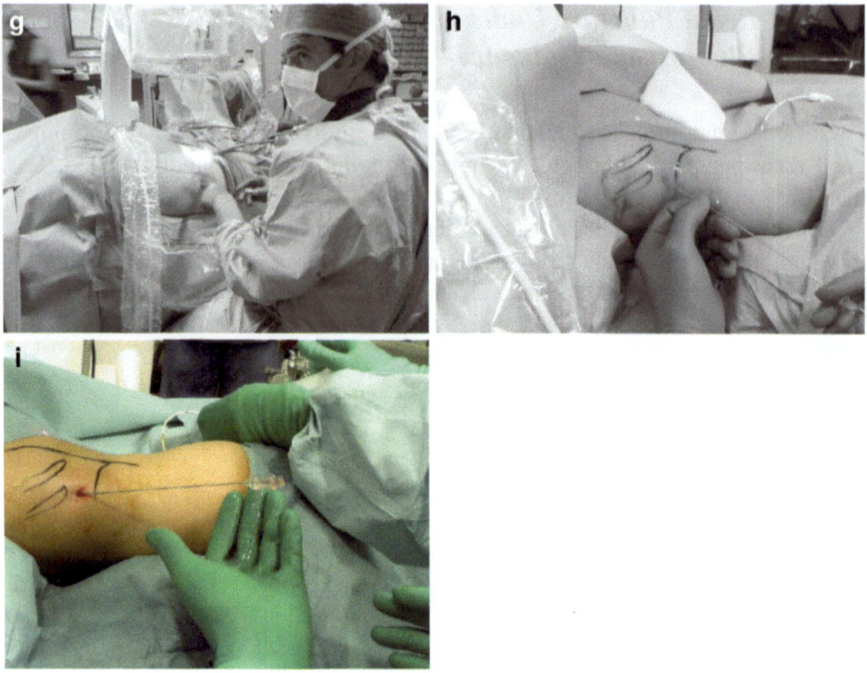

Fig. 13.3 (continued)

stone) with the ultrasound probe, and the probe inclination will reproduce the needle inclination, identifying the third dimension of the puncture and allowing to plan in advance the angle of the needle path (Fig. 13.3b, c). The puncture is then performed under fluoroscopic control, with no need of tilting the C-arm (Fig. 13.3d, e), according to the x/y coordinates on a flat plane on the body of the patient (Fig. 13.3f, g, h), having memorized the inclination of the needle. This method allows a precise puncture of the chosen calyx according to a preplanned three-dimensional "road map" of the needle, reaching its target at the first attempt in more than 80 % of the cases in our series (Fig 13.3i).

13.3.4 Renal Puncture Under Endovision Control

Another kind of renal puncture control to be combined with fluoroscopy and/or ultrasound consists in the Endovision technique [17, 18], advantageous especially for non-dilated systems, complex stone burdens, ectopic or malrotated kidneys, and morbidly obese patients, but valid in general for checking "from inside" the precise exit of the needle through the tip of the chosen papilla (Fig. 13.4a, b). The Endovision puncture consists in the possibility to follow by means of retrograde ureteroscopy (digital or not) associated with a high-definition (HD) video system the

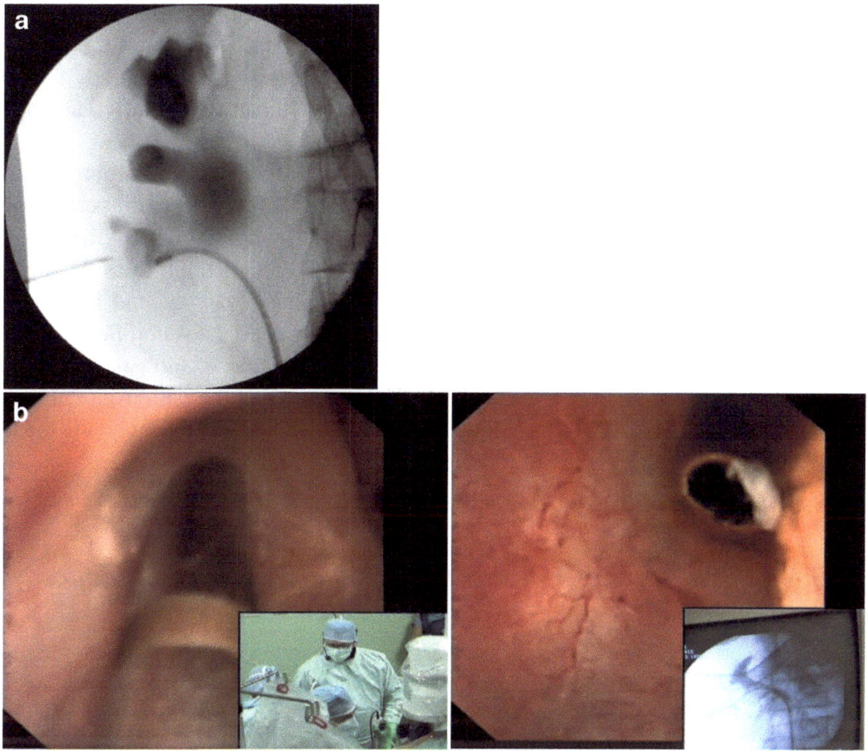

Fig. 13.4 Needle exiting from the tip of the chosen papilla under fluoroscopic (a) and Endovision control (b)

percutaneous renal puncture and the following steps (tract dilation and Amplatz sheath insertion). The Galdakao-modified supine Valdivia position is particularly ergonomic for applying this approach. Of course Endovision puncture is not always possible, especially in case of large staghorn stones, but when feasible it can give a valid support and help in reducing the bleeding risk.

13.3.5 Other Guidance Methods

The "all-seeing" needle has been proposed as a tool for an "eye-guided" renal puncture of the collecting system and as the new frontier of "the smaller the better" philosophy [19] (see also Chap. 24). A 4.85 Ch (1.6 mm) modified needle with an irrigation system and with a micro-optics of 0.6 or 0.9 mm is used. The most important derived application of the all-seeing needle is the Microperc technique, definitely reducing the hemorrhagic risk of the percutaneous approach thanks to the small diameter of the instrumentation. As usual, the problem is that in spite of the "all-seeing needle," the endourologist still needs other guidances to perform a correct renal puncture (fluoroscopy and/or ultrasound), and a further consideration is that you realize to be into the collecting system and in the right part of it containing the stones only when you are already in it, i.e., when you have already found your percutaneous way, while the path from the skin to the upper urinary tract continues to remain a "blind" one.

Following a similar philosophy, the old procedure of the retrograde nephrostomy application (Lawson technique) has been recently revised under flexible ureteroscopy guidance (Ureteroscopy-Assisted Retrograde Nephrostomy = UARN) [20, 21]. This proposal has been made to overcome the reported difficult learning curve of the antegrade renal puncture, especially in non-dilated systems, and to reduce radiation exposure and has also been applied in the Galdakao-modified supine Valdivia position [22]. However, our criticism is that the aid of ultrasound is still absolutely needed in order to avoid visceral damage and that the path from the collecting system to the skin still remains a blind one, exactly as in any antegrade renal puncture, besides being linked to the rigidity of the devices employed.

13.3.6 The Future of Intraoperative Renal Puncture Guidance

Presently we have at our disposal, before going into the operating room, sophisticated imaging tools (for instance, a preoperative multidetector CT pyelography with multiplanar reconstructions and 3D reformatting) for a thorough preoperative planning in any patient requiring a treatment for urolithiasis. Being an optimal renal puncture the crucial step of any percutaneous procedure, in the daily routine endourologists would need even more informative and essential supports during PNL, but as a matter of fact, they can rely only on the basic and simple intraoperative assistance given by fluoroscopy and/or ultrasound (CT and MRI have also been tried, but of course these imaging tools are very expensive, complicated, and difficult to apply from a practical point of view). Nowadays there is a variety of emerging innovative tools for the intraoperative support of PNL/ECIRS [23, 24], aiming at the improvement of the efficacy and safety of such procedure.

13.3.6.1 UroDyna-CT and Laser-Guided Renal Puncture

The UroDyna-CT guidance needs a ceiling-mounted C-arm gaining multiplanar reconstructions (Fig 13.5a, b), which are integrated with 3D digital fluoroscopy after antegrade contrast filling of the collecting system (Fig 13.5c) and CT/MRI images, a specific full-carbon urological interventional table in the operating room, and a Syngo-i-Guide® laser-guided system leading the needle on a preplanned path. At this time this technique is helpful especially for difficult punctures, enhancing precision of the 3D puncture planning, but is very expensive, limited to very selected centers, and, in spite of the effort to reduce radiation and time for the puncture, with a still significant X-ray exposure [25].

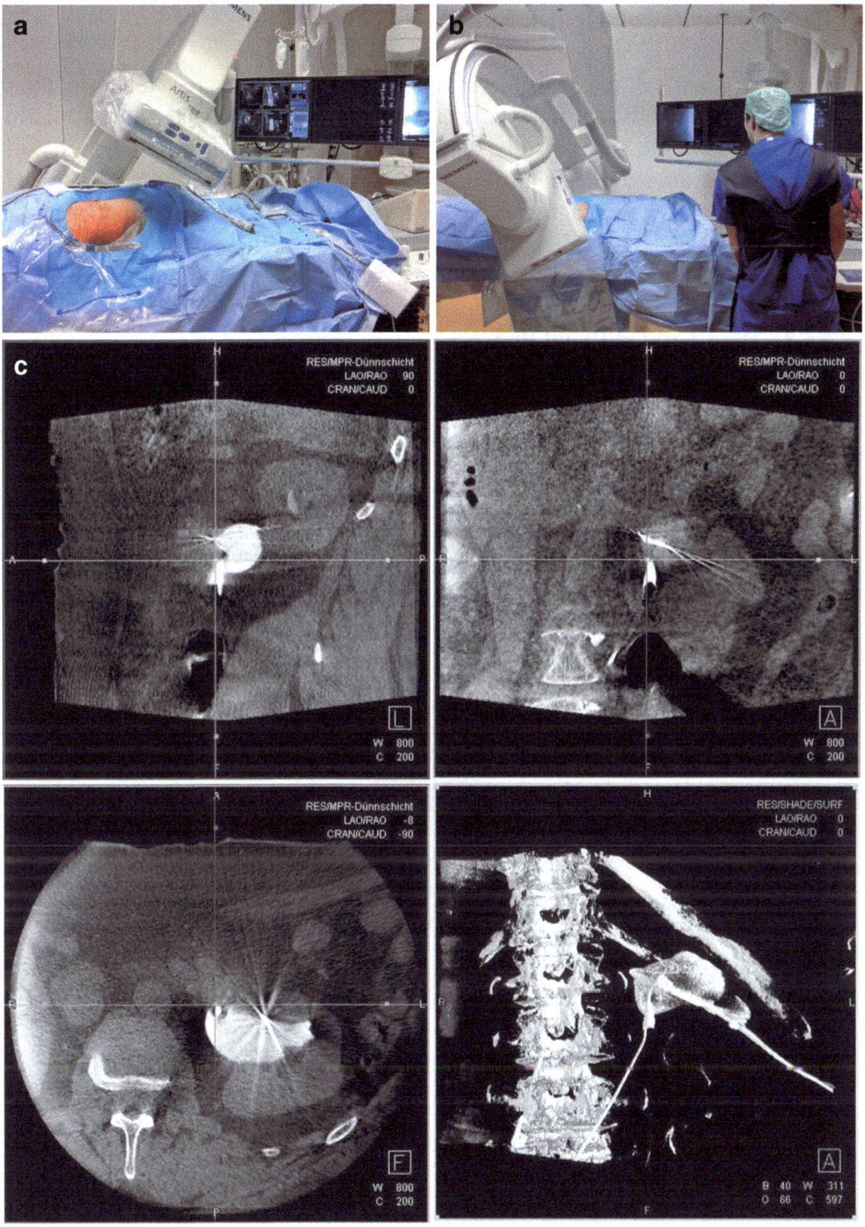

Fig. 13.5 In UroDyna-CT, data acquisition is obtained with ceiling-mounted multidirectional C-arm (**a, b**); multiplanar reconstructions allow to plan the optimal puncture path (**c**) (Courtesy of Prof. Maurice-Stephan Michel and Dr. Manuel Ritter)

13.3.6.2 Other Image-Guided Aids for Renal Puncture

A simplified version of the abovementioned image-guided puncture relies on ultrasound, with evident advantages with regard to costs, ease of management, absence of radiation exposure, and real-time application. The computerized elaboration of CT/MR images after their acquisition by a software allows real-time combined ultrasound scanning for image-guided 3D navigation. The electromagnetic sensor on the tip of the needle helps tracking its path, clearly visualizing its placement [26].

13.3.6.3 iPad-Guided Renal Puncture

Another very appealing new tool is the computer-assisted surgery, already successfully tested in certain settings such as laparoscopic cholecystectomy and, in the urologic field, for laparoscopic procedures on kidney and prostate. Special colored radio-dense markers are applied to the skin of the patient at the time of CT image data capture, which on the surgical bed at the time of surgery will function as navigation aids, ensuring perfect overlapping of the virtual and intraoperative anatomic elements (Fig 13.6a). An innovative DICOM High-Definition Volume-Rendering Software from Favia has been developed by the German

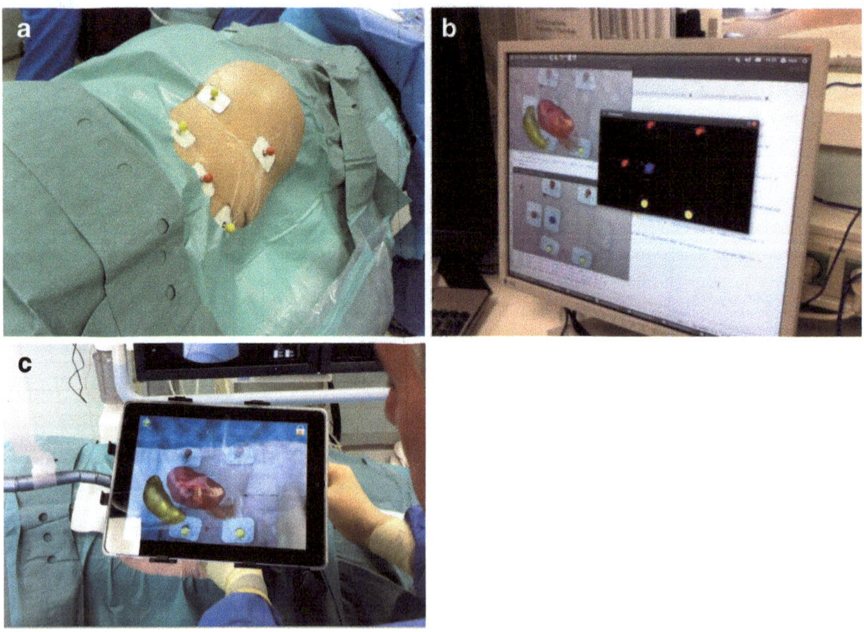

Fig. 13.6 iPad-guided renal puncture: markers placed on the skin serve as spatial reference points (**a**); segmentation is performed by a server using previously obtained CT images (**b**); the camera of the iPad allows identifying the skin markers (**c**); this permits to precisely display the augmented reality images of the kidney on the screen of the iPad (Courtesy of Prof. Jens Rassweiler)

Cancer Research Center. This software allows to overlap 3D images from a 64-thin-sliced CT scan of the collecting system and surrounding organs performed in the same position of the patient as during PNL to the body of the patient undergoing PNL on the surgical bed. The back-facing camera of the iPad obtains images from the access site, compresses, and transmits them via wireless local network to a server located at the control unit of the fluoroscopic table. The server runs the algorithms to analyze the position of the markers in relationship with the iPad and to compute a correct registration of both video image and CT (Fig 13.6b). Finally the server creates the augmented reality-enhanced image and sends it back to the iPad (Fig. 13.6c) [27].

13.3.6.4 Electromagnetic Tracking System for Renal Puncture

To conclude we would like to report a recent interesting proposal, which deserves to be thoroughly developed. The first step consists in the retrograde application of a guidewire with electromagnetic features. The electromagnetic tracking system of the retrogradely inserted guidewire allows the antegrade-guided application of the needle into the renal cavities. As a matter of fact, this approach combines a variety of advantages, including the absence of radiation exposure, the Endovision control of the needle entrance, and the electromagnetic guidance of the needle to the upper urinary tract (with the possible aid of the ultrasound control) [28].

13.3.6.5 Other Aids for Renal Puncture

A novel navigation system to assist percutaneous needle placement, the Locator, has been described and compared with conventional manual techniques. It is a device stabilizing the needle, relying on an adjustable lockable multidirectional head fixed to the operating table, based on fluoroscopy and the bull's eye technique [29].

A telerobotic arm for percutaneous renal puncture combined with ultrasound guidance has also been tested [30, 31].

13.3.7 Single Versus Multiple Renal Punctures

A single percutaneous access seems to be associated with a reduced morbidity (namely, bleeding) when compared to multiple access punctures and comparable stone-free rates using flexible nephroscopic and/or ureteroscopic retrograde approach [18, 32–35]. Multiple accesses additionally have a higher potential for damage or destruction of functioning renal tissue, resulting in diminished global renal function [36]. The CROES study reported multiple punctures in 8 % of the cases [3], which are needed when the stone cannot be approached by the rigid instrument via the primary access or by any flexible instrument. A further Y puncture can be made through the working sheath through the same incision; alternatively, more formal multiple accesses, with separate skin incision and separate tracks, can be performed.

13.3.8 Safety/Working Guidewire Application

Once the collecting system is reached, with outflow of urine from the needle, the following task is to push a guidewire inside the renal cavities, and possibly down the ureter and outside the external urethral meatus, obtaining the so-called "kebab" or "through-and-through" patient, the maximally safe arrangement during a percutaneous procedure (Fig. 13.7a, b). We preferentially use a hydrophilic guidewire

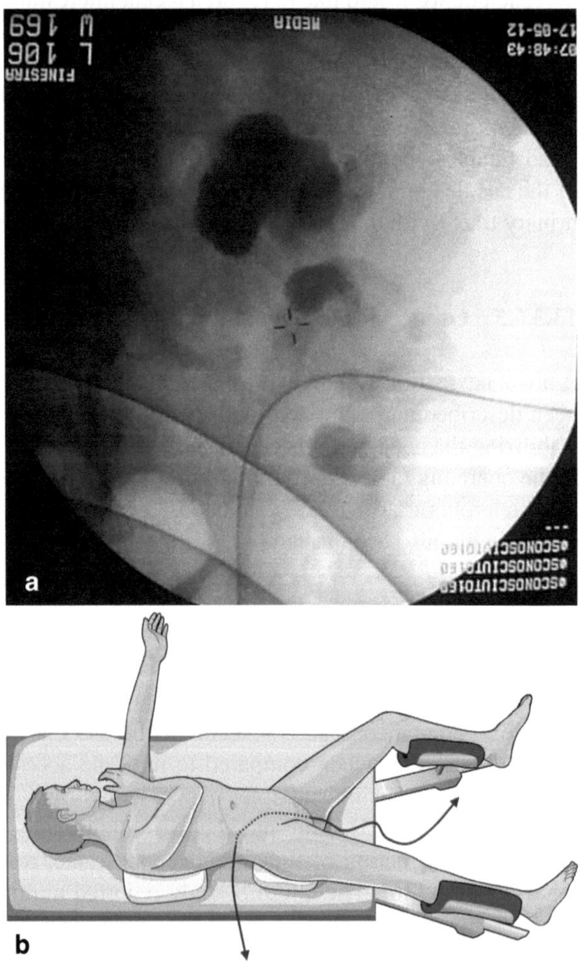

Fig. 13.7 Fluoroscopic image of a descending guidewire (**a**) and the "kebab" patient with the "through-and-through" guidewire, entering through the percutaneous access and exiting through the external urethral meatus (**b**) (© Carole Fumat)

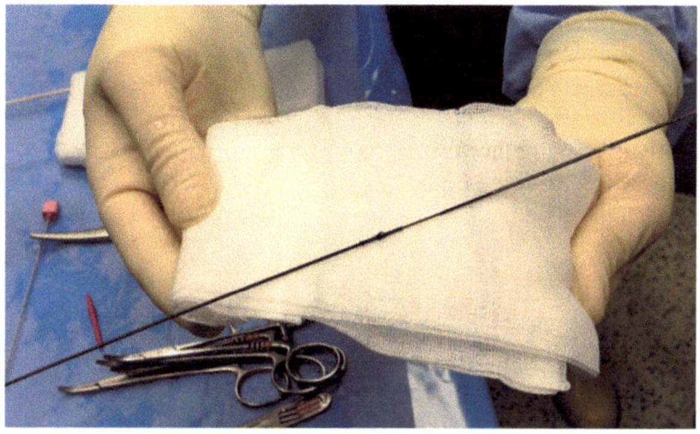

Fig. 13.8 Peeled hydrophilic guidewire after its retraction through the Chiba needle

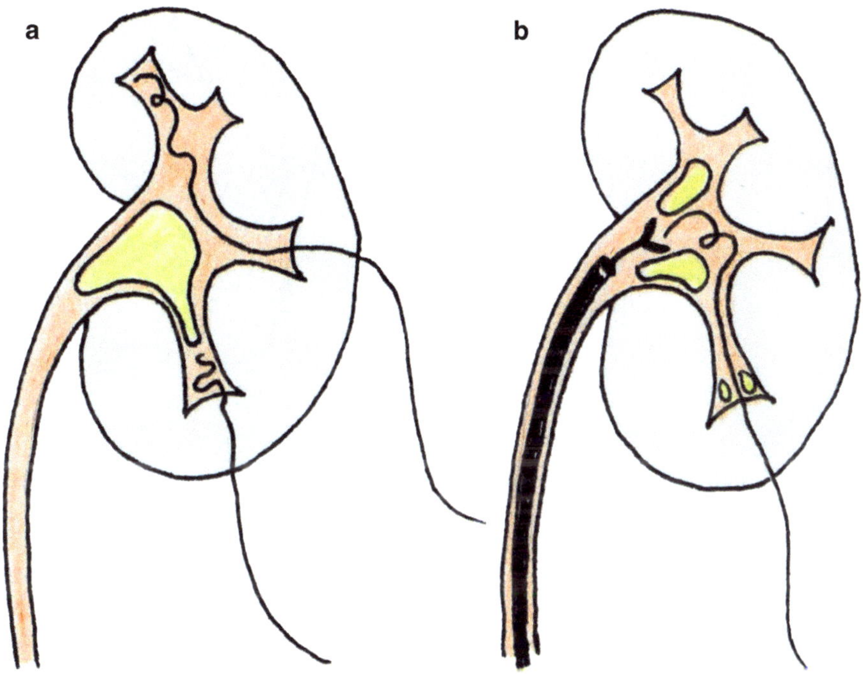

Fig. 13.9 If the guidewire does not descend along the ureter, it may remain coiled within the pelvis or a calyx (**a**) and be subsequently retrieved by means of graspers through a retrogradely inserted ureteroscope (**b**)

because of its easier descent downwards into the ureter, although care should be taken not to peel its coating during its retraction through the needle (Fig. 13.8).

If the guidewire does not pass down into the ureter, it can be coiled into the renal pelvis or a distant calyx and later recovered retrogradely by means of ureteroscope and graspers or nitinol basket (while an additional guidewire can be applied retrogradely via the ureteroscope) (Fig. 13.9a, b). Alternatively, the antegrade retrieval

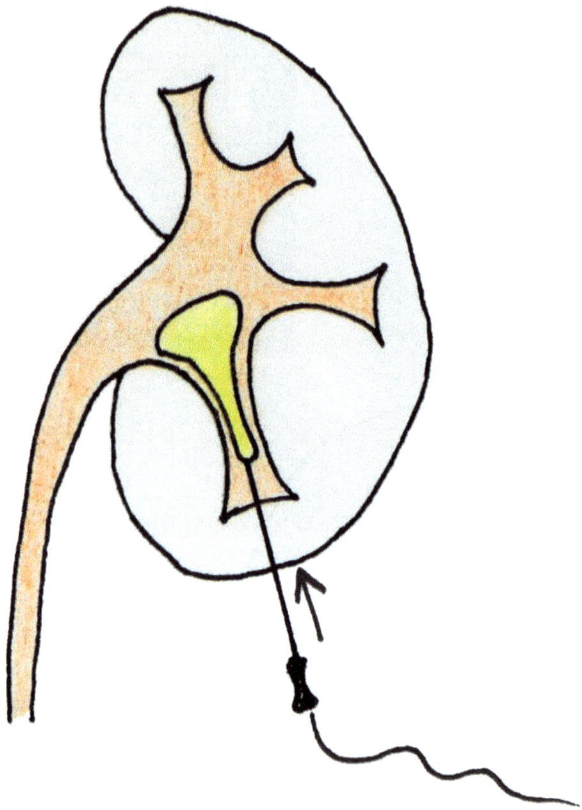

Fig. 13.10 Temptative dislodgement of an impacted stone to create the space for guidewire introduction, gently pushing in the versus of the *arrow* with the Chiba needle on the stone

of a retrogradely inserted guidewire is also possible after the insertion of the Amplatz sheath.

If the guidewire does not enter the collecting system because of a staghorn stone, a useful maneuver consists in the temptative dislodgement of the impacted stone pushing gently on it with the needle (Fig.13.10). Another trick could be the delicate saline injection through the needle and/or the low-pressure irrigation through the flexible ureteroscope, in order to create a sort of "water path" helping its passage (Fig. 13.11).

More rigid guidewires such as a stiff/superstiff hydrophilic or a PTFE one (see also Chap. 12) may be needed in case of difficult introduction, followed by the immediate application of the Alken stylet to stabilize the percutaneous tract if they enter the collecting system only for two/three centimeters (Fig. 13.12).

If a guidewire cannot be applied at least two or three centimeters within the collecting system, tract dilation is not possible and no PNL can be performed.

The loss of the guidewire during tract dilation is one of the worst events which can happen and may cause bleeding and damage to the collecting system. The solution is to start again the renal access from the beginning; otherwise, a double J should be retrogradely applied and PNL stopped and deferred.

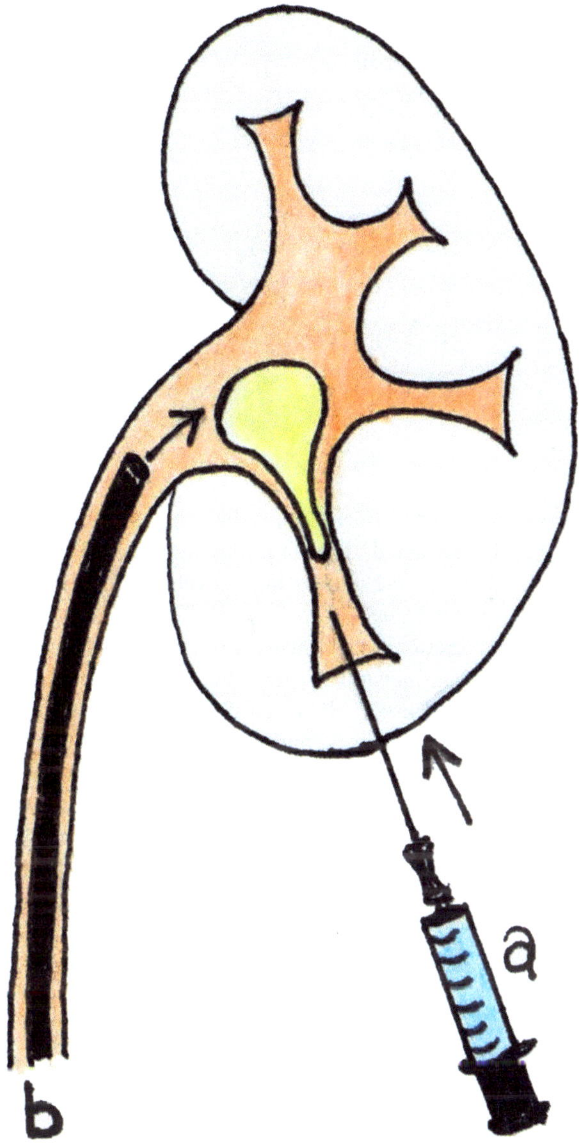

Fig. 13.11 Injection of saline into the needle (*a*) and low-pressure retrograde irrigation by means of the flexible ureteroscope (*b*) to create a "water path" for guidewire introduction and subsequent choice of the dilation method, based upon the space between stone and calyx and stone mobility (*arrows* indicate the versus of saline injection)

13.4 Percutaneous Tract Dilation

13.4.1 Selection of the Method of Dilation

Once the needle is correctly placed and the guidewire inserted, the surgeon can go on with the step of the percutaneous tract dilation. Of course, if turbid or purulent

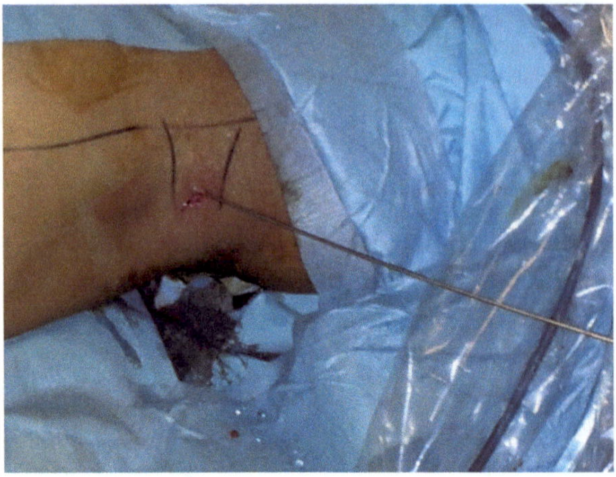

Fig. 13.12 Percutaneous tract stabilization in case the guidewire is inserted only for a short tract within the collecting system, applying the Alken stylet on the guidewire

urines are drained from the needle, a percutaneous nephrostomy should be placed and PNL suspended, until antibiotic therapy and kidney drainage have fulfilled their task. Otherwise the patient may develop infectious complications and even septic shock (see also Chap. 21).

Fascial dilators from 8 to 10 Ch or the Korth device are inserted over the guidewire previous incision of the fascia (Fig. 13.13a, b), then the chosen method of dilation can be used. Alken serial telescopic metallic dilators [37], serial semirigid plastic Amplatz dilators, and balloon dilators [38] of various calibers should be at the surgeon's disposal and ready for use (see Chap. 12).

The features of the urolithiasis (staghorn, stone mobility, entity of space between stone and calyx, Fig. 13.14), of the patient (previous surgeries and BMI) and the shape of the collecting system (especially the diameter of the infundibulum, Fig. 13.15) have a crucial influence on the choice of dilation method and of its size.

Balloon dilators are very convenient because of their one-step application, starting from a small diameter and progressively reaching the desired diameter thanks to the inflation of the balloon. This kind of dilation method should cause less bleeding risk, because the radial force used to spread the renal parenchyma is less traumatic than the shearing or cutting action of sequential Amplatz dilators or metallic telescope dilators [38]. Although, in case of fascial/renal scarring due to previous surgery, balloon dilation may not be successful (Fig. 13.16).

The introduction of serial progressive plastic Amplatz dilators on the stylet also allows to reach the chosen diameter of the Amplatz sheath; however, they require a number of passages extending the duration time of this step and enhancing the risk of exiting from the collecting system. The one-shot technique has been reported to reduce dilation time, radiation exposure, costs, and risk of hemorrhage [39–42]; although, in the short term, it causes more parenchymal damage than the gradual dilation technique [43, 44].

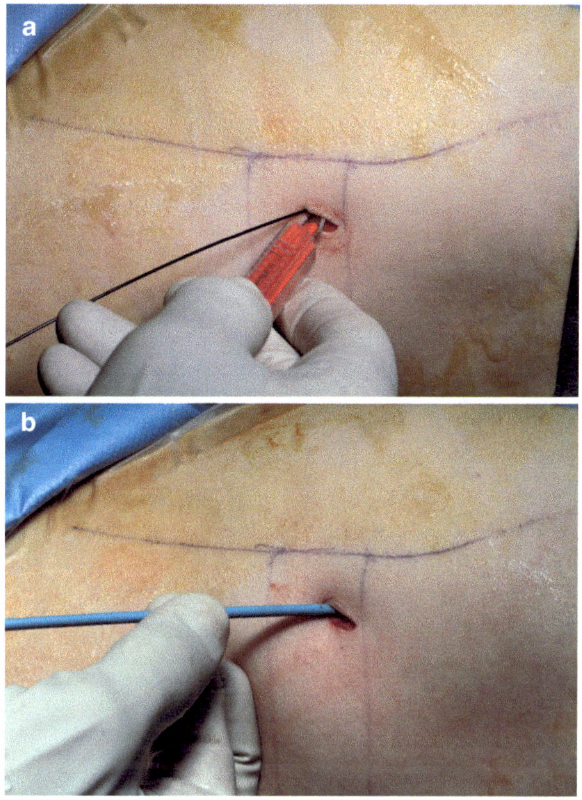

Fig. 13.13 Incision of the fascia with a scalpel (**a**) before starting with the application of the fascial dilators (**b**)

Balloon and progressive serial Amplatz dilators both require a space of at least one centimeter within the collecting system because of the shape of their tip (tapered and flat, respectively), excluding from the dilation of the last centimeter of the device (Fig. 13.17a, b, c). This difference in tract shape is important in case of stones entirely filling the target calyx, for example, in case of staghorn stones. In this particular situation there might be no place in the collecting system to admit the tip of the balloon. A reduced space between stone and papilla, even after saline injection through the needle, and a firmly impacted stone may help in rather choosing Alken telescopic metallic dilators (Fig. 13.18). Also in cases of scarred renal and fascial tissue due to previous surgery, the use of serial dilators might be more successful than balloon dilators [41].

Again, the integrated use of retrograde flexible ureteroscopy during ECIRS can aid the dilation step as well, assisting under Endovision control the correct application of the fascial dilators and of the following devices (balloon (Fig. 13.19) rather than Alken or Amplatz serial dilators), previously checking the space between stone and tip of the papilla and subsequently avoiding insufficient or excessive advancement of the dilators, preventing collecting system damage.

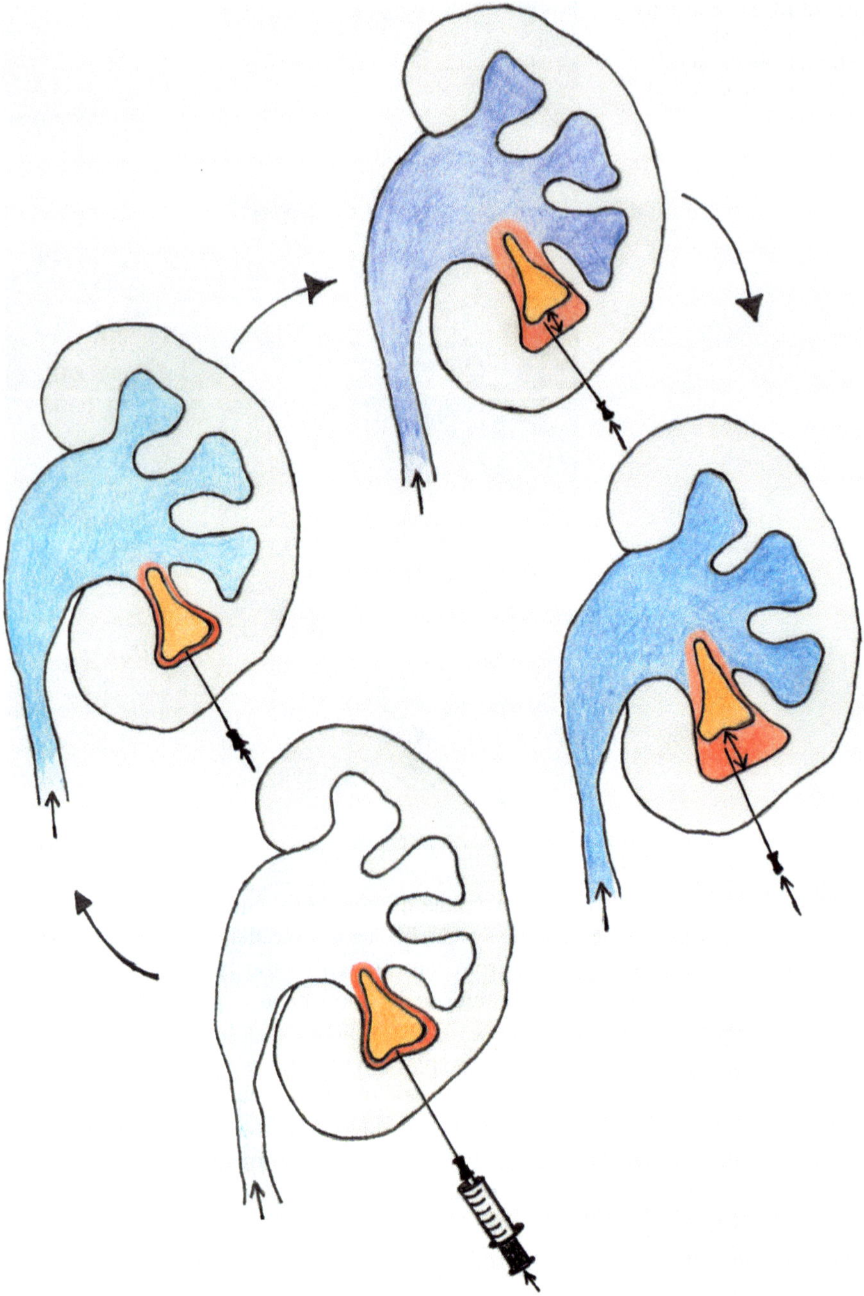

Fig. 13.14 Evaluation of the space between stone and calyx before and after irrigation is fundamental for deciding the dilation method (*small arrows* indicate the versus of saline injection/irrigation)

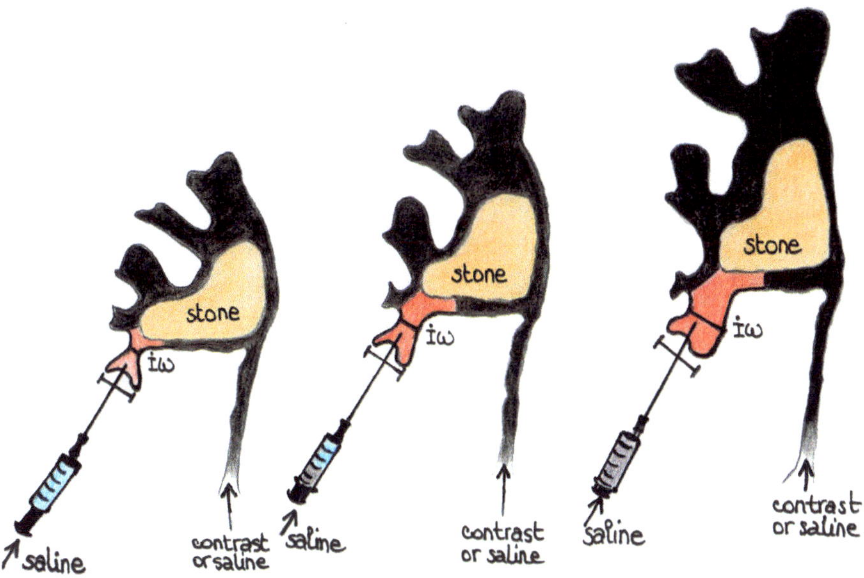

Fig. 13.15 The size of the tract dilation should take into account also the diameter of the calyceal infundibulum, in particular after the injection of saline/contrast medium

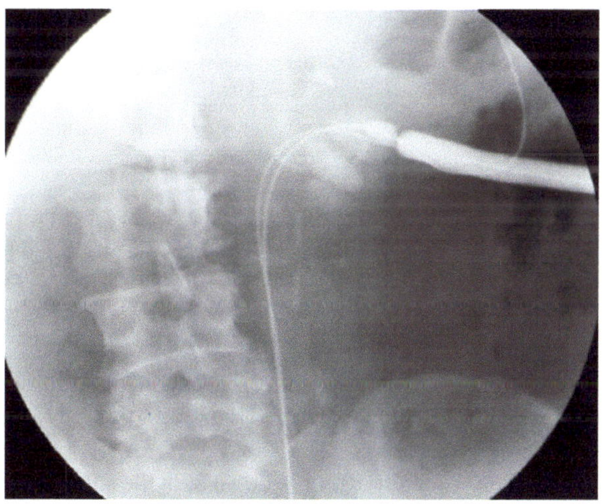

Fig. 13.16 Effect of the fascial postsurgical scarring on the balloon inflation during tract dilation

13.5 Amplatz Sheath Application

Amplatz sheath application after tract dilation has ascertained functions, including stabilization of the percutaneous tract, easy insertion and removal of the nephroscopes, a simple exchange from rigid to flexible nephroscopy, the ability to grasp or

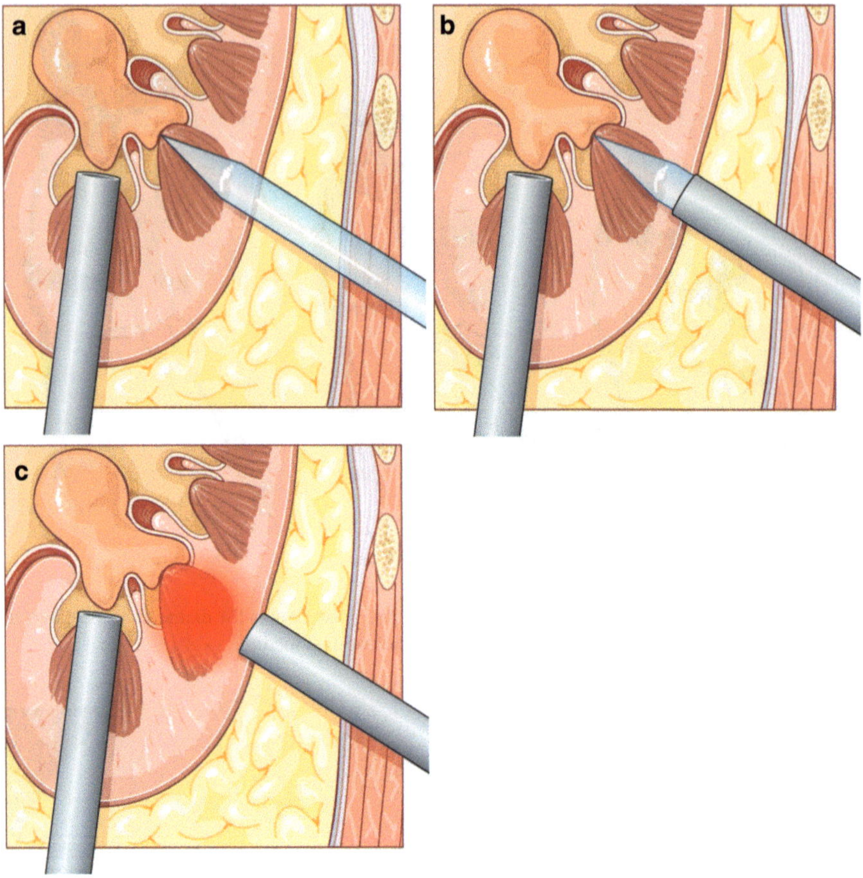

Fig. 13.17 Difference between Alken dilators (*flat end*) and balloon dilators (*tapered end*). When the stone entirely fills the collecting system (**a**), the balloon dilator does not allow the Amplatz sheath to enter the calyx reaching the stone (**b**), thus bleeding may occur after Amplatz removal (**c**) (© Carole Fumat)

basket larger stone fragments, prevention of fluid absorption and extravasation, reduction of intrarenal pressures (below 16 cm H_2O), and prevention of tract bleeding during the procedure.

As already mentioned in Sect. 13.2, in the supine positions the Amplatz sheath is horizontal or slightly inclined downwards (Figs. 13.20 and 13.21a), favoring spontaneous passage of stone fragments. In prone position the Amplatz sheath is more oblique, occasionally even vertical (Fig 13.21b). The choice of the Amplatz sheath diameter follows that dictated by the dilation based upon the many mentioned parameters regarding stone, collecting system and patient's features (smaller sheaths for performing mini- or midi-PNL, in children, …); the length is chosen according to specific features of the patient (longer sheaths in morbidly obese patients) [45–48]. For technical details see Chap. 12.

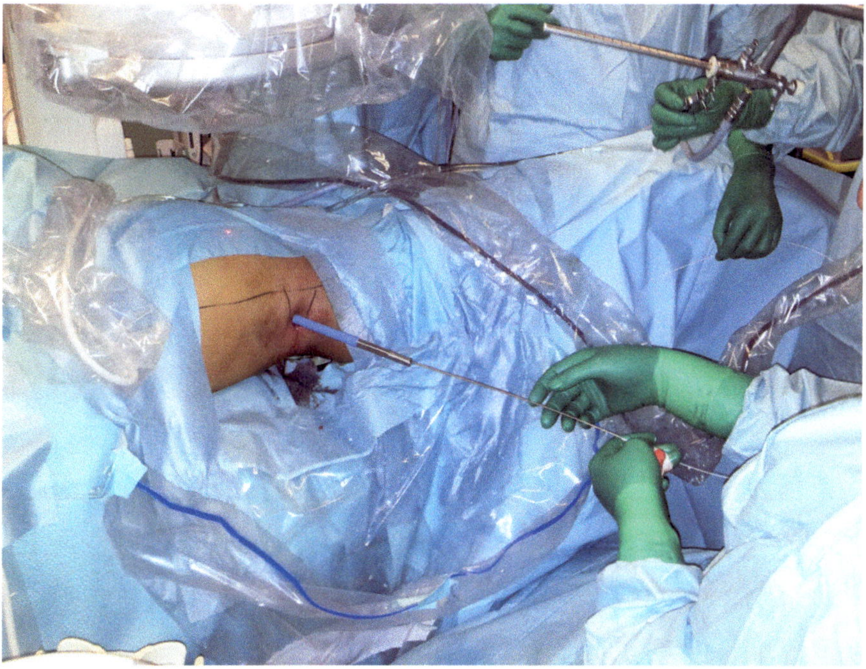

Fig. 13.18 Extraction of the coaxial telescopic metallic Alken dilators after the application of the Amplatz sheath

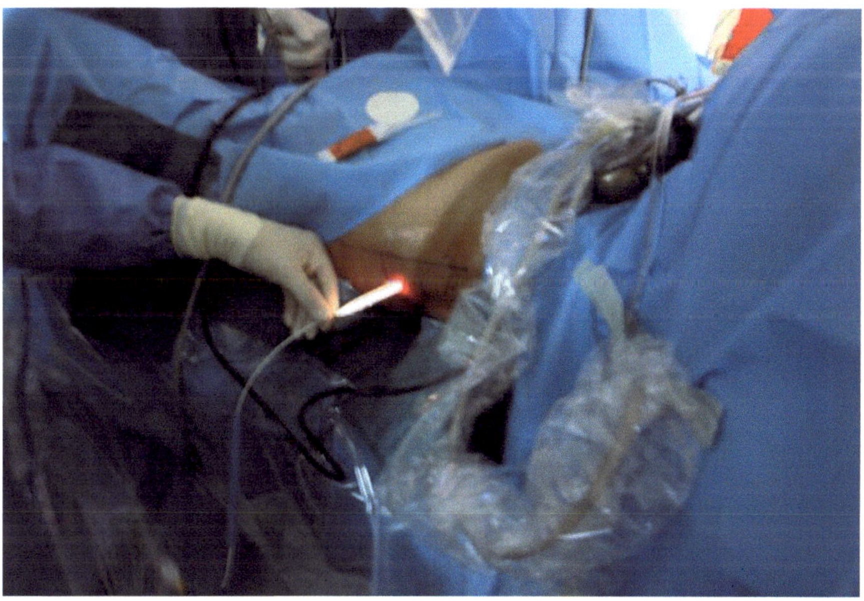

Fig. 13.19 Balloon dilation under Endovision control, retrograde illumination of the balloon

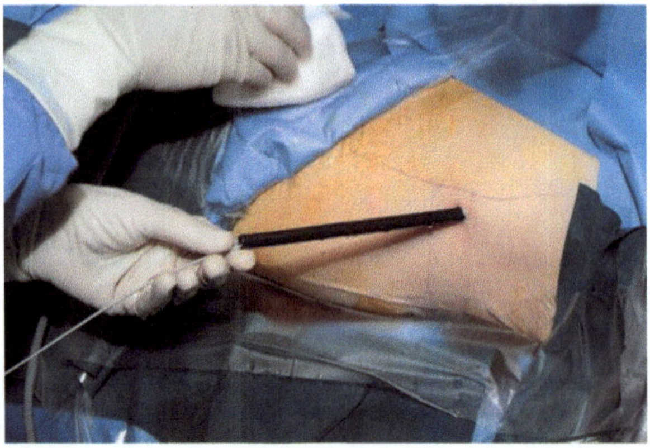

Fig. 13.20 In the supine positions the Amplatz sheath is horizontal or slightly inclined downwards

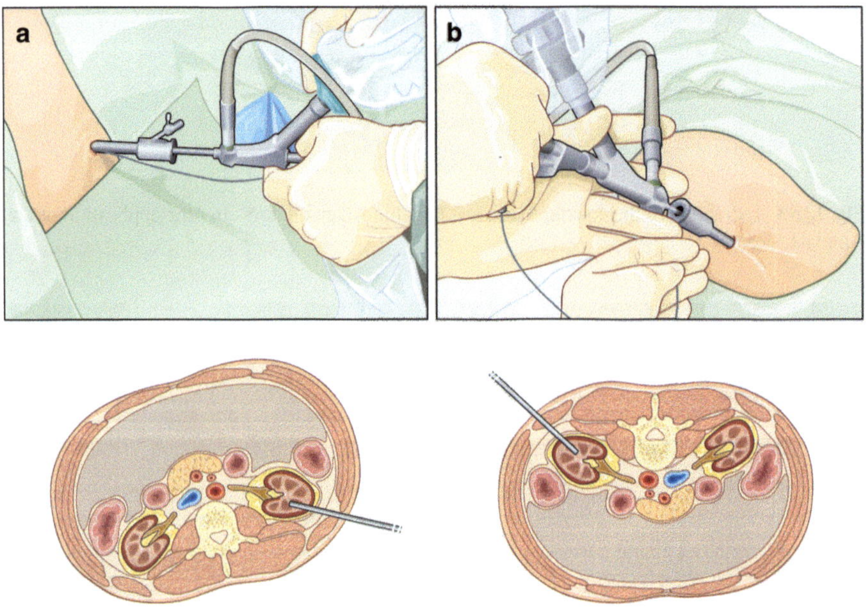

Fig. 13.21 Schematic drawing of the inclination of the Amplatz sheath and of the nephroscope in the supine (**a**) and in the prone (**b**) position (© Carole Fumat)

Care should be taken to avoid the inadvertent over-advancement of the Amplatz sheath, causing bleeding and damage/tear/perforation of the collecting system. Also the opposite problem, i.e., its incomplete application, can be dangerous in terms of fluid resorption and hemorrhagic risk (Fig. 13.22). Also in this case the Endovision technique can be a useful tool, in order to follow its correct insertion under visual control with the tip correctly inserted within the calyx [49].

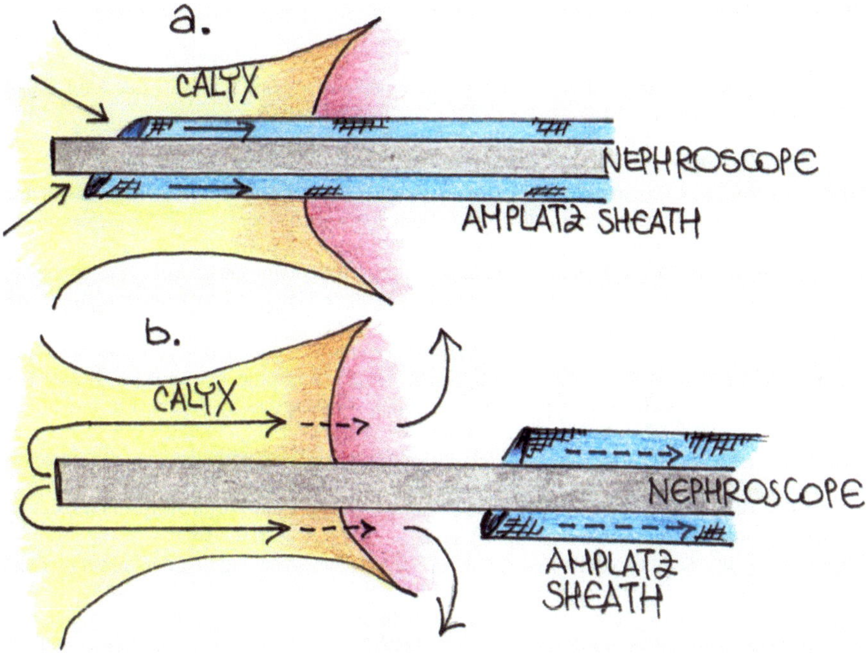

Fig. 13.22 Importance of the correct position of the Amplatz sheath: (**a**) the tip entirely within the calyx allows free efflux of irrigation fluid between sheath and nephroscope; if the Amplatz sheath is incompletely applicated (**b**) the risk to develop high intrarenal pressures is consistent, as well as that of fluid resorption and bleeding

13.6 How We Do It: The Authors' Point of View

- Our preference goes either to the fluoroscopic-guided access with the 30° cephalad tilting of the C-arm or to the ultrasound-assisted fluoroscopic access.
- This combined technique of renal puncture is further ameliorated by the Endovision control of the puncture by means of retrograde flexible ureteroscopy, assessing the entry of the needle through the tip of the papilla, to maximally prevent hemorrhagic complications.
- Also the subsequent steps, i.e., percutaneous tract dilation and Amplatz sheath application, can take advantage of the Endovision assistance.
- We use an 18 gauge Chiba needle, in which we can introduce a 0.038″ hydrophilic stiff guidewire (kebab patient!), once the collecting system has been correctly reached, but the choice of the guidewire is a very personal matter of preference.
- The choice of the dilation technique and the size of the tract should be tailored on specific parameters regarding the patient, the features of its urolithiasis, and the morphology of its collecting system. For this reason, the different dilation devices should be at the surgeon's disposal and ready to be used.

References

1. Ritter M, Krombach P, Michel MS (2011) Percutaneous stone removal. Eur Urol Suppl 10:433–439
2. Miller NL, Matlaga BR, Lingeman JE (2007) Techniques for fluoroscopic percutaneous renal access. J Urol 178:15–23
3. De La Rosette J, Assimos D, Desai M et al (2011) The Clinical Research Office of the Endourological Society percutaneous nephrolithotomy global study: indications, complications, and outcomes in 5803 patients. J Endourol 25:11–17
4. Spann A, Poteet J, Hyatt D et al (2011) Safe and effective obtainment of access for percutaneous nephrolithotomy by urologists: the Louisiana State University experience. J Endourol 25:1421–1425
5. Watterson JD, Soon S, Jana K (2006) Access related complications during percutaneous nephrolithotomy: urology versus radiology at a single academic institution. J Urol 176:142–145
6. Tomaszewski JJ, Ortiz TD, Gayed BA et al (2010) Renal access by urologist or radiologist during percutaneous nephrolithotomy. J Endourol 24:1733–1737
7. Lang E, Thomas R, Davis R et al (2009) Risks, advantages, and complications of intercostal versus subcostal approach for percutaneous nephrolithotripsy. Urology 74:751–755
8. Soria F, Delgado MI, Sanchez FM et al (2009) Effectiveness of three-dimensional fluoroscopy in percutaneous nephrostomy: an animal model study. Urology 73:649–652
9. Steinberg PL, Semins MJ, Wason SE et al (2009) Fluoroscopy-guided percutaneous renal access. J Endourol 23:1627–1631
10. Hoznek A, Ouzaid I, Gettman M et al (2011) Fluoroscopy-guided renal access in supine percutaneous nephrolithotomy. Urology 78:221–224
11. Desai M (2009) Ultrasonography-guided punctures – with and without puncture guide. J Endourol 23:1641–1643
12. Basiri A, Mohammadi Sichani M, Hosseini SR et al (2010) X-ray-free percutaneous nephrolithotomy in supine position with ultrasound guidance. World J Urol 28:239–244
13. Hopper KD, Sherman JL, Luethke JM et al (1987) The retrorenal colon in the supine and prone patient. Radiology 162:443–446
14. Tuttle DN, Yeh BM, Meng MV et al (2005) Risk of injury to adjacent organs with lower-pole fluoroscopically guided percutaneous nephrostomy: evaluation with prone, supine, and multiplanar reformatted CT. J Vasc Interv Radiol 16:1489–1492
15. Brancaforte A, Serantoni S, Silva Barbosa F et al (2011) Renal volume assessment with 3D ultrasound. Radiol Med 116:1095–1104
16. Tranquart F, Mercier L, Frinking P et al (2012) Perfusion quantification in contrast-enhanced ultrasound (CEUS) – ready for research projects and routine clinical use. Ultraschall Med 33(Suppl 1):S31–S38
17. Khan F, Borin JF, Pearle MS et al (2006) Endoscopically guided percutaneous renal access: seeing is believing. J Endourol 20:451–455
18. Scoffone CM, Cracco CM, Cossu M et al (2008) Endoscopic combined intrarenal surgery in Galdakao-modified supine Valdivia position: a new standard for percutaneous nephrolithotomy? Eur Urol 54:1393–1403
19. Bader MJ, Gratzke C, Seitz M et al (2011) The "all-seeing needle": initial results of an optical puncture system confirming access in percutaneous nephrolithotomy. Eur Urol 59:1054–1059
20. Kawahara T, Ito H, Terao H et al (2012) Ureteroscopy assisted retrograde nephrostomy: a new technique for percutaneous nephrolithotomy. BJU Int 110:588–590
21. Wynberg JB, Borin JF, Vicena JZ et al (2012) Flexible-ureteroscopy-directed retrograde nephrostomy for percutaneous nephrolithotomy: description of a technique. J Endourol 26:1268–1274

22. Kawahara T, Ito H, Terao H et al (2012) Effectiveness of ureteroscopy-assisted retrograde nephrostomy (UARN) for percutaneous nephrolithotomy (PCNL). PLoS ONE 7:e52149. doi:10.1371/journal.pone.0052149
23. Kalogeropoulou C, Kallidonis P, Liatsikos EN (2009) Imaging in percutaneous nephrolithotomy. J Endourol 23:1571–1577
24. Chen ML, Shukla G, Jackman SV et al (2011) Real-time tomographic reflection in facilitating percutaneous access to the renal collecting system. J Endourol 25:743–745
25. Ritter M, Rassweiler MC, Haecker A, Michel MS (2013) Laser-guided percutaneous kidney access with the UroDyna-CT: first experience of three-dimensional puncture planning with an ex-vivo model. World J Urol 31:1147–1151
26. Appelbaum L, Solbiati L, Sosna J et al (2013) Evaluation of an electromagnetic image-fusion navigation system for biopsy of small lesions: assessment of accuracy in an in vivo swine model. Acad Radiol 20:209–217
27. Mueller M, Rassweiler MC, Klein J et al (2013) Mobile augmented reality for computer-assisted percutaneous nephrolithotomy. Int J Comput Assist Radio Surg 8:663–675
28. De Lima REA, Oliveira C, Rodrigues P et al (2013) Percutaneous renal collecting system access using a novel electromagnetic tracking: first experience in vivo pig model. Eur Urol Suppl 12:e968
29. Lazarus J, Willams J (2011) The Locator: novel percutaneous nephrolithotomy apparatus to aid collecting system puncture – a preliminary report. J Endourol 25:747–750
30. Challacombe B, Patriciu A, Glass J et al (2005) A randomized controlled trial of human versus robotic and telerobotic access to the kidney as the first step in percutaneous nephrolithototomy. Comput Aided Surg 10:165–171
31. Bruyère F, Ayoub J, Arbeille P (2011) Use of a telerobotic arm to perform ultrasound guidance during renal biopsy in transplant recipients: a preliminary study. J Endourol 25:231–234
32. Landman J, Venkatesh R, Ragab M et al (2002) Comparison of intrarenal pressure and irrigant flow during percutaneous nephroscopy with an indwelling ureteral catheter, ureteral occlusion balloon, and ureteral access sheath. Urology 60:584–587
33. Landman J, Venkatesh R, Lee DL et al (2003) Combined percutaneous and retrograde approach to staghorn calculi with application of the ureteral access sheath to facilitate percutaneous nephrolithotomy. J Urol 169:64–67
34. Marguet CG, Springhart WP, Tan YH et al (2005) Simultaneous combined use of flexible ureteroscopy and percutaneous nephrolithotomy to reduce the number of access tracts in the management of complex renal calculi. BJU Int 96:1097–1100
35. Williams SK, Leveillee RJ (2008) Management of staghorn calculus: single puncture with judicious use of the flexible nephroscope. Curr Opin Urol 18:224–228
36. Akman T, Binbay M, Sari E et al (2011) Factors affecting bleeding during percutaneous nephrolithotomy: single surgeon experience. J Endourol 25:327–333
37. Alken P (1981) Telescopbougierset zur perkutanen Nephrostomie. Aktuel Urol 12:216–219
38. Clayman RV, Castaneda-Zuniga WR, Hunter DW et al (1983) Rapid balloon dilatation of the nephrostomy track for nephrostolithotomy. Radiology 147:884–885
39. Frattini A, Barbieri A, Salsi P et al (2001) One shot: a novel method to dilate the nephrostomy access for percutaneous nephrolithotripsy. J Endourol 15:919–923
40. Rusnak B, Castaneda-Zuniga W, Kotula F et al (1982) An improved dilator system for percutaneous nephrostomies. Radiology 144:174
41. Gonen M, Istanbulluoglu OM, Cicek T et al (2008) Balloon dilatation versus Amplatz dilatation for nephrostomy tract dilatation. J Endourol 22:901–904
42. Yamaghuci A, Skolarikos A, Buchholz NPN et al (2011) Operating times and bleeding complications in percutaneous nephrolithotomy: a comparison of tract dilation methods in 5537 patients in the Clinical Research Office of the Endourological Society percutaneous nephrolithotomy global study. J Endourol 25:933–939

43. Aminsharifi A, Alavi M, Sadeghi G et al (2011) Renal parenchymal damage after percutaneous nephrolithotomy with one-stage tract dilation technique: a randomized clinical trial. J Endourol 25:927–931
44. Handa RK, Evan AP, Willis LR et al (2009) Renal functional effects of multiple-tract percutaneous access. J Endourol 23:1951–1956
45. Chan DY, Jarrett TW (2000) Mini-percutaneous nephrolithotomy. J Endourol 14:269–273
46. Lahme S, Bichler KH, Strohmaier WL, Gotz T (2001) Minimally invasive PCNL in patients with renal pelvic and calyceal stones. Eur Urol 40:619–624
47. Giusti G, Piccinelli A, Taverna G et al (2007) Miniperc? No, thank you! Eur Urol 51:810–814
48. Abdelhafez MF, Amend B, Bedke J et al (2013) Minimally invasive percutaneous nephrolithotomy: a comparative study of the management of small and large renal stones. Urology 81:241–245
49. Clayman RV (2000) Nephroscopy sheath characteristics and intrarenal pressure: human kidney model. J Urol 163:1616

Chapter 14
Stone Fragmentation and Extraction

András Hoznek, Michael N'Tege Kimuli, and Cesare Marco Scoffone

Abstract Once an adequate percutaneous tract is created, the next step is to clear the stone. The fragmentation and extraction strategies should be tailored according to stone (hardness, location, size, and burden) and instrument (chosen size of the Amplatz sheath, diameter of the working channel of the endoscope in use) factors. Such strategies are similar in both prone and supine position, in spite of the fact that the slightly downward inclination of the Amplatz sheath in the supine position favors fragments' spontaneous evacuation. Various tips and tricks, like the variety of laser settings with their different effects or the vacuum-cleaner effect, are described.

14.1 Introduction

Once an adequate tract is created, the next step is to clear the stone. Stones with a diameter smaller than that of the Amplatz sheath can be simply extracted without being fragmented. Cutting the Amplatz longitudinally allows to extract even larger stones. Bulky stones need to be fragmented into smaller pieces until sufficiently small to pass the nephrostomy tract.

A. Hoznek, MD (✉)
Department of Urology, CHU Henri Mondor, 51. Av. du Ml. de Lattre de Tassigny, 94010 Créteil Cedex, France
e-mail: andras.hoznek@gmail.com

M.N. Kimuli
Pyrah Department of Urology, St James's University Hospital, Beckett Street, Leeds, LS9 7TF, UK
e-mail: nkimuli@hotmail.com

C.M. Scoffone, MD
Department of Urology, Cottolengo Hospital, Via Cottolengo 9, 10152 Torino, Italy
e-mail: scoof@libero.it

C.M. Scoffone et al. (eds.), *Supine Percutaneous Nephrolithotomy and ECIRS*,
DOI 10.1007/978-2-8178-0459-0_14, © Springer-Verlag France 2014

The process of fragmentation is dealt together with extraction in this chapter because some devices like ultrasonic lithotripters, with or without combination of the pneumatic system, perform the two functions simultaneously.

The fragmentation and extraction strategy should be tailored according to stone and instrument factors:

- Stone factors include hardness, location, stone size, and burden.
- Instrument factors include the caliber of the working channel of the nephroscope, the size of the Amplatz sheath, and whether a rigid or flexible instrument is used.

The currently available fragmentation devices and their principles have already been described in Chap. 12.

14.2 Strategies of Stone Fragmentation and Extraction

There are two main strategies available:

- The first consists in vaporizing the stone, washing the debris out through the Amplatz sheath, or aspirating the sand with the ultrasonic probe or with a combined device (like CyberWand or Swiss LithoClast Master). With a pneumatic device, "multiple pulse setting" is preferable to obtain pulverization. Obviously, if a flexible instrument has to be used, fragmentation with laser is the only option, and adequate settings of energy and frequency should be chosen in order to obtain pulverization (low energy and high frequency for dusting the stone, Fig. 14.1) rather than rough fragmentation (higher energy and lower frequency, Fig. 14.2).

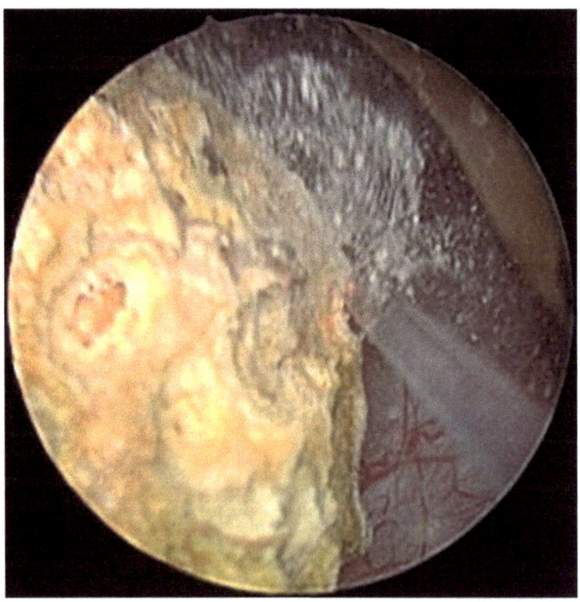

Fig. 14.1 Laser vaporization of a stone (high frequency and low energy)

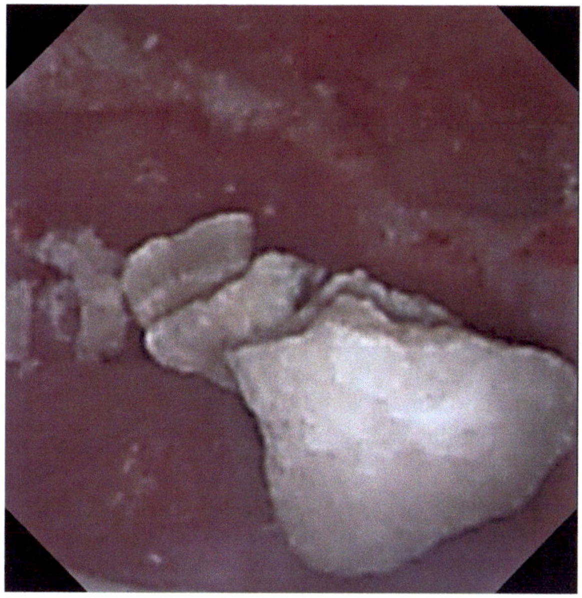

Fig. 14.2 Laser fragmentation of a stone (low frequency and high energy)

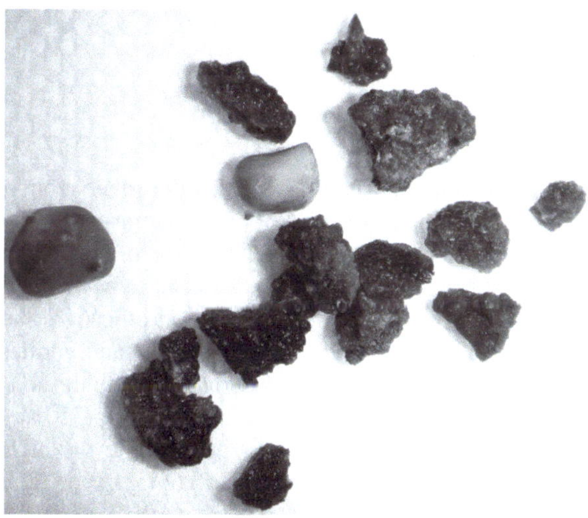

Fig. 14.3 Ballistic fragmentation of a stone in large fragments

- The second one aims at obtaining bigger pieces with a pneumatic device until reaching a diameter allowing their passage through the Amplatz sheath (Fig. 14.3). "Single pulse setting" has been found more efficient to obtain such a controlled stone disintegration. Reportedly, this latter method allows to obtain better stone free rates because it prevents small fragments to migrate into unreachable parts of the collecting system [1].

14.3 Stone Factors

14.3.1 Stone Hardness

14.3.1.1 Soft Stones

Soft stones like struvite (magnesium ammonium phosphate) or weddellite (calcium oxalate dihydrate) respond well to pulverization with ultrasound. They are quickly transformed into sand and aspirated through the ultrasound probe. To increase fragmentation efficacy, ultrasound can be combined with simultaneous ballistic lithotripsy, like in the LithoClast Master device or potentiated like in the CyberWand device. However, the large 10 Ch ultrasound probes necessitate nephroscopes with a larger working channel, allowing not only the passage of the probe but also a sufficient irrigation flow.

An abundant irrigation is crucial, especially in the supine position: in fact, due to the roughly horizontal or downward axis of the Amplatz sheath (see Chap. 13) and to the efficient aspiration, the collecting system tends to collapse and visibility deteriorates. To guarantee a high flow, the irrigation fluid containing bag should be elevated (Fig. 14.4). Alternatively, some urologists use hyperpressurized irrigation or peristaltic pumps to increase irrigation flow, although continuous or intermitted high intrarenal pressures should be avoided in order to prevent the uroseptic risk more marked in case of infectious stones.

14.3.1.2 Hard Stones

Hard stones such as whewellite (calcium oxalate monohydrate), cystine, or brushite (calcium phosphate) respond poorly to ultrasonic fragmentation. Pneumatic lithotripters (Swiss LithoClast) or combination of pneumatic and ultrasound (like Swiss LithoClast Master) is recommended. The CyberWand device uses only ultrasound, but due to the two different frequencies, its efficacy is similar to that of the LithoClast Master. Recently, a compact, autonomous, and cordless handheld lithotripter has also been developed. The StoneBreaker is highly efficient in case of hard stones because it produces a high amount of pressure (31 bar, compared with the 3 bar of standard pneumatic lithotripters) and despite the high energy of the mechanical shock minimal displacement at the tip of the probe [2, 3].

14.3.2 Location

As previously mentioned, the nephrostomy tract should pass through a calyx that allows dealing with the major stone burden. In this case, rigid and straight fragmentation tools such as ultrasound or pneumatic or combined lithotripters can be used.

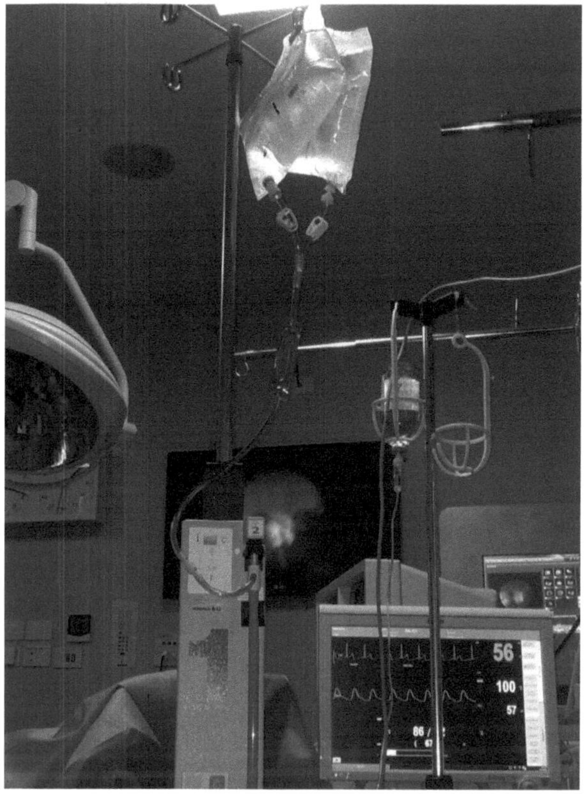

Fig. 14.4 Elevation of the fluid bags in order to increase the irrigation pressure

However, in case of complex or multiple calculi, not all calyces can be reached with the rigid nephroscope. In such circumstances, if multiple percutaneous tracts are not a routine choice, a flexible nephroscope via the Amplatz sheath (Fig. 14.5a) or a transurethrally passed uretero-nephroscope (Fig. 14.5b) should be used. Obviously, such instruments necessitate the use of laser fiber technology, to be employed in situ or to help stone dislocation into more reachable locations by means of a basket.

14.3.3 Stone Size and Burden

Staghorn stones necessitate a specific fragmentation strategy. A step-by-step description was recently given by Peter Alken for prone PNL [4] (Fig. 14.6). This method is also valid for supine position, with the difference that in the latter the whole procedure can be assisted by retrograde ureteroscopic laser fragmentation of stone portions difficult to reach with the rigid nephroscope.

Usually, staghorn stones are constituted of struvite which is characterized by softness and fragility. Therefore, fragmentation of such stones with ultrasound can

Fig. 14.5 For complex urolithiasis flexible nephroscope (**a**) or flexible ureteroscope (**b**) are fundamental aids for a better stone clearance

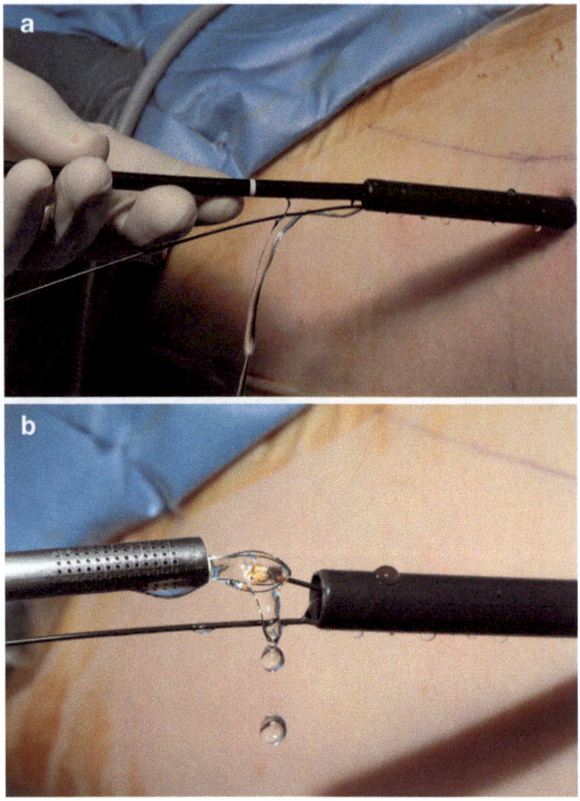

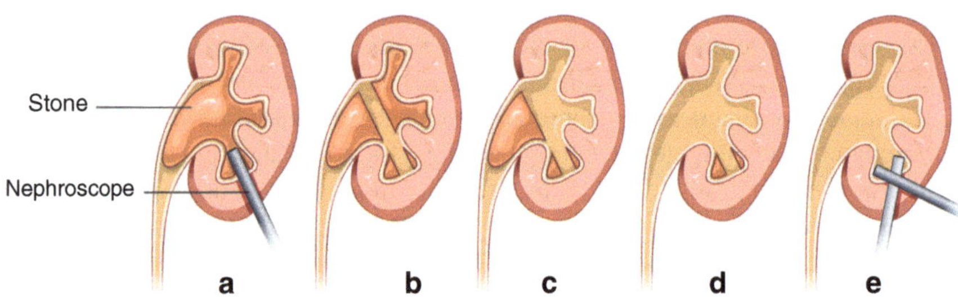

Fig. 14.6 (**a**) Start fragmentation in the puctured calix except laterally because of the risk of injury to forniceal veins. (**b**) Carry on fragmentation until the medial wall of the kidney pelvis is reached. (**c**) Clear distant calices. The fragment in the ureteropelvic junction prevents fragment migration into the ureter. (**d**) Remove the remaining stone from the ureteropelvic junction. (**e**) Complete fragment extraction in the punctured calix in the forniceal region. Lithotripsy strategy (courtesy of professor Peter Alken) for a staghorn stone (© Carole Fumat)

be spectacularly quick. In case of infectious stones, care should be taken to maintain the irrigation fluid pressure as low as possible to prevent septicemia. Obviously, patients having struvite stone should have preoperative antibiotic therapy according to antibiogram of urine analysis. A couple of prospective randomized studies suggest that a 1-week preoperative antibiotic therapy with ciprofloxacin or nitrofurantoin significantly diminishes infectious complications (see also Chap. 21). Occasionally, in case of an exceptionally high metabolic lithogenic activity, cystin or uric acid can give birth to particularly hard staghorn stones.

When dealing with staghorn stones entirely filling the collecting system, it can be difficult to insert the tip of the Amplatz sheath into the renal cavities immediately after dilation. Some bleeding may occur during this initial step. Therefore, the first objective is to clear the punctured calyx and create a working space in order to be able to push the Amplatz sheath further into the collecting system. If this goal is achieved, bleeding immediately stops due to the compressive effect of the Amplatz on renal parenchyma, and the risk of fluid resorption also decreases. At this point, it is not recommended to try to clear fragments laterally to the original tract because this may result in tearing forniceal veins due to the required angulation of the nephroscope (Fig. 14.6a).

Instead, stone disintegration should be carried on straightforward, following the direction of the original puncture axis until the median kidney pelvis wall is reached (Fig. 14.6b). This allows in case of complication to insert at least a nephrostomy and postpone the procedure.

Next, the whole pelvic portion of the stone is removed, except the portion extending into the ureteropelvic junction. This prevents stone fragments to migrate into the ureter. However, this concern is less important in supine position because of the possibility of avoiding the migration of the fragments into the ureter thanks to the retrograde ureteroscopic access.

The following step is to remove the stones in the distant calyces and the kidney pelvis (Fig. 14.6c, d). For calyces difficult to reach with the rigid nephroscope, a flexible nephroscope or ureterorenoscope is necessary. Stone fragments smaller than the diameter of the Amplatz sheath can be grasped with different types of nitinol baskets inserted via the flexible instrument. Such fragments can be pulled out from the calyx and delivered through the Amplatz sheath. Bigger fragments should first be disintegrated with laser.

The last step of the procedure is the complete clearance of the punctured calyx, which is done during the progressive withdrawal of the Amplatz sheath (Fig. 14.6e). Again, a flexible ureterorenoscope can be particularly efficient to reach stones in calyces parallel or with a difficult angle with respect to the Amplatz sheath.

14.4 Instrument Factors

14.4.1 Size of the Working Channel of the Nephroscope and Fragmentation Devices

The nephroscope design determines which fragmentation device can be used with a given instrument. Pneumatic probes are of different caliber. If a miniature nephroscope (12 Ch) is used, only the thinnest probe is able to pass through the working channel. Usually, this diameter is used with rigid ureteroscopes, and therefore, the probe is originally too long and its use is poorly ergonomic. It is better to shorten the probe to a length compatible with the length of the miniature nephroscope. The larger pneumatic probes pass through the midi and standard nephroscopes.

Ultrasound necessitates a larger working channel, superior or equal to 10 Ch. Since through the probe irrigation fluid and sand are continuously aspirated, a good irrigation is mandatory.

14.4.2 Size of the Amplatz Sheath and Fragments Removal

As previously mentioned, ultrasonic lithotripters simultaneously remove sand with aspiration. In addition, due to irrigation and the roughly horizontal axis of the Amplatz, a considerable amount of sand is simply washed out during a supine procedure. Some urologists use peristaltic pumps to increase irrigation flow. Otherwise, a pneumatic device can be employed with multiple pulse setting in alternative to ultrasound. To prevent high pressures within the renal cavities, it is advisable to use an Amplatz sheath which is significantly larger in diameter than the nephroscope, so that excess irrigation flow can easily evacuate [5].

A second mechanism to clear fragments is called the "vacuum-cleaner" effect. This occurs when using midi (22 Ch) nephroscope with a 24 Ch Amplatz sheath or a mini (12 Ch) through a 16.5 Ch Amplatz sheath. The explanation of this phenomenon is the Bernoulli's principle: decrease of cross section in a tube leads to the acceleration of flow and drop of fluid pressure (Fig. 14.7). This is the case in mini- or midi-PNL, where the cross section of the Amplatz sheath is diminished by the nephroscope (Fig. 14.8). Stone fragments are attracted to the tip of the nephroscope and can be simply pulled out. This makes mini- and midi-PNL a particularly time- and cost-efficient procedure: there is often no need for an expensive stone retrieval basket, and the use of disposable material is limited to the minimum [6–8]. Of course, the Bernoulli's principle is more pronounced and efficient in supine PNL compared to prone PNL, because of the more horizontal axis of the Amplatz sheath.

Different types of stone graspers have been proposed to aid the removal of larger stone fragments (Fig. 14.9). Basically, two types can be discerned: active and passive graspers. In active graspers opening and closing is operated with a handle. In passive graspers like the tripod, a spring mechanism is used to close the jaws.

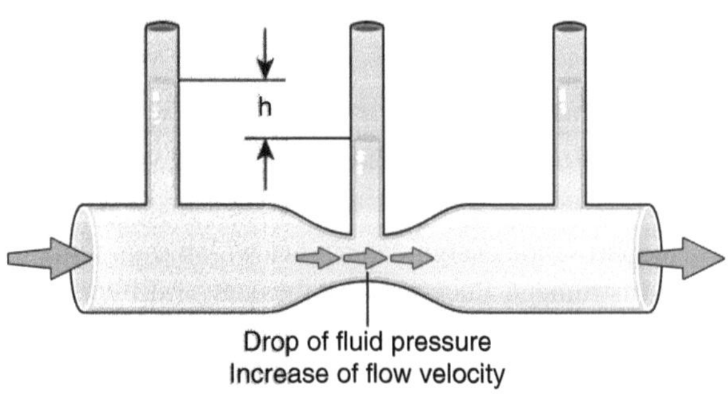

Fig. 14.7 Scheme explaining the Bernoulli's principle (© Carole Fumat)

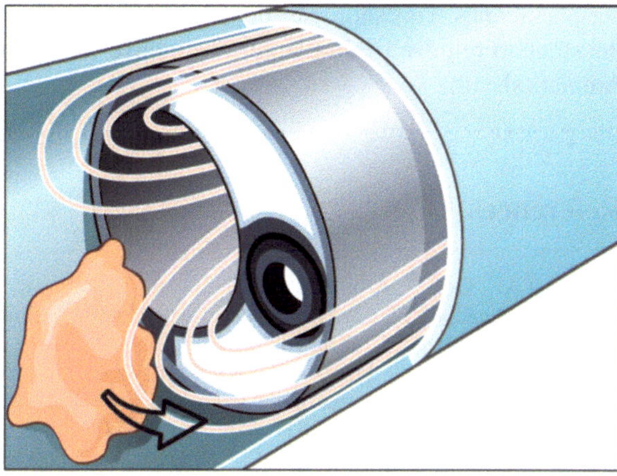

Fig. 14.8 Practical application of the Bernoulli's principle during PNL (© Carole Fumat)

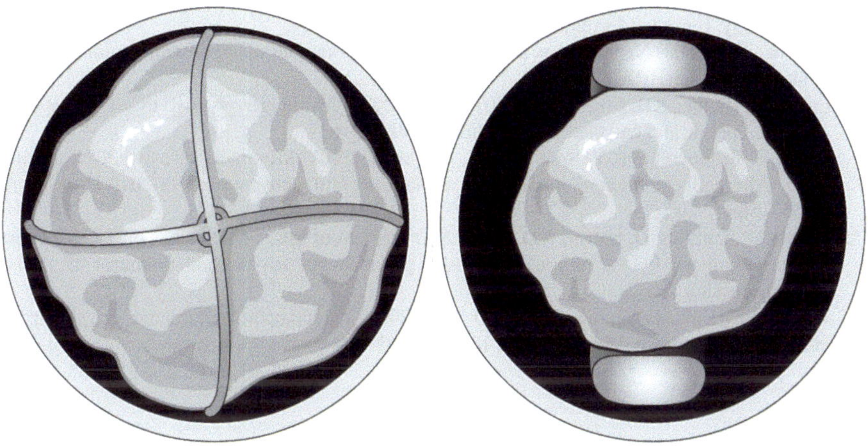

Fig. 14.9 Graspers occupy more space within the Amplatz sheath than a nitinol basket (© Carole Fumat)

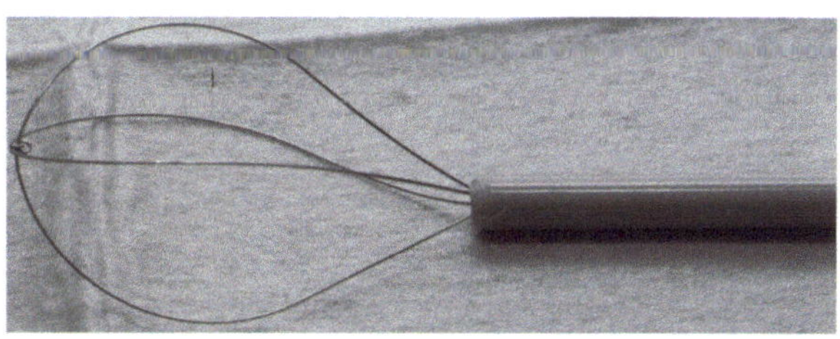

Fig. 14.10 A nitinol basket is very ergonomic and easy to use for fragment extraction

Specific nitinol baskets for PNL have also been developed. The advantage of the Perc N-Circle is its ability to remove larger stone fragments than with the classic stone graspers (Fig. 14.10) [9]. Stone fragments should be removed starting from the most anterior ones and progressively going backwards to catch the most peripheral ones. This should be done in order to avoid entrapment of the basket with the stone to remove behind larger obstructive stones, hindering the passage to the Amplatz sheath.

References

1. Hemal AK, Goel A, Aron M et al (2003) Evaluation of fragmentation with single or multiple pulse setting of Lithoclast for renal calculi during percutaneous nephrolithotripsy and its impact on clearance. Urol Int 70:265–268
2. Nerli RB, Koura AC, Prabha V et al (2008) Use of LMA Stonebreaker as an intracorporeal lithotrite in the management of ureteral calculi. J Endourol 22:641–644
3. Chew BH, Arsovska O, Lange D et al (2011) The Canadian StoneBreaker trial: a randomized, multicenter trial comparing the LMA StoneBreaker and the Swiss LithoClast(R) during percutaneous nephrolithotripsy. J Endourol 25:1415–1419
4. Alken P (2010) PNL for staghorn stones. In: Rane AM, Desai M, Keeley FX (eds) Top tips in endourology. Euromed Communications, Passfield, pp 20–24
5. Clayman RV (2000) Nephroscopy sheath characteristics and intrarenal pressure: human kidney model. J Urol 163:1616
6. Lahme S, Bichler KH, Strohmaier WL, Gotz T (2001) Minimally invasive PCNL in patients with renal pelvic and calyceal stones. Eur Urol 40:619–624
7. Lahme S, Zimmermanns V, Hochmuth A, Janitzki V (2008) Minimally invasive PCNL (mini-perc). Alternative treatment modality or replacement of conventional PCNL? Urologe A 47:563–568
8. Nagele U, Schilling D, Sievert KD (2008) Management of lower-pole stones of 0.8 to 1.5 cm maximal diameter by the minimally invasive percutaneous approach. J Endourol 22:1851–1853, discussion 7
9. Hoffman N, Lukasewycz SJ, Canales B et al (2004) Percutaneous renal stone extraction: in vitro study of retrieval devices. J Urol 172:559–561

Chapter 15
Kidney Drainage and Percutaneous Tract Closure

Cesare Marco Scoffone, András Hoznek, and Cecilia Maria Cracco

Abstract Exit strategy after PNL, irrespective to the patient's position, is an area of continuous innovation to improve its outcomes and minimize its morbidity. Traditionally, a nephrostomy tube at the conclusion of a PNL was left for kidney drainage, hemostasis and tract healing, and allowance for postoperative renal access. During the years, various modifications have been made in the design and size of the nephrostomy tubes. Recently, the possibility of avoiding nephrostomy tube placement (tubeless but stented or totally tubeless PNL) has become real, according to definite inclusion criteria. The various techniques to establish hemostasis of a tubeless access tract are also reported, with particular reference to the use of hemostatic agents.

15.1 Kidney Drainage

15.1.1 Standard PNL with Final Nephrostomy Tube Placement

Exit strategy after percutaneous nephrolithotomy (PNL), irrespective to the patient's position during the procedure, is an area of continuous innovation to improve its outcomes and minimize its postoperative morbidity.

C.M. Scoffone, MD (✉) • C.M. Cracco, MD, PhD
Department of Urology, Cottolengo Hospital, via Cottolengo 9, 10152 Torino, Italy
e-mail: scoof@libero.it; cecilia.cracco@libero.it

A. Hoznek, MD
Department of Urology, CHU Henri Mondor, 51. Av. du Ml. de Lattre de Tassigny, 94010 Créteil Cedex, France
e-mail: andras.hoznek@gmail.com

C.M. Scoffone et al. (eds.), *Supine Percutaneous Nephrolithotomy and ECIRS*,
DOI 10.1007/978-2-8178-0459-0_15, © Springer-Verlag France 2014

Traditionally, it has been standard practice for years to insert and leave in place a nephrostomy tube at the conclusion of a PNL with the following intended purposes:

1. Drainage of the kidney (facilitating elimination of clots and small stone debris, otherwise possibly obstructing the edematous ureter and causing renal colics, urine extravasation, and urinoma formation).
2. Hemostasis and healing of the fresh percutaneous tract (through a supposed compressive mechanism on the percutaneous tunnel).
3. Allowance for postoperative access to the collecting system (planned reentry procedures in a staged PNL, antegrade contrast studies, percutaneous chemolitholysis).

During the years, various modifications have been made in the design of the nephrostomy tubes (self-retaining pigtail catheters, Cope loops, Foley catheters, Malecot catheters, reentry nephrostomy tubes, circle nephrostomy tubes, the specially designed Council-tip or Kaye tamponade catheters in case of significant hemorrhage), to aid appropriate management of different clinical situations, decrease complications, and improve cost-effectiveness [1, 2].

Subsequently, efforts have been also expended to reduce the size of the nephrostomy tube in order to minimize postoperative morbidity of PNL, mainly pain perception and analgesic requirements. The use of double-J stents brought out from the flank or of small-bore nephrostomy tubes (7–10F) (Fig. 15.1) was introduced instead of the large-bore (18–26F) nephrostomy tubes [3–11] (Table 15.1).

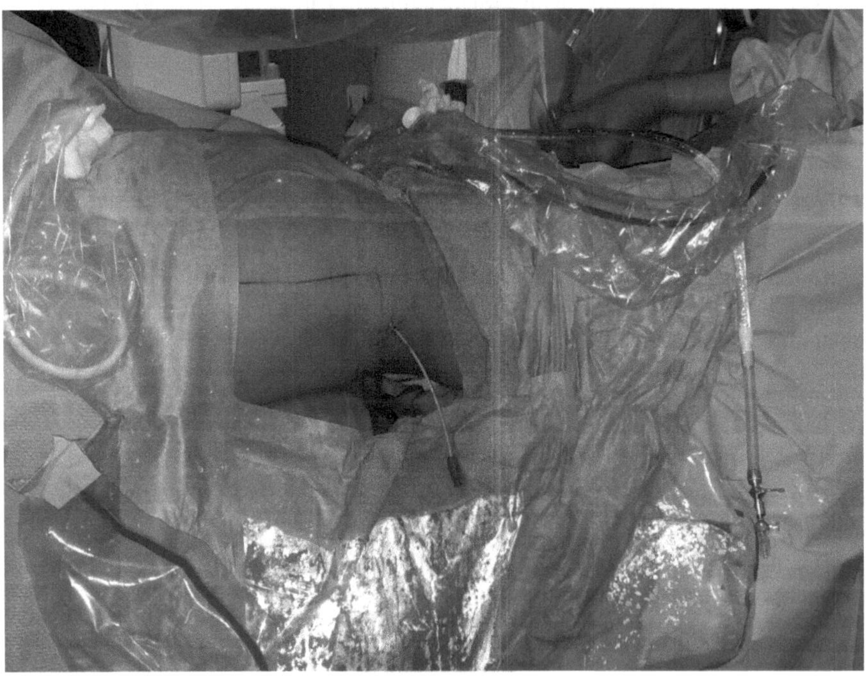

Fig. 15.1 Final 8 Ch pyelostomy placement after ECIRS

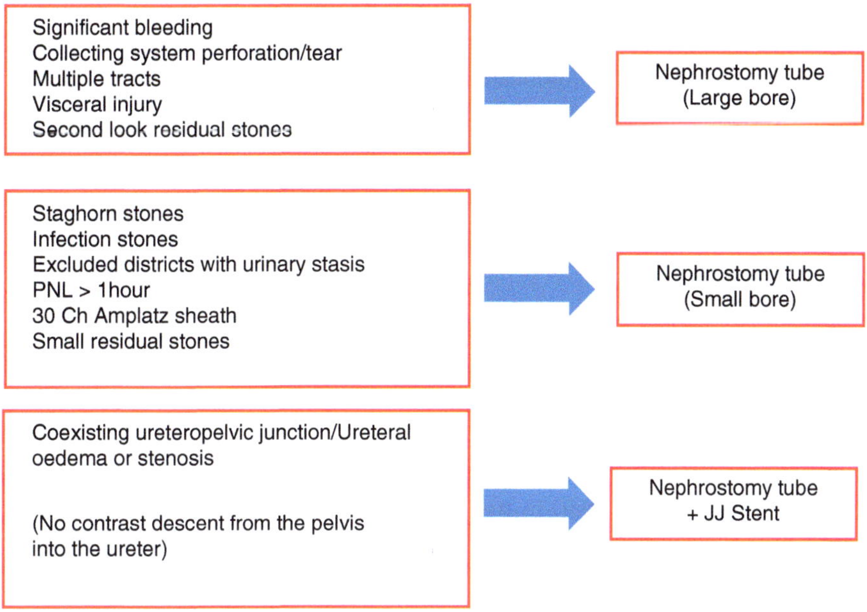

Table 15.1 Criteria suggesting nephrostomy tube application according to our experience in a standard PNL

According to our experience, small-bore nephrostomies are very well tolerated and guarantee an optimal drainage of the treated collecting system per the first post-operative 24–48 h, with minimal analgesic requirements and no increased risk of bleeding (1 % Clavien 2 in our series). Nephrostomy tube can be immediately closed and possibly opened again if the patient suffers from colic pain in absence of a ureteral drainage, which in case of urinary leakage should be applied. Our experience is similar to that reported on a large series of PNL patients (more than 1,000) in the United Kingdom, where the percentage of nephrostomy tube application was 76 % [12].

15.1.2 Tubeless PNL

Recently, the possibility of avoiding nephrostomy tube placement has become real, with the alternative of eliminating it altogether. In fact, the absolute need for post-operative renal drainage after PNL has been definitely questioned and challenged in recent years:

1. The prolonged tube permanence in the percutaneous tract somehow matures tissues and establishes an anomalous path, leading to prolonged urine leakage (up to about 11 % in the literature) [13].

2. The supposed compressive hemostatic mechanism on the percutaneous tunnel is lost in case of small-bore nephrostomies, demonstrating that most bleedings are self-limiting [14, 15]. Additionally, the absence of a nephrostomy tube, together with tract closure and conservative measures, might even aid in self-tamponade of the tract, thanks to the thrombolytic effect of urokinase present in the urine [16, 17]. It should also be reported that, going against the tide, the CROES group recently published a paper based on almost 4,000 patients from 96 centers worldwide, concluding that large-bore nephrostomy tubes (≥18F) after PNL seem to reduce bleeding and overall complication rates [18].

15.1.3 Tubeless or Nephrostomy-Free (but Stented) PNL

The description of a conventional PNL without the final application of a nephrostomy tube was first published in 1997 by Bellman and coworkers and has now been accepted as a safe and effective alternative. In both standard [14, 19] and miniaturized PNL [20–22], the tubeless procedure is in any case a stented PNL. In fact, alternative ureteral drainage to prevent urine leakage through the percutaneous tract is provided by the retrograde application of a ureteral catheter or a double-J stent with external string for few days (reducing costs and stent-related morbidity and avoiding endoscopic procedure for its removal) or the placement of a double-J stent for longer periods (one or more weeks, depending upon postoperative stone clearance status, with sometimes significant stent-related symptoms and the need for a postoperative cystoscopy for its removal).

15.1.4 Totally Tubeless (Unstented) PNL

The true totally tubeless PNL (tubeless and stentless), proposed by Wickham and colleagues almost 30 years ago, has no postoperative drainage of the operated collecting system at all and may be put into practice with success in very selected cases [23–25].

15.1.5 Advantages of Tubeless PNL

Randomized studies, carried out mainly with the patient in prone position [13, 26] and only in a couple of studies in the supine position [27, 28], demonstrated that tubeless procedures imply:

1. Better patient comfort.
2. Less pain with reduced postoperative need for analgesics (especially in patients with supracostal access, where the tube irritates the periosteum of the rib).

3. Quicker recovery and shorter hospital stay in comparison even with small nephrostomy tubes.
4. Comparable outcomes in terms of stone clearance.
5. No differences for fever, bleeding complications/blood transfusions, or other complications.
6. Less urinary leakage.
7. No chance of a second-look procedure in case of residual fragments.

A tubeless procedure seems feasible with reduced postoperative morbidity even in particular cases, including large stone burdens, children, elderly, obese patients, after previous ipsilateral open surgery, patients with a solitary kidney, horseshoe or ectopic pelvic kidneys, raised serum creatinine levels, on antiplatelet therapy or cirrhotic patients, and bilateral synchronous PNL [19, 29–37].

15.1.6 Inclusion Criteria for Tubeless PNL

Various authors [2, 13, 37] suggested a number of inclusion criteria for tubeless procedures, from which we can argue that one universal solution is not applicable for all patients undergoing PNL and that the optimal renal drainage method should be individualized, depending upon patient features, operative course, procedural complexity, stone burden:

1. Less than two access tracts.
2. Stone size less than 3 cm.
3. No infected stones.
4. Less than two (one)-hour procedure.
5. An uncomplicated procedure (no significant intraoperative bleeding, no intrathoracic violation, no significant perforation of the collecting system).
6. No added procedures (as endopyelotomy or opening of the calyceal diverticulum).
7. No ureteral/ureteropelvic junction obstruction.
8. No need for a second-look procedures.
9. No particular situations (congenital abnormalities, bilateral procedures, children or elderly, ASA score >2, renal failure, etc.).

There is no general consensus about the wisdom of tubeless PNL. Some authors demonstrated equivalent results with early removal of small-bore nephrostomy tubes, anywhere carried out from 1 to 2 days postoperatively and in any case before the patient is discharged home [38, 39].

The European Association of Urology guidelines suggest: in uncomplicated cases tubeless PNL, with or without application of a sealant or double-J stenting (LE 1b, grade of recommendation A); in complicated cases or when a second intervention is necessary a standard PNL with a nephrostomy tube in place.

15.2 Closure of the Percutaneous Tract

Alternative or innovative techniques to establish hemostasis of the tubeless access tract have been reported, from the simple mechanical compression of the percutaneous tract for few minutes at the end of the procedure [7] to the application of deep fascial stitches [40] and from the cryoablation of the tract with a single 10-min freeze-thaw cycle to −20 °C, in which the cryoprobe traverses the nephrostomy tract [38], to its monopolar or bipolar cauterization using a blunt electrocautery loop mounted on a 26F resectoscope [41, 42]. The last frontier is the application of absorbable hemostatic agents (including Surgicel from Ethicon, a blood clot-inducing material made up of oxidized cellulose polymers), with the additional aim to prevent urine leakage [37, 43–45].

Absorbable hemostatic agents include:

1. Liquid products like fibrin sealants, containing all the components that are necessary to produce a fibrin clot independent of patient-derived factors (Tisseel from Baxter, Evicel from Ethicon, TachoSil from Takeda, thrombin from several companies). Fibrin sealants display both hemostatic and adhesive properties, being the mechanical strength of the fibrin matrix determined by the relative concentration of fibrinogen versus thrombin plus possibly factor XIII and/or an antifibrinolytic agent such as bovine aprotinin or tranexamic acid. Higher thrombin concentrations produce more rapid meshworks, higher fibrinogen concentrations, and stronger but slower meshworks.
2. Flowable or gelatin matrix products, providing a matrix for platelet adhesion and aggregation, aiding in the formation of a clot when mixed with thrombin and in augmenting the clotting cascade (FloSeal and CoSeal synthetic from Baxter, Surgiflo from Johnson & Johnson, the absorbable gelatin Spongostan). They contain no fibrinogen and allow the thrombin present in the sealant to activate the patient's natural one. Gelatin materials will additionally swell within the tract from 19 to 400 % greater than the applied volume, adding to hemostasis by means of a compressive effect.

Fibrin glues are expensive and their use raised concerns for a possible lithogenic effect. According to experimental studies in a porcine model, hemostatic gelatin matrix was found to be the most optimal because it remains in fine particulate suspension in urine, whereas fibrin maintains a semisolid gelatinous state and may persist in the tract for up to 30 days, thus inhibiting wound healing [46–50].

15.3 How We Do It: The Authors' Point of View

- Final combined (antegrade and retrograde) flexible evaluation of the stone-free status.

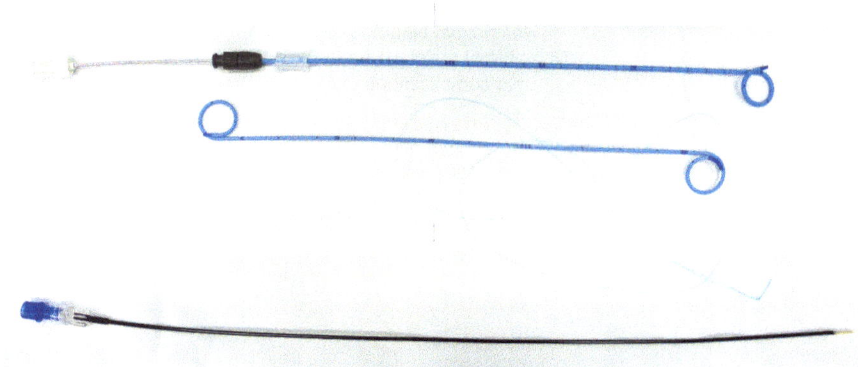

Fig. 15.2 8 Ch pyelostomy and double-J stent we usually adopt after ECIRS

- Final endoscopic evaluation of the entity of bleeding from the percutaneous tract.
- No bleeding, no residual stone fragments, and no other complicating elements = *tubeless PNL feasible* (simple mechanical compression of the percutaneous tract).
- Final combined endoscopic inspection and antegrade pyeloureterography to evaluate the absence of perforation of the collecting system and the free passage of the contrast medium down the ureter to the bladder through the ureteropelvic junction = *totally tubeless* (*tubeless and stentless*) *PNL feasible*.
- In case of modest bleeding with risk of clot formation, small stone fragments not be treated by a second-look procedure, ureteral/ureteropelvic junction edema, ureteral spasm, or stenosis = *nephrostomy-free but stented PNL*, with a ureteral catheter or a double-J stent with the string left attached, if it has to be removed within few days, and without string if the double-J stent has to be left for 20 days or more.
- In case of problematic/complicated PNL = *standard procedure*, *with both nephrostomy and ureteral drainage*. The nephrostomy tube can be left closed immediately after PNL, to contribute to tamponade, or opened in case of renal colics, to aid urine drainage.
- *Most of the times*, we apply a small-bore nephrostomy, which is immediately closed, and a double J with string (Fig. 15.2). The order of tube removal will be 1) closed nephrostomy after 1–2 days; 2) urethral catheter after one more day, if the percutaneous tract remains dry; and 3) double-J stent after a few days (if it has the string) or after 2–6 weeks with cystoscopy (Table 15.2).

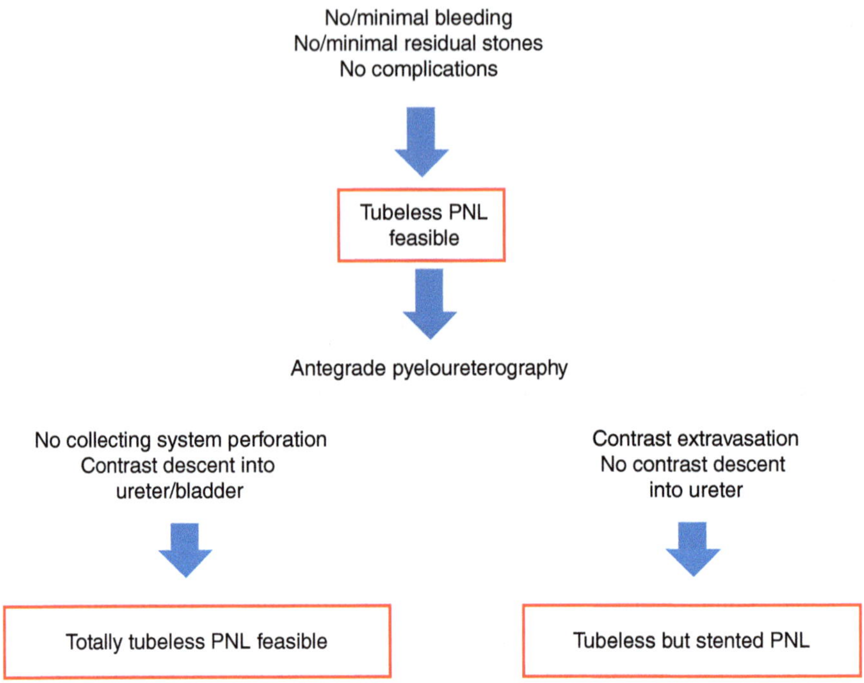

Table 15.2 Criteria for choosing a tubeless or a totally tubeless PNL

References

1. Paul EM, Marcovich R, Lee BR, Smith AD (2003) Choosing the ideal nephrostomy tube. BJU Int 92:672–677
2. Srinivasan AK, Herati A, Okeke Z, Smith AD (2009) Renal drainage after percutaneous nephrolithotomy. J Endourol 23:1743–1749
3. Maheshwari PN, Andankar MG, Bansal M (2000) Nephrostomy tube after percutaneous nephrolithotomy: large-bore or pigtail catheter? J Endourol 14:735–737
4. Liatsikos EN, Hom D, Dinlenc CZ et al (2002) Tail stent versus re-entry tube: a randomized comparison after percutaneous stone extraction. Urology 59:15–19
5. Pietrow PK, Auge BK, Lallas CD et al (2003) Pain after percutaneous nephrolithotomy: impact of nephrostomy tube size. J Endourol 17:411–414
6. Desai MR, Kukreja RA, Desai MM et al (2004) A prospective randomized comparison of type of nephrostomy drainage following percutaneous nephrostolithotomy: large bore versus small bore versus tubeless. J Urol 172:565–567
7. Kukreja R, Desai M, Patel S, Bapat S (2004) Factors affecting blood loss during percutaneous nephrolithotomy: prospective study. J Endourol 18:715–722
8. Choi M, Brusky J, Weaver J et al (2006) Randomized trial comparing modified tubeless percutaneous nephrolithotomy with tailed stent with percutaneous nephrostomy with small-bore tube. J Endourol 20:766–770
9. De Sio M, Autorino R, Quattrone C et al (2011) Choosing the nephrostomy size after percutaneous nephrolithotomy. World J Urol 29:707–711
10. Dirim A, Turunc T, Kuzgunbay B et al (2011) Which factors may affect urinary leakage following percutaneous nephrolithotomy? World J Urol 29:761–766

11. Shen P, Liu Y, Wang J (2012) Nephrostomy tube-free versus nephrostomy tube for renal drainage after percutaneous nephrolithotomy: a systematic review and meta-analysis. Urol Int 88:298–306
12. Armitage JN, Irving SO, Burgess NA (2012) Percutaneous nephrolithotomy in the United Kingdom: results of a prospective data registry. Eur Urol 61:1188–1193
13. Borges CF, Fregonesi A, Silva DC, Sasse AD (2010) Systematic review and meta-analysis of nephrostomy placement versus tubeless percutaneous nephrolithotomy. J Endourol 24:1739–1746
14. Giusti G, Piccinelli A, Taverna G et al (2007) Miniperc? No, thank you! Eur Urol 51:810–815
15. Etemadian M, Soleimani MJ, Haghighi R et al (2011) Does bleeding during percutaneous nephrolithotomy necessitate keeping the nephrostomy tube? A randomized controlled clinical trial. Urol J 8:21–26
16. Crook TJ, Lockyer CR, Keoghane SR et al (2008) Totally tubeless percutaneous nephrolithotomy: our experience. J Endourol 22:25–28
17. Shoma AM, Elshal AM (2012) Nephrostomy tube placement after percutaneous nephrolithotomy: critical evaluation through a prospective randomized study. Urology 79:771–776
18. Cormio L, Preminger G, Saussine C et al (2012) Nephrostomy in percutaneous nephrolithotomy (PCNL): does nephrostomy tube size matter? Results from the Global PCNL Study from the Clinical Research Office of Endourology Society. World J Urol PMID 23073656 (in press)
19. Agrawal MS, Agrawal M (2010) Tubeless percutaneous nephrolithotomy. Indian J Urol 26:16–24
20. Lahme S, Zimmermanns V, Hochmuth A, Liske P (2008) Stones of the upper urinary tract. Update on minimal-invasive endourological treatment. Arch Ital Urol Androl 80:13–17
21. Knoll T, Wezel F, Michel MS et al (2010) Do patients benefit from miniaturized tubeless percutaneous nephrolithotomy? A comparative prospective study. J Endourol 24:1075–1079
22. Kruck S, Anastasiadis AG, Herrmann TR et al (2012) Minimally invasive percutaneous nephrolithotomy: an alternative to retrograde intrarenal surgery and shockwave lithotripsy. World J Urol 30:639–646
23. Karami H, Gholamrezaie HR (2004) Totally tubeless percutaneous nephrolithotomy in selected patients. J Endourol 18:475–476
24. Aghamir SM, Hosseini SR, Gooran S (2004) Totally tubeless percutaneous nephrolithotomy. J Endourol 18:647–648
25. Istanbulluoglu MO, Ozturk B, Gonen M et al (2009) Effectiveness of totally tubeless percutaneous nephrolithotomy in selected patients. A prospective randomized study. Int Urol Nephrol 41:541–545
26. Marchant F, Recabal P, Fernandez MI et al (2011) Postoperative morbidity of tubeless versus conventional percutaneous nephrolithotomy: a prospective comparative study. Urol Res 39:477–481
27. Falahatkar S, Khosropanah I, Roshani A et al (2008) Tubeless percutaneous nephrolithotomy for staghorn stones. J Endourol 22:1447–1451
28. Rana AM, Bhojwani JP, Junejo NN, Das Bhagla S (2008) Tubeless PCNL with patient in supine position: procedure for all seasons? With comprehensive technique. Urology 71:581–585
29. Shah HN, Kausik VB, Hedge SS et al (2005) Safety and efficacy of bilateral simultaneous tubeless percutaneous nephrolithotomy. Urology 66:500–504
30. Shah H, Khandkar A, Sodha H et al (2009) Tubeless percutaneous nephrolithotomy: 3 years of experience with 454 patients. BJU Int 104:840–846
31. Kara C, Resorlu B, Bayndir M, Unsai A (2010) A randomized comparison of totally tubeless and standard percutaneous nephrolithotomy in elderly patients. Urology 76:289–294
32. Zilberman DE, Lipkin ME, de la Rosette JJ et al (2010) Tubeless percutaneous nephrolithotomy – the new standard of care? J Urol 184:1261–1266
33. Aghamir SM, Hamidi M, Aloosh M et al (2011) Efficacy and morbidity following PCNL in patients with renal anomalies: the outcome from a randomized study comparing different imaging modalities for assessment. Minerva Urol Nefrol 63:207–212

34. Jou YC, Shen CH, Lin CT et al (2011) Safety and efficacy of tubeless percutaneous nephrolithotomy in patients on anti-platelet therapy and cirrhotic patients. Urol Res 39:393–396
35. Resorlu B, Kara C, Sahin E, Unsal A (2011) Comparison of nephrostomy drainage types following percutaneous nephrolithotomy requiring multiple tracts: single tube versus multiple tubes versus tubeless. Urol Int 87:23–27
36. Amer T, Ahmed K, Bultitude M et al (2012) Standard versus tubeless percutaneous nephrolithotomy: a systematic review. Urol Int 88:373–382
37. Wang J, Zhao C, Zhang C et al (2011) Tubeless vs standard percutaneous nephrolithotomy: a meta-analysis. BJU Int 109:918–924
38. Okeke Z, Andonian S, Srinivasan A et al (2009) Cryotherapy of the nephrostomy tract: a novel technique to decrease the risk of hemorrhage after tubeless percutaneous renal surgery. J Endourol 23:417–420
39. Mishra S, Sabnis RB, Kurien A et al (2010) Questioning the wisdom of tubeless percutaneous nephrolithotomy (PCNL): a prospective randomized controlled study of early tube removal vs tubeless PCNL. BJU Int 106:1045–1049
40. Li R, Louie MK, Lee HJ et al (2010) Prospective randomized trial of three different methods of nephrostomy tract closure after percutaneous nephrolithotripsy. BJU Int 107:1660–1665
41. Jou YC, Cheng MC, Sheen JH et al (2004) Electrocauterization of bleeding points for percutaneous nephrolithotomy. Urology 64:443–447
42. Aron M, Goel R, Kesarwani PK, Guota NP (2004) Hemostasis in tubeless PNL. Point of technique. Urol Int 73:244–247
43. Choe CH, L'Esperance JO, Auge BK (2009) The use of adjunctive hemostatic agents for tubeless percutaneous nephrolithotomy. J Endourol 23:1733–1738
44. Lipkin ME, Mancini JG, Simmons WN et al (2011) Pathologic evaluation of hemostatic agents in percutaneous nephrolithotomy tracts in a porcine model. J Endourol 25:1353–1357
45. Aghamir SM, Khazaeli MH, Meisami A (2006) Use of Surgicel for sealing nephrostomy tract after totally tubeless percutaneous nephrolithotomy. J Endourol 20:293–295
46. Lee DI, Uribe C, Eichel L et al (2004) Sealing percutaneous nephrolithotomy tracts with gelatin matrix hemostatic sealant: initial clinical use. J Urol 171:575–578
47. Kaufmann OG, Sountoulides P, Kaplan A et al (2009) Skin treatment and tract closure for tubeless percutaneous nephrolithotomy: University of California, Irvine, Technique. J Endourol 23:1739–1741
48. Eden CG, Sultana SR, Murray KH, Carruthers RK (1997) Extraperitoneal laparoscopic dismembered fibrin-glued pyeloplasty: medium-term results. BJU Int 80:382–389
49. Kim IY, Eichel L, Edwards R et al (2007) Effects of commonly used hemostatic agents on the porcine collecting system. J Endourol 21:652–654
50. Uribe CA, Eichel L, Khonsari S et al (2005) What happens to hemostatic agents in contact with urine? An in vitro study. J Endourol 19:312–317

Chapter 16
Supine and Supine Modified PNL in Special Situations

Cecilia Maria Cracco, Cesare Marco Scoffone, Arvind P. Ganpule, Amit Doshi, and Mahesh R. Desai

Abstract PNL is a safe and effective procedure not only in a standard patient (adult with normal body mass index (BMI) and body habitus, no renal malformations, first procedure for urolithiasis, no previous renal or abdominal surgery, normal anaesthesiological risk) but also in a variety of particular situations regarding the patient's physical and clinical features. The only exception is pregnancy; in fact, although anecdotical cases performed during early pregnancy have been reported, PNL regardless to patient positioning is not advised in this case and should be delayed till after delivery. Elderly, obese, and high-risk patients, children, patients with skeletal malformations or urinary anomalies, previous surgery, and urinary diversions may greatly benefit from PNL in the supine position, which may even be obliged in ectopic pelvic or transplanted kidneys. Of course, not all musculoskeletal deformities can be easily arranged in the supine position, and bilateral procedures or certain renal stones in calyceal diverticula of the superior district might rather benefit from the prone position.

C.M. Cracco, MD, PhD (✉) • C.M. Scoffone, MD
Department of Urology, Cottolengo Hospital, Via Cottolengo 9, 10152 Torino, Italy
e-mail: cecilia.cracco@libero.it; scoof@libero.it

A.P. Ganpule • A. Doshi • M.R. Desai
Department of Urology, Muljibhai Patel Urological Hospital, Nadiad, Gujarat 387001, India
e-mail: doctorarvind1@gmail.com; dr.doshiamit@gmail.com; mrdesai@mpuh.org

C.M. Scoffone et al. (eds.), *Supine Percutaneous Nephrolithotomy and ECIRS*,
DOI 10.1007/978-2-8178-0459-0_16, © Springer-Verlag France 2014

16.1 Introduction

PNL is a safe and effective procedure not only in a standard patient (adult with normal body mass index (BMI) and body habitus, no renal malformations, first procedure for urolithiasis, no previous renal or abdominal surgery, normal anaesthesiological risk) but also in a variety of particular situations regarding the patient's physical and clinical features. The only exception is pregnancy; in fact, although anecdotical cases performed during early pregnancy have been reported, PNL regardless to patient positioning is not advised in this case and should be delayed till after delivery.

16.2 Elderly and High-Risk Patients

Urolithiasis is an increasing problem in patients over 80 years. In fact, the frequent lack of the classic symptoms of a renal colic may lead to a later presentation with larger and more complex stone disease. Being elderly often also high-risk patients because of their multiple comorbidities (high ASA scores) [1], treatment of their renal stones might be challenging. In such cases, prone PNL implies some concerns like difficult airway control and suboptimal ventilation in case of pulmonary disease [2–4], whereas under these respects supine PNL is safe and effective [5].

PNL in elderly patients might imply a theoretical higher risk of hemorrhage, since arteriosclerosis causes the loss of normal muscle and elastin layers of the blood vessels and thus a decreased ability to close when lacerated [6, 7]. However, it has been demonstrated that PNL can be safely performed in elderly patients with no increased complication rates, and totally tubeless procedures have been carried out as well [4, 8].

The large category of high-risk patients also includes those with poor preoperative renal function, and particular attention should be paid to chronic kidney disease stages IV/V. In fact, it has been demonstrated that such patients have statistically significant worse postoperative outcomes after PNL [9].

16.3 Children

Urolithiasis in children is frequently metabolic or infectious in origin, associated with kidney anomalies and previous history of stone intervention, requiring repeated surgical procedures [10]. In spite of all this, PNL can be safely and effectively applied to children of any age group [11, 12]. The percutaneous approach (possibly tubeless and with single access) seems even better than open surgery and of reiterated ESWL, often requiring anaesthesia without guarantee of a complete stone clearance [13, 14]. In children, the supine position is increasingly and successfully employed (12 % in the CROES series) [12] (see Chap. 17) (Fig. 16.1).

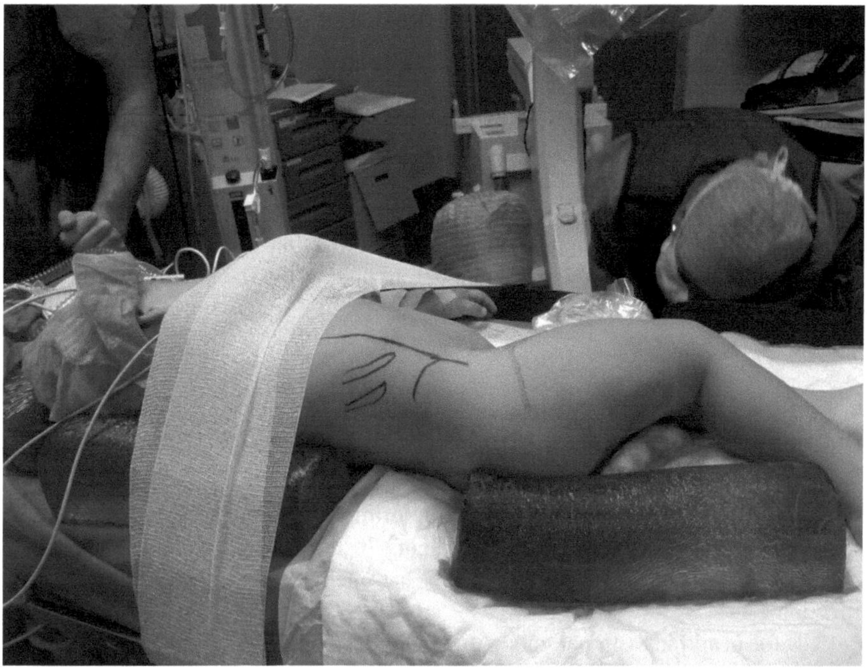

Fig. 16.1 Child arranged in the Galdakao-modified supine Valdivia position with reference lines for the renal puncture

16.4 Obese Patients

Obesity has been identified as an independent risk factor for stone formation in the United States. Obesity (BMI >35) also places surgical patients at a greater risk of complications, because of the increased incidence in this group of diabetes, hypertension, ischemic heart disease, postoperative deep venous thrombosis, and pulmonary embolism and because of poor radiographic visualization, obscure anatomic landmarks, more difficult renal access, and inferior stone-free rates [15].

Because of a greater perceived difficulty in performing percutaneous surgery in obese patients, investigators have theorized in the past that PNL in such patients may be less effective, technically difficult, and associated with higher complication rates [16]. On the contrary, there are no adverse effects of obesity on PNL outcomes in terms of stone-free rates, complication rates, and length of hospital stay [17–19], apart from a slightly longer operative time [20]. Therefore, morbid obesity is no sufficient reason for choosing multisession retrograde endoscopic lithotripsy instead of PNL for the treatment of large renal calculi, obtaining low stone-free rates as 33 % [21].

We agree that there are some tips and tricks and modifications of the standard PNL technique and instrumentation to bear in mind when planning a PNL in an obese patient [17, 22], like the use of larger and longer access sheaths and nephroscopes as effective additions to the urologist's armamentarium, the suture of the Amplatz sheath to the skin to prevent its loss beneath it or the muscle fascia, and the trick to pull abdominal fat opposite to the operated side, possibly putting the patient in the supine/supine-modified position.

Supine PNL has been proven to be very ergonomic and suitable in obese patients (Fig. 16.2), also considered high-risk ones for the abovementioned reasons. The supine decubitus has the advantages of a significant shorter operative time (the 2008 CROES study reported the opposite, with the bias that they did not take into account all the preliminary retrograde procedure before puncturing the kidney) and hospital stay [5, 20, 23–25].

16.5 Skeletal Malformations

Scoliosis involves a lateral and rotational deformity of the thoracolumbar spine and occurs in less than 4 % of the population, being 70 % idiopathic and 30 % secondary to congenital, neuromuscular disease, mesenchymal disorders, trauma, or infection.

PNL for urolithiasis in patients with spinal deformities, such as kyphoscoliosis or severe hip ankylosis, might be challenging from an anaesthesiological (respiration impaired, mainly restrictive pulmonary deficit), surgical (anatomic variations and accurate preoperative planning to avoid visceral damage), and technical point of view. A thorough preoperative imaging study should be carried out, especially to choose the best therapeutic approach and, in case of PNL, the more fit position [26]. The supine position improves anesthesiological assistance from a cardioventilatory point of view and implies less risk of postural damage, more comfort of the patient, and the possibility of a combined approach, although supine position may not be applicable to all skeletal malformations and may leave a very reduced space between ribs and iliac crest when the stone is located on the concave side of the spine (Fig. 16.3).

16.6 Previous Surgery

Urolithiasis has been often previously treated by means of extracorporeal shock wave lithotripsy (ESWL) and percutaneous, ureteroscopic, open, or laparoscopic surgery [27, 28]. Given the equivalence prone/supine, safe and effective PNL can be performed in such patients, with no higher risk of complications, except the need for more attempts to access the pelvicalyceal system and the difficulty in tract dilation secondary to fascial and retroperitoneal scarring (and in this case the use of Alken coaxial dilators is of the utmost importance) [29] (Fig. 16.4).

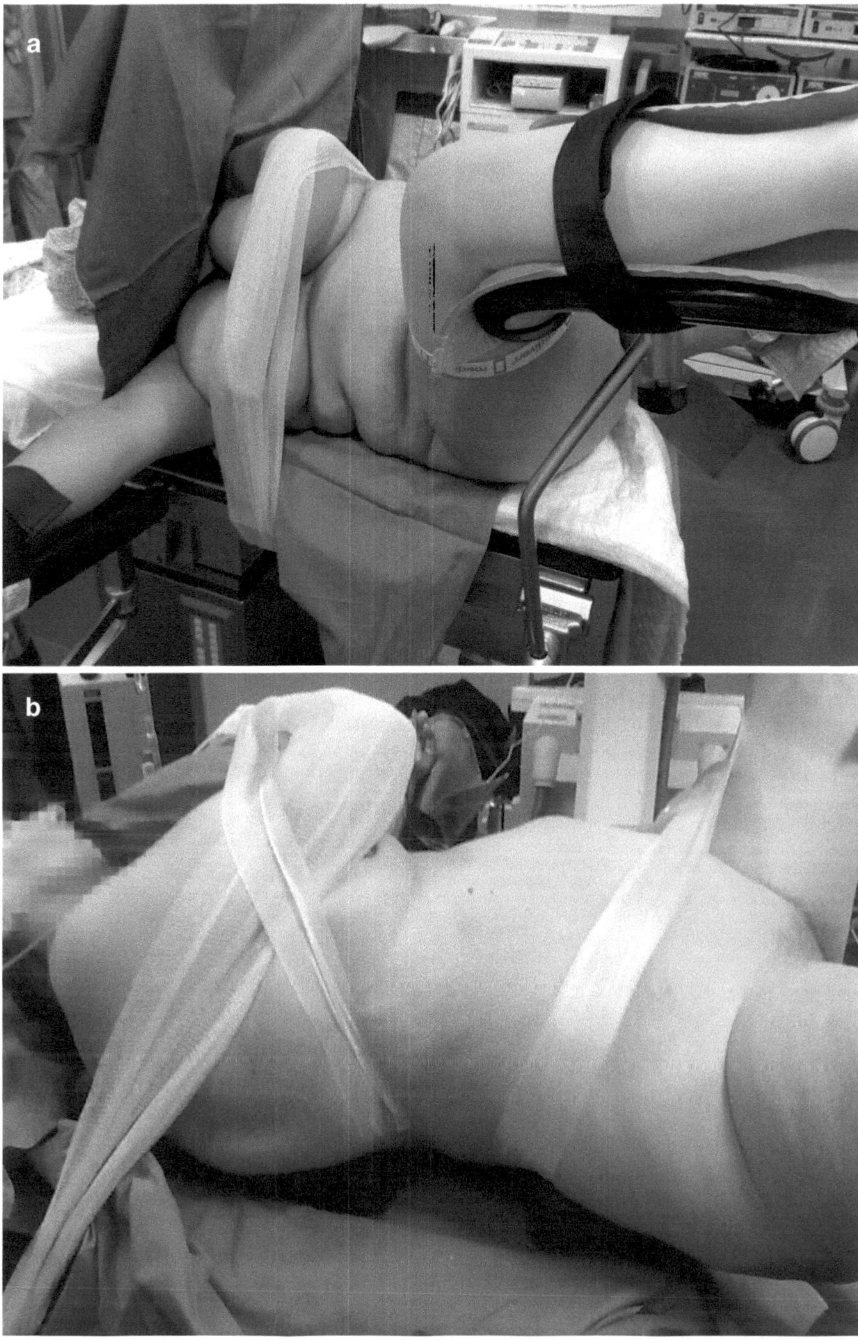

Fig. 16.2 Obese patient in the Galdakao-modified supine Valdivia position, ready for ECIRS (**a**) and prepared with adhesive strips in order to move the fat towards the side that does not need to be operated (**b**)

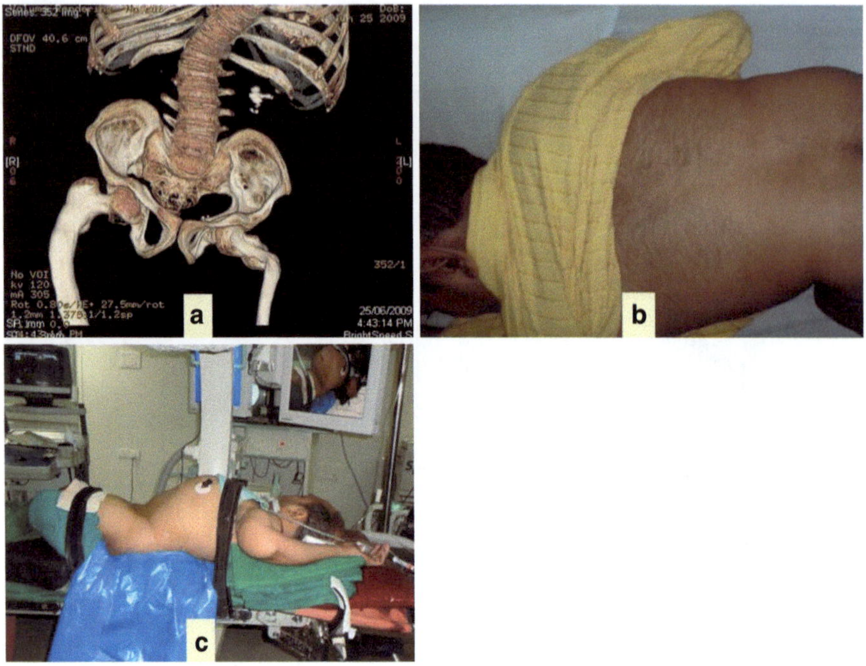

Fig. 16.3 Patient with kyphoscoliosis and osteogenesis imperfecta. CT scan for the study of the staghorn urolithiasis and of the anatomy (**a**) It was impossible to put the patient in the prone position (**b**) and thus the supine position was employed (**c**)

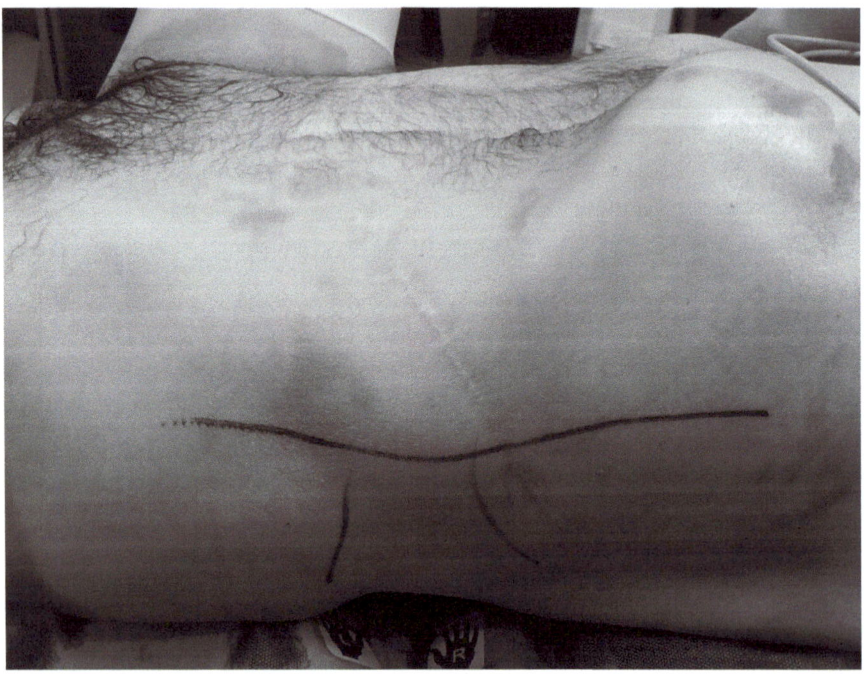

Fig. 16.4 Post-pyelolithotomy scar in a patient undergoing ECIRS

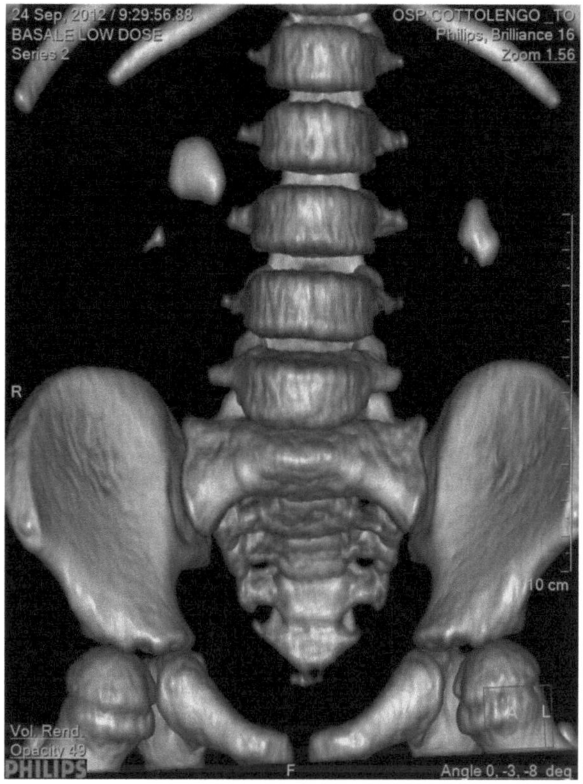

Fig. 16.5 3D CT scan reconstruction of a bilateral urolithiasis

16.7 Bilateral Urolithiasis

Prone position seems more adapt for performing synchronous bilateral percutaneous procedures, in spite of the increased hemorrhagic risk [30, 31] (Fig. 16.5).

16.8 Upper Pole Puncture

During ECIRS performed in the Galdakao-modified supine Valdivia position, upper pole puncture is seldom required because of the use of flexible antegrade/retrograde endoscopes. Under this respect, a patient suffering from upper calyceal stone disease is the ideal one for ECIRS in this position.

In any case, if a subcostal access to the renal superior calyx is required in a supine position, renal displacement technique should be carried out, with lung inflation to facilitate the puncture and to reduce intrathoracic morbidity. Alternatively, the kidney could be pulled down with a balloon catheter [32], or, according to our personal experience, the inclination of the patient on the operating table can be further increased.

16.9 Urinary Congenital Malformations

A variety of developmental abnormalities of the kidney can present in adulthood. Anomalous kidneys (solitary, horseshoe, ectopic, and malrotated kidneys) often have abnormal renal position, anatomy, calyceal orientation, relationships of the calyces to the renal pelvis and upper ureter, rotation, aberrant vasculature, relative renal immobility, atypical relationships between kidney and other organs, and all elements causing urinary stasis with stone formation, often associated with concomitant infection and metabolic alterations. The same reasons causing an increased risk of stone formation contribute to an increased risk of renal stone management in anomalous kidneys [7, 33, 34].

PNL in anatomically abnormal kidneys is challenging for fear of inaccessibility, and of vascular and visceral injury, but can be safely and effectively performed, sometimes with an extended operative time. Even more than usual it deserves a meticulous preoperative assessment of the anatomy of the collecting system and of visceral relationships for planning an optimal renal puncture, intraoperatively aided by real-time ultrasound assistance. The supine and oblique positions may be particularly favorable, especially in ectopic pelvic and malrotated kidneys [35, 36], with the bolster below the hemipelvis pushing the kidney closer to the anterior abdominal wall, while the bowel loops are displaced cephalad both by the position and by the pressure of the ultrasound probe itself. Also in horseshoe kidneys (Fig. 16.6), the supine position may be particularly useful to improve safety and efficacy of the percutaneous procedure. All the same, universal application of PNL may also be challenged with alternative and creative solutions, like the combination with the laparoscopic approach (personal experience) (Fig. 16.7) or the alternative use of single port laparoscopic access for pyelolithotomy surgery [37, 38].

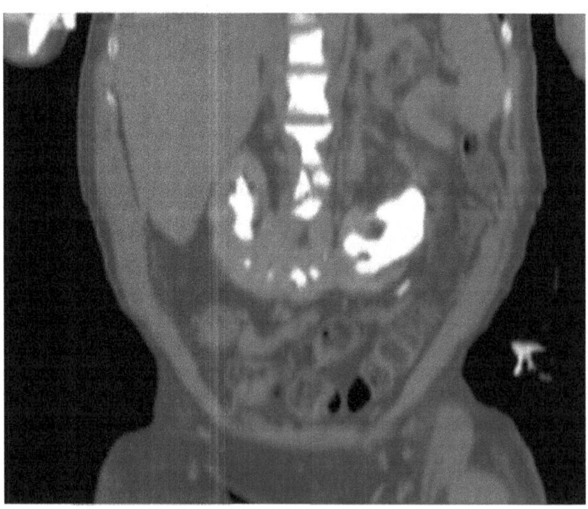

Fig. 16.6 CT scan without contrast of a paraplegic patient with a horseshoe kidney

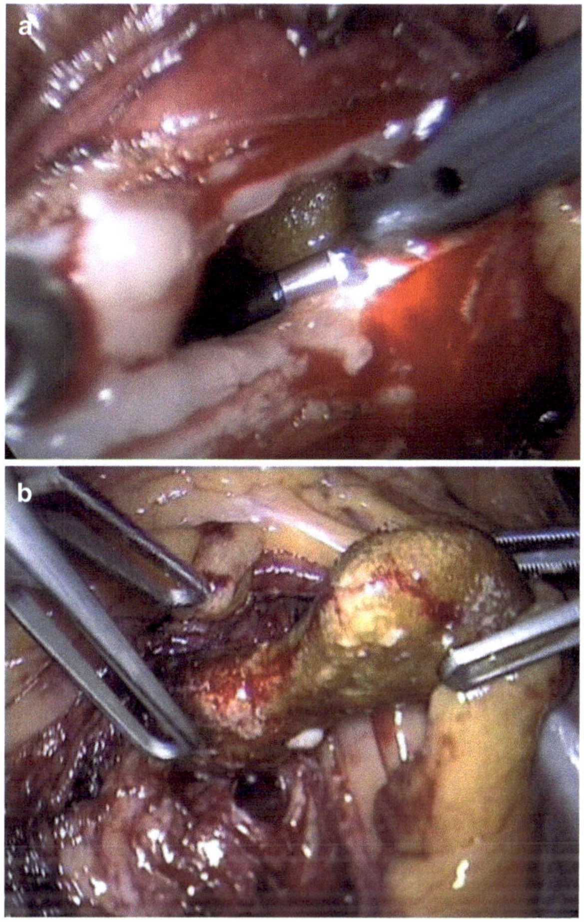

Fig. 16.7 Combination of laparoscopy and ECIRS in the same paraplegic patient. Flexible RIRS phase (**a**) and litholapaxy (**b**)

As to UPJ stricture, similar to what happens in pediatric patients, concomitant laparoscopic correction should be performed; thus, associated stones, often candidates to a percutaneous approach, may be extracted during the laparoscopic procedure, with graspers or combining trans-trocar lithotripsy. This is also our personal experience.

16.10 Transplanted Kidney

Nephrolithiasis is an unusual (0.2–3 % of all urological complications) but challenging late complication of transplanted kidneys, due to hyperparathyroidism and nonabsorbable sutures, as well as to other predisposing causes identical to patients with native kidneys (obstructive uropathy, recurrent urinary tract infections, metabolic abnormalities like hyperuricosuria).

Renal stones in transplanted kidneys need prompt recognition and management, as they can be an important cause of deterioration of the graft function. PNL is most often the best modality to render patients stone-free, being effective and safe. Allograft superficial location close to the skin and its proximity to the bony pelvis, peritoneum, and iliac vessels makes the supine position a valid option, also allowing combined antero-retrograde approach with the use of flexible scopes [39–42].

16.11 After Urinary Diversions

Complications related to urinary-intestinal diversions are numerous and rather frequent (up to 11 % within 3 years after surgery) because of anatomic and metabolic factors including refluxing ureteroileal anastomoses, upper urinary tract dilation, urinary stasis, and heightened risk of stone formation. The hyperchloremic metabolic acidosis from reabsorption of solutes across the intestinal mucosa results in an increased burden of urinary titratable acids, with an increased risk of hyperoxaluria, calcium oxalate stone formation in patients with ileal resection, and higher recurrence of urinary tract infections. Urea-splitting organisms elevate urinary pH and increase the risk of forming calcium phosphate and struvite stones [43]. Renal and ureteral calculi may be approached antegradely or with a combined approach, if the ureteroileal anastomosis is compliant enough to allow a retrograde approach [44], being the supine position particularly beneficial in this setting.

16.12 Pregnancy

Normal anatomic and physiological changes of the urinary tract during pregnancy (mechanical compression of the ureter, effect of the circulating progesterone on the ureteral smooth muscle with reduced peristalsis and increased dilation, gestational hypercalciuria secondary to a combination of increased GFR, dietary and fetal factors) may predispose to stone formation. Thus, nephrolithiasis is a not infrequent complication in pregnancy (the incidence of symptomatic nephrolithiasis during pregnancy varies between 1 in 244 and 1 in 2,000 pregnancies, but the actual incidence is likely to be higher), representing a clinical dilemma because of potential risks to both mother and fetus [45].

Most cases of urolithiasis in pregnancy are managed conservatively either with ureteral stents or percutaneous nephrostomy tubes, which need to be changed at regular intervals. Definitive management of the stone should be reserved to after delivery. Otherwise, X-ray-free ureteroscopy in pregnant patients can be carried out in the appropriate setting and with a multidisciplinary approach [46].

PNL is not advised during pregnancy, in spite of the fact that supine positions and X-ray-free percutaneous approaches might be employed. General anaesthesia, length of the procedure, use of fluoroscopy, and prone position make PNL a hazardous procedure [45, 47], although anecdotical cases have been reported [48, 49].

16.13 Conclusions

Once PNL is the indicated treatment for a definite urolithiasis, the choice of patient positioning should not be dogmatic and aprioristic but rather tailored on the patient's features. A supine PNL may be obliged in ectopic pelvic or transplanted kidneys; might be a very good option for elderly, high-risk, or obese patients, especially those with an impaired cardiopulmonary function; and can be a valid alternative for children with renal anomalies or previous surgeries. On the contrary, not all musculoskeletal deformities can be easily arranged in the supine position, and bilateral procedures or certain renal stones in calyceal diverticula of the superior district might rather benefit from the prone position.

References

1. Toksoz S, Dirim A, Kizilkan Y, Ozkardes H (2012) The effect of American Society of Anesthesiology scores on percutaneous nephrolithotomy outcomes. Urol Int 89:301–306
2. Patel SR, Haleblian GE, Pareek G (2010) Percutaneous nephrolithotomy can be safely performed in the high-risk patient. Urology 75:51–55
3. Karami H, Mazloomfard MM, Golshan A et al (2010) Does age affect outcomes of percutaneous nephrolithotomy? Urol J 7:17–21
4. McCarthy JP, Skinner TA, Norman RW (2011) Urolithiasis in the elderly. Can J Urol 18:5717–5720
5. Manohar T, Jain P, Desai M (2007) Supine percutaneous nephrolithotomy: effective approach to high-risk morbidly obese patients. J Endourol 21:44–49
6. Handa RK, Willis LR, Connors BA et al (2010) Time-course for recovery of renal function after unilateral (single-tract) percutaneous access in the pig. J Endourol 24:283–288
7. Akman T, Binbay M, Sari E et al (2011) Factors affecting bleeding during percutaneous nephrolithotomy: single surgeon experience. J Endourol 25:327–333
8. Kara C, Resorlu B, Bayindir M, Unsai A (2010) A randomized comparison of totally tubeless and standard percutaneous nephrolithotomy in elderly patients. Urology 76:289–294
9. Sairam K, Scoffone CM, Alken P et al (2012) Percutaneous nephrolithotomy and chronic kidney disease: results from the CROES PCNL global study. J Urol 188:1195–1200
10. Frattini A, Ferretti S, Salvaggio A (2010) Percutaneous nephrolithotripsy (PCNL) in children: experience of Parma. Arch Ital Urol Androl 82:51–52
11. Dogan HS, Kilicarsian H, Kordan Y et al (2011) Percutaneous nephrolithotomy in children: does age matter? World J Urol 29:725–729
12. Guven S, Frattini A, Onal B, Desai M et al (2013) Percutaneous nephrolithotomy in children of different age groups: data from the Clinical Research Office of the Endourological Society (CROES) percutaneous nephrolithotomy global study. BJU Int 111:148–156
13. Gonen M, Turunc T, Ozturk B et al (2009) Outcome of percutaneous nephrolithotomy in children having complex stones. Urol Int 83:416–419
14. Bayrak O, Seckiner I, Ertorhan S et al (2012) Comparative analyses of percutaneous nephrolithotomy versus open surgery in pediatric urinary stone disease. Pediatr Surg Int 28:1025–1029

15. Tomaszewski JJ, Smaldone MC, Schuster T et al (2010) Outcomes of percutaneous nephrolithotomy stratified by body mass index. J Endourol 24:547–550
16. Faerber GJ, Goh M (1997) Percutaneous nephrolithotripsy in the morbidly obese patients. Tech Urol 3:89–95
17. Pearle MS, Nakada SY, Womack JS, Kryger JV (1998) Outcomes of contemporary percutaneous nephrostolithotomy in morbidly obese patients. J Urol 160:669–673
18. El-Hassmy AM, Shokeir AA, El-Nahas AR et al (2007) Outcome of percutaneous nephrolithotomy: effect of body mass index. Eur Urol 52:199–204
19. Alyami FA, Skinner TA, Norman RW (2012) Impact of body mass index on clinical outcomes associated with percutaneous nephrolithotomy. Can Urol Assoc J 15:1–5
20. Falahatkar S, Moghaddam KG, Kezemnezhad E et al (2011) Factors affecting operative time during percutaneous nephrolithotomy: our experience with the complete supine position. J Endourol 25:1831–1836
21. Wheat JC, Roberts WW, Wolf JS Jr (2009) Multi-session retrograde endoscopic lithotripsy of large renal calculi in obese patients. Can J Urol 16:4915–4920
22. Bugeja S, Zammit P, German K (2009) Use of a modified syringe barrel to ensure control of the Amplatz sheath during percutaneous nephrolithotripsy in obese patients. J Endourol 23:1817–1819
23. De La Rosette JJ, Tsakiris P, Ferrandino MN et al (2008) Beyond prone position in percutaneous nephrolithotomy: a comprehensive review. Eur Urol 54:1262–1269
24. Ferena Perez LA, Zungri Telo ER, Valdivia JG (2005) Supine position as the best option for percutaneous surgery of renal calculi in morbidly patients. Actas Urol Esp 29:997–1000
25. Mazzucchi E, Vicentini FC, Marchini GS et al (2012) Percutaneous nephrolithotomy in obese patients: comparison between prone and total supine position. J Endourol 26:1437–1442
26. Goumas-Kartalas I, Montanari E (2010) Percutaneous nephrolithotomy in patients with spinal deformities. J Endourol 24:1081–1089
27. Falahatkar S, Panahandeh Z, Ashoori E et al (2009) What is the difference between percutaneous nephrolithotomy in patients with and without previous open surgery? J Endourol 23:1107–1110
28. Resorlu B, Kara C, Senocak C et al (2010) Effect of previous open renal surgery and failed extracorporeal shockwave lithotripsy on the performance and outcomes of percutaneous nephrolithotomy. J Endourol 24:13–16
29. Gupta R, Gupta A, Singh G et al (2011) PCNL – a comparative study in nonoperated and in previously operated (open nephrolithotomy/pyelolithotomy) patients –a single-surgeon experience. Int Braz J Urol 37:739–744
30. Williams SK, Hoenig DM (2009) Synchronous bilateral percutaneous nephrostolithotomy. J Endourol 23:1707–1712
31. Bagrodia A, Raman JD, Bensalah K et al (2009) Synchronous bilateral percutaneous nephrostolithotomy: analysis of clinical outcomes, cost and surgeon reimbursement. J Urol 181:149–153
32. Falahatkar S, Enshael A, Afsharimoghaddam A et al (2010) Complete supine percutaneous nephrolithotomy with lung inflation avoids the need for a supracostal puncture. J Endourol 24:213–218
33. Liatsikos EN, Kallidonis P, Stolzenburg JU et al (2010) Percutaneous management of staghorn calculi in horseshoe kidneys. A multi-institutional experience. J Endourol 24:531–536
34. Osther PJ RH, Liatsikos E et al (2011) Percutaneous nephrolithotomy among patients with renal anomalies: patient characteristics and outcomes; a subgroup analysis of the Clinical Research Office of the Endourological Society global percutaneous nephrolithotomy study. J Endourol 25:1627–1632
35. Desai MR, Jasani A (2000) Percutaneous nephrolithotomy in ectopic kidneys. J Endourol 14:289–292
36. Mosavi-Bahar SH, Amirzargar MA, Rahnavardi M et al (2007) Percutaneous nephrolithotomy in patients with kidney malformations. J Endourol 21:520–524

37. Rana AM, Bhojwani JP (2009) Percutaneous nephrolithotomy in renal anomalies of fusion, ectopia, rotation, hypoplasia, and pelvicalyceal aberration: uniformity in heterogeneity. J Endourol 23:609–614
38. Pérez-Lanzac A, Soto-Villalva J, Ledo Cepero MJ et al (2013) Transumbilical single port surgery with conventional laparoscopic instruments in horseshoe kidney. Actas Urol Esp 37(5):311–315
39. Francesca F, Felipetto R, Boggi U et al (2002) Percutaneous nephrolithotomy of transplanted kidney. J Endourol 16:225–227
40. Rifaioglu MM, Berger AD, Penguine W, Stoller ML (2008) Percutaneous management of stones in transplanted kidneys. Urology 72:508–512
41. Oliveira M, Branco F, Martins L, Lima E (2011) Percutaneous nephrolithotomy in renal transplants: a safe approach with a high stone-free rate. Int Urol Nephrol 43:329–335
42. Stravodimos KG, Adamis S, Tyritzis S, Georgios Z, Costantinides CA (2012) Renal transplant lithiasis: analysis of our series and review of the literature. J Endourol 26:38–44
43. Fernandez A, Foell K, Nott L, Denstedt JD, Razvi H (2011) Percutaneous nephrolithotripsy in patients with urinary diversions: a case–control comparison of perioperative outcomes. J Endourol 25:1615–1618
44. Okhunov Z, Duty B, Smith AD, Okeke Z (2011) Management of urolithiasis in patients after urinary diversions. BJU Int 108:330–336
45. Semins MJ, Matlaga BR (2010) Management of stone disease in pregnancy. Curr Opin Urol 20:174–177
46. Scarpa RM, De Lisa A, Usai E (1996) Diagnosis and treatment of ureteral calculi during pregnancy with rigid ureteroscopes. J Urol 55:875–877
47. Srirangam JJ, Hickerton B, Van Cleynenbreugel B (2008) Management of urinary calculi in pregnancy: a review. J Endourol 22:867–875
48. Shah A, Chandak P, Tiptaft R et al (2004) Percutaneous nephrolithotomy in early pregnancy. Int J Clin Pract 58:809–810
49. Toth C, Toth G, Varga A et al (2005) Percutaneous nephrolithotomy in early pregnancy. Int Urol Nephrol 37:1–3

Chapter 17
PNL in Paediatric Patients

Antonio Frattini, Cesare Marco Scoffone, and Stefania Ferretti

Abstract Incidence and indications of urolithiasis treatment in children are revised in this chapter. In particular, the authors afford the issue of paediatric PNL, with particular reference to the operative armamentarium needed, patient positioning and advantages of the supine position in children, renal anatomical features and technical aspects of ECIRS (Endoscopic Combined IntraRenal Surgery) in young age (with details regarding renal access and tract dilation). Paediatric ECIRS is as safe and effective as in adults, especially in case of concomitant congenital urinary malformations.

17.1 Introduction

Incidence of urolithiasis, stone location and composition vary among different geographic areas. In Southeast Asia and Africa, bladder stones are widespread. On the other hand upper urinary tract stones are much more frequent in Europe and the USA, with a shift of this disease from the lower to the upper urinary tract in developed countries and a marked predominance of male gender in adults.

Urinary stone disease in children is relatively rare if compared to adult population, representing about 1 % of all patients affected by this disease. However, the

A. Frattini, MD (✉)
Department of Urology, Guastalla Hospital, via Donatori Sangue 1, 42016 Guastalla, (Reggio Emilia), Italy
e-mail: afrattini@ausl.re.it

C.M. Scoffone, MD
Department of Urology, Cottolengo Hospital, Via Cottolengo 9, 10152 Torino, Italy
e-mail: scoof@libero.it

S. Ferretti, MD
Department of Surgery, Urology Unit, University Hospital of Parma, via Gramsci 14, 43125 Parma, Italy
e-mail: stefaniaferretti@icloud.com

C.M. Scoffone et al. (eds.), *Supine Percutaneous Nephrolithotomy and ECIRS*,
DOI 10.1007/978-2-8178-0459-0_17, © Springer-Verlag France 2014

epidemiology of paediatric urolithiasis has quite changed in the last three decades. Incidence rates tend to increase and range between 0.3 and 0.94 of cases per 1,000 hospitalizations in the western countries. Stone formation is uncommon in children younger than two years of age, and boys seem to be affected only slightly more than girls. Calcium oxalate and calcium phosphate are the most common types, accounting for more than 75 % of all paediatric urolithiasis. Bladder stones are commonly encountered in developing countries and mostly depend upon dietary factors; primary bladder stones in developed countries are usually related to bladder malformations.

As to the etiological modifications of lithogenesis, the most significant evidence in Europe is the apparent reduction in infection stones (made up by organic matrix and struvite) in favour of those related to metabolic abnormalities, increased from 16 % of the 1980s up to 44 % nowadays. This epidemiological phenomenon is probably linked to the prompt and early identification and treatment of the urinary tract infections in children living in developed countries. On the other hand, it may also be due to the improved etiopathogenetic knowledge of the paediatric urolithiasis worldwide, with a similar incidence of European and US metabolic defects (due to inherited genetic causes and environmental factors such as obesity, high daily salt consumption, inadequate overall hydration. Metabolic alterations (hypercalciuria, hyperoxaluria, cystinuria, hyperuricosuria, hypocitraturia) account for more than 50 % of diagnoses in children; thier prompt identification is fundamental to prevent the development of relevant and often recurrent stone burdens.

Several studies demonstrated a high incidence of urolithiasis (20–44 %) in association with urinary malformations. Many children suffering from kidney stones also have urinary malformations, but the opposite cannot be demonstrated; in fact, a survey on 618 children with urinary malformations showed that only 3.6 % suffered from renal stones. Probably other environmental factors contribute to the development of renal stones [1].

17.2 Stone Management in Children: Treatment Options

The objective of stone management in children should be complete stone clearance along with prevention of stone recurrence, preservation of renal function, control of urinary infections, correction of anatomical abnormalities and of associated metabolic alterations. Thus, any surgery should be planned after a thorough and comprehensive medical evaluation and followed by planned medical treatments as well as by long-term follow-up.

17.2.1 Extracorporeal Shock Wave Lithotripsy (ESWL)

ESWL was successfully introduced into the paediatric setting in 1986 and very appreciated because of its minimal invasiveness, safety and effectiveness. For a very long time, ESWL remained the first-line treatment for single or multiple stones of both kidney and ureter. Nowadays, ESWL is the preferred approach for little patients with renal calculi <20 mm (<15 mm in case of cystine stones), as reported in the European Association of Urology guidelines. Stone-free rates range between 57 and 92 %. It's well known that ESWL treatment of lower calyceal stones has a rather low success rate (50–62 %), depending upon that specific anatomical site and gravity; it depends on the length of the calyceal infundibulum, the infundibulopelvic angle (cut-off 40°) and of course on the stone burden [1, 2]. Spontaneous stone expulsion is easier in children than in adults (except for some urinary malformations); thus, the need for ancillary procedures (5–38 %) such as ureteral stenting or retrograde ureteroscopy is not so frequent as in adults [3, 4].

17.2.2 Semirigid and Flexible Ureteroscopy for Retrograde IntraRenal Surgery (RIRS)

Semirigid ureteroscopy is recommended for proximal and mid-ureteral stones as first choice in experienced hands or after a single session of failed ESWL. Rigid and flexible instruments on the market have a larger working channel than years ago. Flexible endoscopes can bend up to 270° and are especially useful for removing stones from the lower pole. The incidence of postoperative ureteral strictures or vesico-ureteral reflux is low (ostium dilation is very rare nowadays, owing to the miniaturization of the instruments). Complication rates of RIRS in children and in adults are similar (0–7 %), and the success rate in different paediatric published series ranges from 86 to 100 %, with a mean value of 90 % with a single procedure for ureteral calculi.

The evolution and miniaturization of flexible instruments and the introduction of L.A.S.E.R. as energy source for lithotripsy have strongly supported the retrograde ureterorenoscopic approach among the therapeutic opportunities in the treatment of paediatric urolithiasis. RIRS is a minimally invasive approach, high efficient in the treatment of stones of 2 cm or less [1, 2].

Since the ureter in children aged <3 years is not always compliant enough to allow the insertion of a ureteral access sheath, ureteral pre-stenting few days before RIRS might represent a good strategy. RIRS should be preferred to PNL when its mini-invasiveness does not compromise its effectiveness. The supine position of the child allows to modify the surgical technique from RIRS to Endovision PNL when needed, with no intraoperative changes in patient positioning.

17.2.3 Percutaneous Nephrolithotomy (PNL)

The percutaneous approach is reserved to bigger and more complex stones, in case of ESWL-refractory stones or in the presence of anatomical abnormalities like calyceal diverticula, representing a problem for lithotripsy or expulsion of the stone fragments. PNL is more invasive than ESWL and RIRS, but stone-free rates are about 90 % and complication rates very low [1, 2, 5–7].

17.2.4 Laparoscopic/Open Surgery

Open surgery remains the treatment of choice for 0.3–5.4 % of the paediatric population in developed countries, while it is used in 14 % of cases in developing countries because of its cost-effectiveness [8, 9]. The combination of stone removal and simultaneous correction of anatomical abnormalities is the gold standard [2].

17.3 Indications of PNL in Children

Based on our personal experience and on the world literature, the indications of PNL could be summarized as follows:

Kidney stones >2 cm
Cystine kidney stones ≥1.5 cm
Lower pole stones >1.5 cm or with an unfavourable infundibular angle
Stones in anatomical abnormalities suitable for percutaneous resolution (calyceal diverticula, ureteral stenosis, recurrence after UPJ stenosis surgery)
ESWL-refractory stones when RIRS is not suitable for difficult retrograde approach

In the end, the indications are substantially identical to adults, in the absence of congenital urinary malformations requiring open or laparoscopic reconstructive surgery, but the child safeguard needs the following essential requirements:

1. Minimal invasiveness (small calibre of the endoscopes).
2. Minimal anaesthetic time.
3. Minimal X-ray exposure.
4. Maximal stone clearance in one session.
5. Shortest duration of post-operative drainage (possibly tubeless PNL), leading to more comfort and less pain.

17.4 Operative Armamentarium

17.4.1 Endoscopes

The instruments are the same as in adult procedures but with reduced calibre and length. It's mandatory to have all paediatric endoscopic sets for performing PNL in a child, especially if aged <3 years.

There are semirigid ureteroscopes with a very small calibre on the market (like the Wolf 4.8 Ch), allowing to enter virtually any ureter, even the smaller ones. The harmless shape of the tip of the ureteroscope, exactly as in the adult, is an essential feature of such instruments (see Chap. 12). The new generation of semirigid ureteroscopes includes 7 Ch instruments with a large 4.8 Ch operating channel, sometimes suitable also for older children and adolescents as well as for adults (Fig. 17.1).

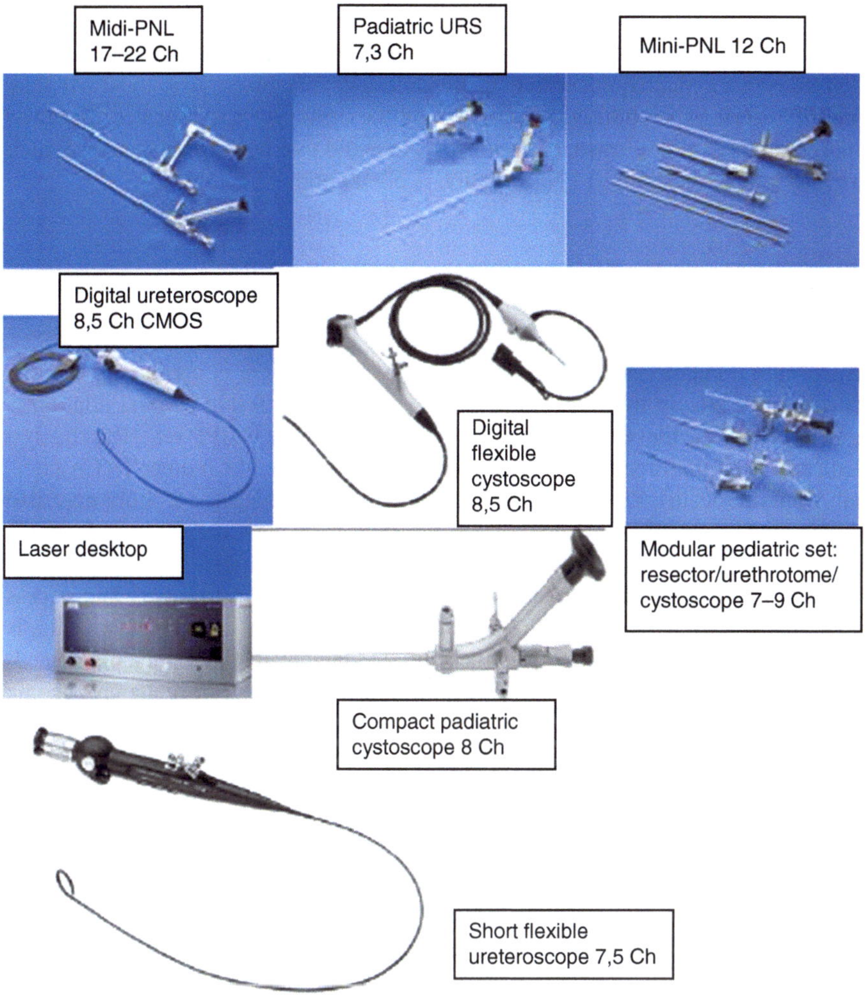

Fig. 17.1 Endoscopes used in a paediatric setting (RIRS/PNL)

Also flexible ureteroscopes, representing an important support for all percutaneous/endoscopic maneuver, need to be suitable for paediatric urinary systems in terms of calibre and length. In our department, we use standard 7.5 Ch Flex-X2 ureteroscope by Storz, allowing also the paediatric approach, upon application of a very small ureteral access sheath (9.5 Ch) when possible (Fig. 17.1).

As to the nephroscopes, those used for mini-PNL can be very handy, since their calibre is 12 Ch and their operative channel allows the introduction of ballistic probes and laser fibres, the intracorporeal lithotripsy energies most commonly employed during this kind of procedure. Larger nephroscopes (17–20 Ch) may also be used, when a 24 Ch Amplatz sheath can be applied.

As to the flexible instruments, both nephroscopes and ureteroscopes also in their digital version can be used, depending upon the diameter of the Amplatz sheath.

Warmed irrigation fluid should be used for all the endoscopes. In fact, another relevant issue in the child is hypothermia. Being their body so small, heath dispersion takes place much quicker than in an adult; thus, the anaesthesiologist will take care of covering the child with warmers and the urologist to use heated irrigation fluids (except during ultrasound lithotripsy, to avoid overheating), measures which are mandatory especially if PNL duration is 60–90 min.

17.4.2 Dilation Set

The usual percutaneous renal access in very small children is commonly the one called mini-PNL. In the mini-percutaneous approach, a Teflon coaxial dilation is used in order to achieve the 14/19 Ch Amplatz calibre (e.g. MIPP set – Rüsch – is a dedicated set with three coaxial hydrophilic dilators and a 14 Ch inner/19 Ch external Amplatz sheath). The mini-PNL set conceived by U. Nagele for Storz may also be employed, as well as a pneumatic set for dilation of the renal access (18–24 Ch Cook pneumatic balloon set or larger ones by Cook or Boston).

The leading concept of operative endoscopy, i.e. that instruments and access must adapt to the collecting system anatomy of the patient and not vice versa, is valid for the child even more than in the adult. In fact, any damage (including bleeding or urinary extravasation) may cause long-term consequences which may become difficult to manage with time.

The choice of the Amplatz sheath should be modulated on the calibre of the instruments we want to use in order to leave some space between Amplatz and endoscope, allowing the irrigation fluid to pour out freely, avoiding dangerous high intrarenal pressures, septic risk and liquid resorption. In fact, even minimal fluid resorption may cause hydro-electrolytic alterations and relevant metabolic consequences in children. This is also the reason why we consider 60–90 min as the maximal duration of a percutaneous procedure in a child, in spite of all due precautions, and we rather prefer an early second look to a prolonged PNL.

17.5 Technical Aspects

17.5.1 Positioning on Surgical Table

The supine positioning is employed because of the related anaesthesiological and management advantages [7], and in particular the Galdakao-modified supine Valdivia position is obtained as follows (Figs. 17.2, 17.3, and 17.4):

- The use of antidecubitus cushions nearby the costal arch and the gluteus in order to lift and expose the flank involved.
- The contralateral leg is lifted in semiflexed position.

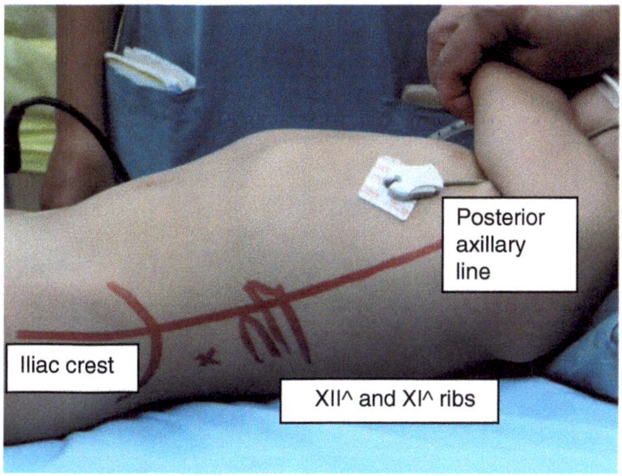

Fig. 17.2 Percutaneous puncture landmarks are the posterior axillary line, the lower margin of costal arch and the upper margin of iliac crest

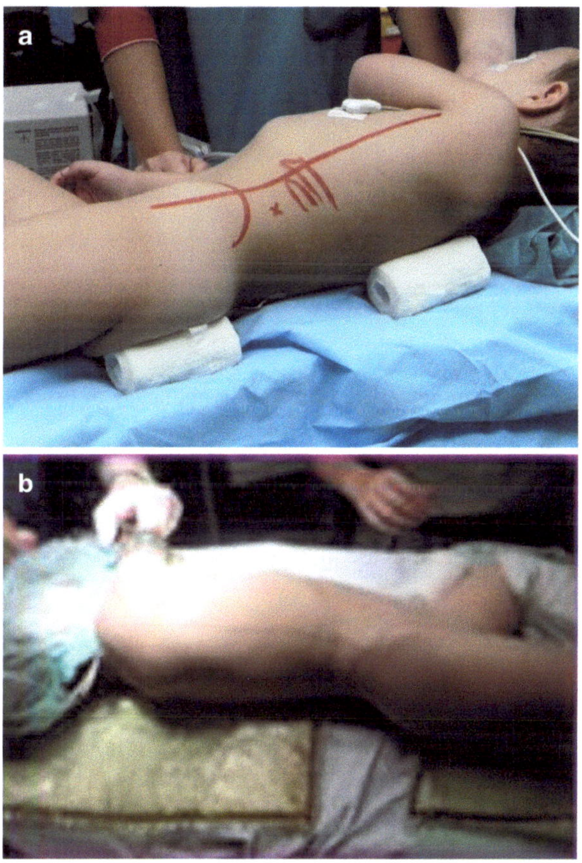

[AU3]

Fig. 17.3 Double support under the thorax and the ankle for supine position. Jelly supports can be used as well

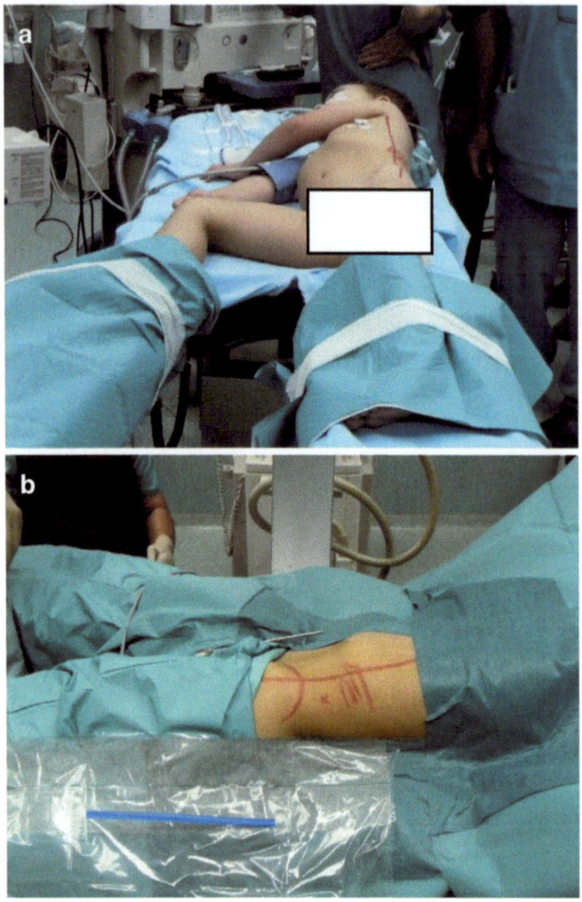

Fig. 17.4 Child in the Galdakao-modified supine Valdivia position, frontal view (**a**) and surgical percutaneous field (**b**)

- The homolateral leg is slightly abducted in order to allow the introduction of cystoscope and ureteroscope.
- The homolateral arm is adducted and laid on the chest in order to allow a further elevation of the posterior axillary line.
- The contralateral arm is abducted and fixed horizontally for venous accesses.
- Reference lines are marked on the skin.

17.5.2 Renal Access and Endovision Procedure

The puncture of the chosen renal calyx follows the same rules applied in adults (Figs. 17.5) (see also Chap. 13). It depends on the surgeon's habit and preference (X-ray and/or ultrasound guided). When possible, the puncture of the renal papilla under direct vision (Endovision procedure) allows more security of the correct (in-line) axis of the puncture with a lower hemorrhagic risk. Furthermore, it's possible to follow all phases of the tract dilation with less X-ray exposure time for the child.

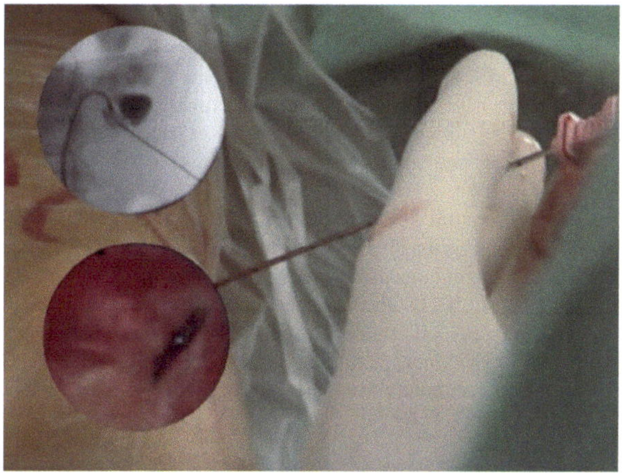

Fig. 17.5 Radiological and endoscopic view of renal puncture

17.6 Final Remarks

1. PNL in the child is a safe and effective procedure but requires particular attention and experience.
2. The paediatric kidney is not "so small" as generally thought, but the hypochondriac viscera are proportionally larger than in adults. Before renal puncture, ultrasound guidance could be useful for a general checking.
3. The use of all the armamentarium you have for an optimal renal puncture (fluoroscopy, ultrasound, Endovision technique) is fundamental to avoid hemorrhagic complications. In any case, the use of radiations should be limited to the minimum.
4. It is essential to have the availability of all the instruments required to adapt our surgery to the anatomy of the child.
5. In children <3 years old, the ureter is less compliant than after 3 years of age. Therefore, insertion of a double J stent few days before the endourological procedure should be considered.
6. The maximal duration of a percutaneous procedure in a child is 60–90 min in order to minimize complications and resorption risks; hypothermia should be minimized using warmed irrigation fluids.
7. Since paediatric urolithiasis is frequently related to urinary malformations, a thorough diagnostic evaluation and a preoperative planning with a paediatric surgeon is mandatory.

References

1. Sarica K, Horuz R (2013) In: Knoll T, Pearle MS (eds) Clinical management of urolithiasis. Springer, Berlin/Heidelberg, pp 133–154
2. Straub M, Gschwend J, Zorn C (2010) Pediatric urolithiasis: the current surgical management. Pediatr Nephrol 25:1239–1244
3. Sternberg K, Greenfield SP, Williot P, Wan J (2005) Pediatric stone disease: an evolving experience. J Urol 174:1711–1714

4. Rhee K, Palmer JS (2006) Ungated extracorporeal shock wave lithotripsy in children: an initial series. Urology 67:392–393
5. Dawaba MS, Shokeir AA, Hafez A, Shoma AM et al (2004) Percutaneous nephrolithotomy in children: early and late anatomical and functional results. J Urol 172:1078–1081
6. Ozden E, Mercimek MN, Yakapoglu YK, Ozkaya O, Sarikaya S (2011) Modified Clavien classification in percutaneous nephrolithotomy: assessment of complications in children. J Urol 185:264–268
7. Guven S, Frattini A, Onal B, Desai M et al (2013) Percutaneous nephrolithotomy in children in different age groups: data from the Clinical Research Office of the Endourological Society (CROES) percutaneous nephrolithotomy global study. BJU Int 111:148–156
8. Zargooshi J (2011) Open stone surgery in children: is it justified in the era of minimally invasive therapies? BJU Int 88:928–931
9. Bayrak O, Seckiner I, Erthrhan S, Duzgun I, Yagci F (2012) Comparative analyses of percutaneous nephrolithotomy versus open surgery in pediatric urinary stone disease. Pediatr Surg Int 28:1025–1029

Chapter 18
Technical Aspects of Percutaneous Management of Ureteral Stenosis and Upper Urinary Tract Transitional Cell Carcinomas (UUT-TCC)

Marianne Brehmer

Abstract The present chapter deals with the technical aspects of percutaneous management of ureteral stenosis and upper urinary tract (UUT) tumours, where the preoperative investigations are usefully integrated by the preliminary retrograde endoscopic assessment of ureteral and pyelocalyceal features allowed by ECIRS in the Galdakao-modified supine Valdivia position. Antegrade treatment details are also given, as well as follow-up advices, according to the current guidelines.

18.1 Investigations Before the Procedure

18.1.1 Stenosis

If the patient has a normal renal function and there is some passage of urine through the stenosis, a computed tomography (CT) scan in native and excretory phase is useful to map both localization and length of the stricture. This exam will also give some information about the renal function.

A reduced renal parenchyma means that the kidney has been obstructed for some time. However, to get a clear picture of the separated function of each kidney, the glomerular filtration rate (GFR) should be checked and a renogram with split function performed.

In case of severe stenosis with significant or complete obstruction, the renal unit requires to be urgently decompressed applying a nephrostomy tube. In such a case, a renogram should be repeated some weeks after decompression.

M. Brehmer
Department of Urology, Institution of Oncology and Pathology, Karolinska Institutet, Aarhus University Hospital, 8200 Aarhus N, Denmark
e-mail: marianne.brehmer@rm.dk, marianne.brehmer@ki.se, mail@mbrehmer.com

C.M. Scoffone et al. (eds.), *Supine Percutaneous Nephrolithotomy and ECIRS*, DOI 10.1007/978-2-8178-0459-0_18, © Springer-Verlag France 2014

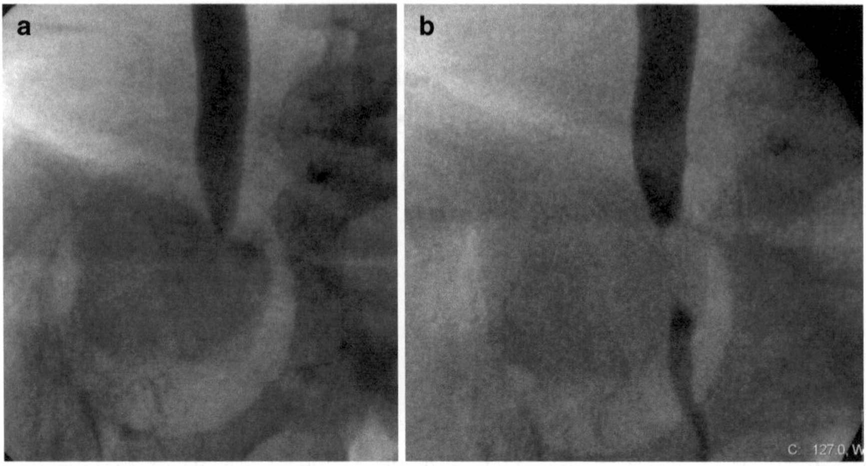

Fig. 18.1 (**a**) Contrast from antegrade approach only; (**b**) contrast added from combined antegrade and retrograde approaches helps to map the length and severity of a ureteral stenosis

A tight stenosis causing partial obstruction may seem longer than it is because of the very small amount of contrast passing. Contrast administrated only through an antegrade approach is not able to evidentiate correctly the length of the stricture. To map a stenosis precisely, an antegrade pyelography in combination with a retrograde one is the method of choice (Fig. 18.1).

Moreover, a reconstruction of a CT scan in arterial and excretory phases will reveal the presence of a vessel causing a stenosis (Fig. 18.2) or the presence of vessels located posterolaterally to a ureteral pelvic stricture, which is important to know before laser incision.

18.1.2 Transitional Cell Cancer (TCC) in the Upper Urinary Tract (UUT)

The preoperative planning of the percutaneous access route is of utmost importance. The chosen calyx should give access to the calyces needed or to the ureter. Moreover, in case of TCC of the renal pelvis, it is crucial not to puncture through the tumour. The access should always be placed through a calyx containing no tumour.

A computerized tomography with three-dimensional reconstruction (3D-CT) is a good tool for a thorough preoperative planning. Even though some tumours will not be revealed by CT (see also Chap. 5), this is probably the best radiographic method to map out the UUT-TCC. By rotating 3D images in different directions, one can get a good idea on accessibility through a punctured calyx to other calyces and to the ureter.

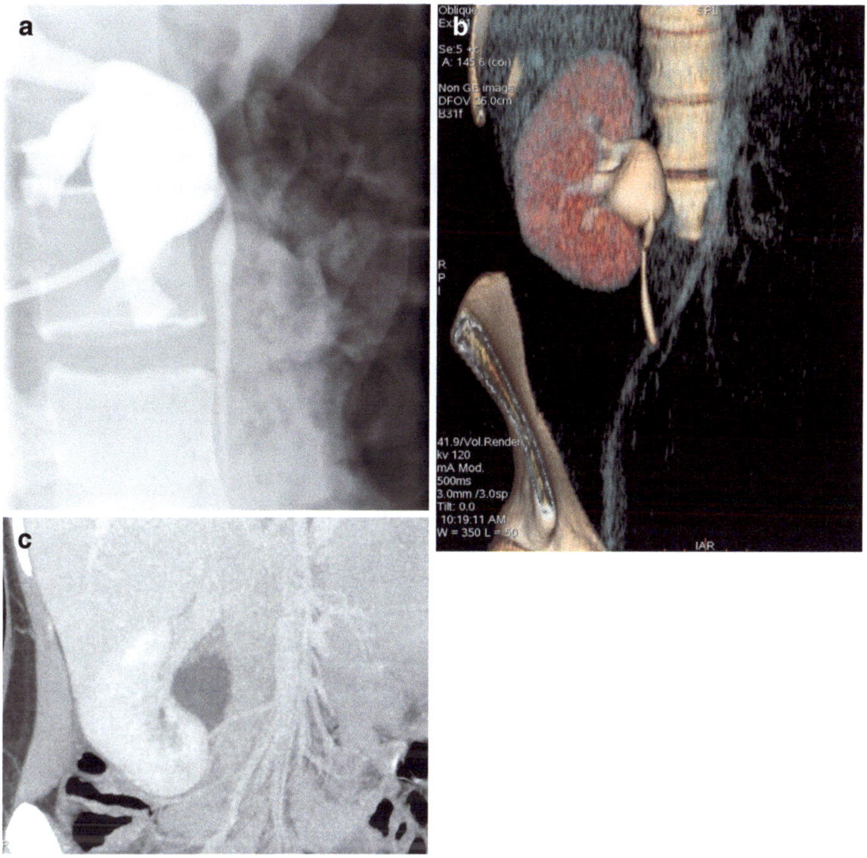

Fig. 18.2 (**a**) Antegrade pyelography showing a stenosis of the UPJ. However, the underlying cause is not clear. (**b**) 3D-CT scan, excretory phase, again illustrating UPJ obstruction. (**c**) CT artery phase visualizes a polar artery. By putting figure (**b**) and (**c**) together, it is clear that the stenosis is caused by a polar artery

18.2 Preparation and Positioning of the Patient

Ureterorenoscopy (retrograde, antegrade and combined approach) can be performed under general or spinal anaesthesia. General anaesthesia has the advantage of the patient being spared of the discomfort that may occur from manipulation and irrigation of the renal pelvis and the possibility to obtain breathing control if needed.

For the possibility of a combined antegrade and retrograde approach, the patient is placed in a supine position. One or two wedge cushions are placed under the flank so that a desired calyx can be punctured or the nephrostomy tube becomes accessible (Fig. 18.3). Placing a nephrostomy tube a few days prior to the percutaneous procedure could be an advantage because bleeding caused by the puncture will not disturb the endoscopic evaluation of renal pelvis and ureter. On the other hand,

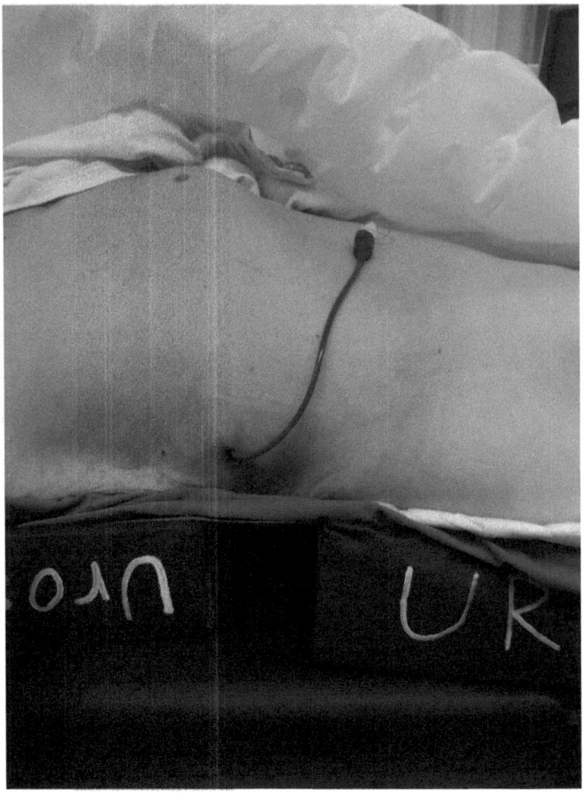

Fig. 18.3 Positioning on operating table, with wedge cushions under the flank to expose the nephrostomy tube

if the patient has a tumour, an indwelling nephrostomy tube may increase the risk of tumour cell seeding. Irrespective of the timing of the renal puncture (performed at the time of percutaneous surgery or beforehand for the placement of a nephrostomy tube), the choice of the calyx for renal access has to be planned thoroughly.

18.3 Accessing and Investigating the Renal Pelvis and Ureter

When the patient is punctured on the operating table during the percutaneous procedure, a ureteral catheter is placed whenever possible. This will allow to inject contrast and distend the renal pelvis. By using a combination of ultrasound and fluoroscopy guidance, the desired calyx can then be punctured. In case the patient has a suitable nephrostomy tube placed at the tip of a desired calyx, that access can be used.

If access to the renal pelvis is needed for the treatment of a calyceal diverticulum, a large renal pelvic tumour or a UPJ stenosis, it is advisable to dilate the access tract and to place an Amplatz sheath. If the ureter is the target, it is usually not

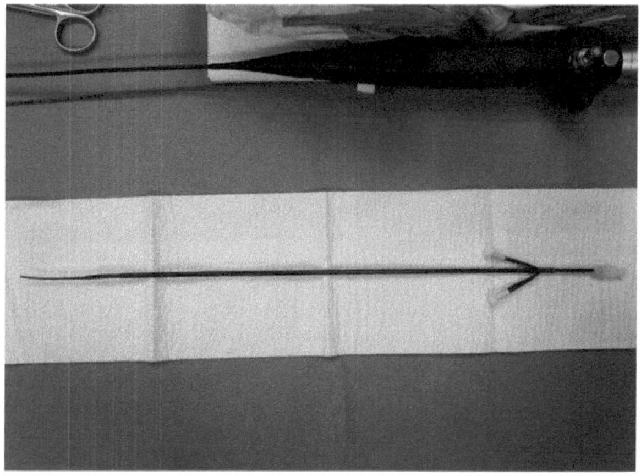

Fig. 18.4 Peel-away sheath

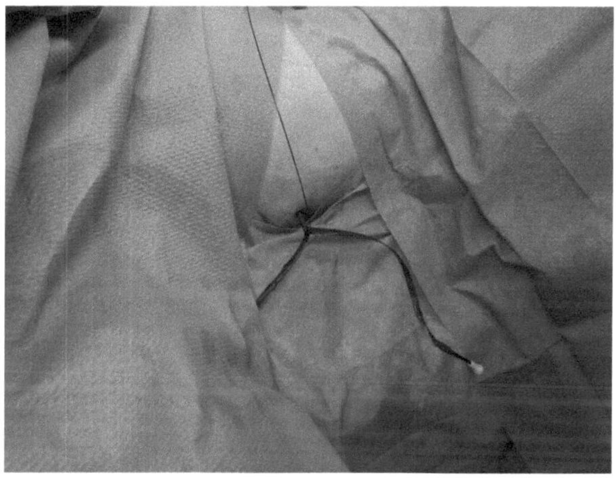

Fig. 18.5 Peel-away sheath with guidewire

needed to dilate up to 26–30. In those situations, it is handy to use a ureteral access sheath (UAS) or a peel-away sheath. A peel-away sheath has the advantage of being adjustable in length, decreasing the risk of slipping out of the body (Figs. 18.4, and 18.5) as compared to a UAS. A flexible ureteroscope can then be introduced, beside the safety guidewire, through the peel-away sheath (Fig. 18.6).

In case of a ureteral stricture or of a patient with a urinary diversion, a guidewire is placed all the way from the renal pelvis through the urethra or urine reservoir stoma, so that traction can be added through the wire (Figs. 18.7, and 18.8). An additional guidewire is placed using a dual-lumen catheter in order to have both a safety and a working guidewire (Figs. 18.9, and 18.10). A flexible ureteroscope can then be introduced antegradely or retrogradely (Fig. 18.11).

In the presence of suspicious lesions, selected cytology and biopsies are taken. Biopsies are taken out together with the instrument. If the biopsy is extracted through the scope, valuable material will be lost when the small biopsy forceps is

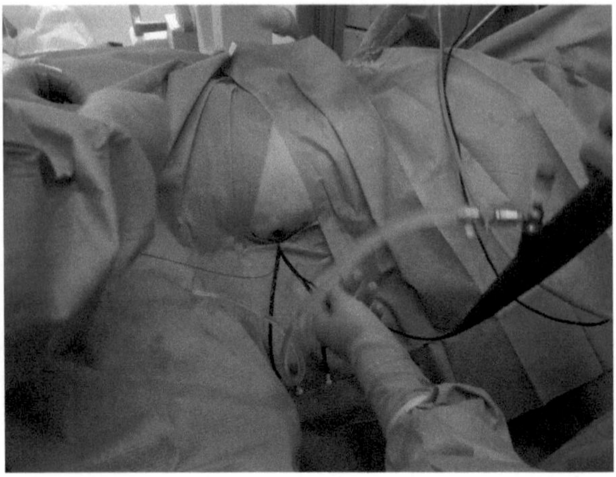

Fig. 18.6 Flexible ureteroscope introduced through a peel-away sheath

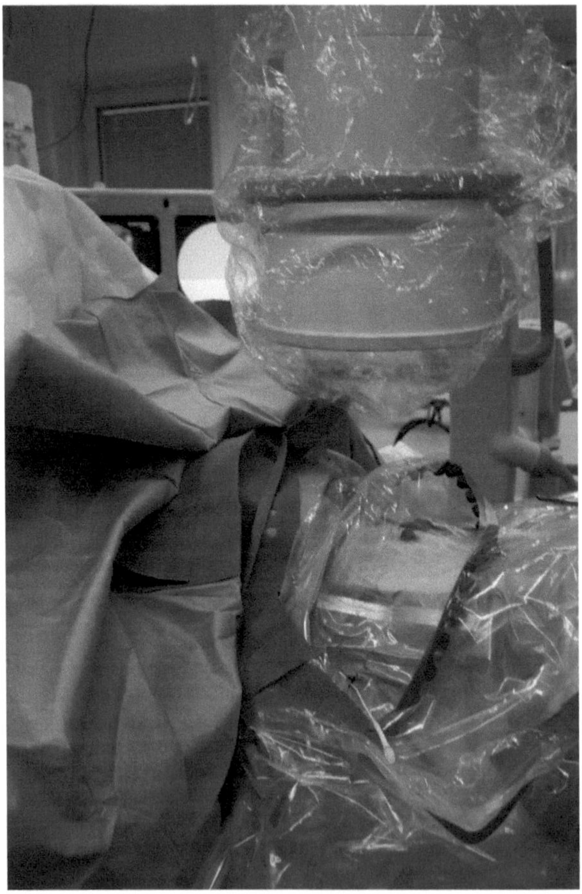

Fig. 18.7 Positioning of urine-deviated patient with nephrostomy tube

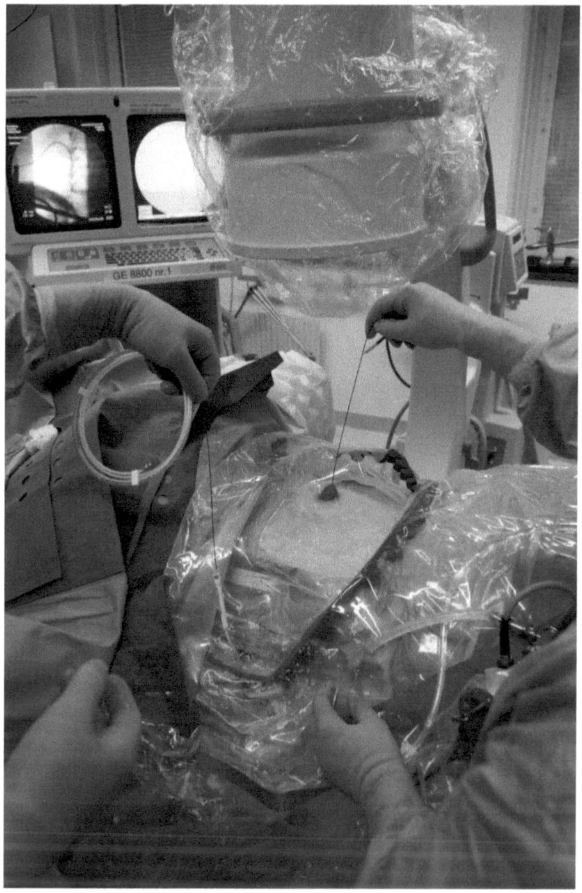

Fig. 18.8 Guidewire entered through a nephrostomy tube, grabbed with forceps and brought out through the stoma

dragged through the tight working channel in the instrument (Fig. 18.12). The biopsy, usually very small, is placed in a tube containing saline and treated as cytology material [1]. Larger biopsies can be obtained using the BIGopsy® forceps (Cook Medical); however, it needs to be backloaded into the ureteroscope and consequently requires a ureteral access sheath to avoid damage to the ureter.

18.4 Treatment

18.4.1 Stenosis

Access to a calyceal diverticulum can be obtained using a small balloon (3 Ch) (Fig. 18.13) or performing a holmium:YAG laser incision. Before cutting with the laser, it is advisable to insert a safety guidewire through the opening into the

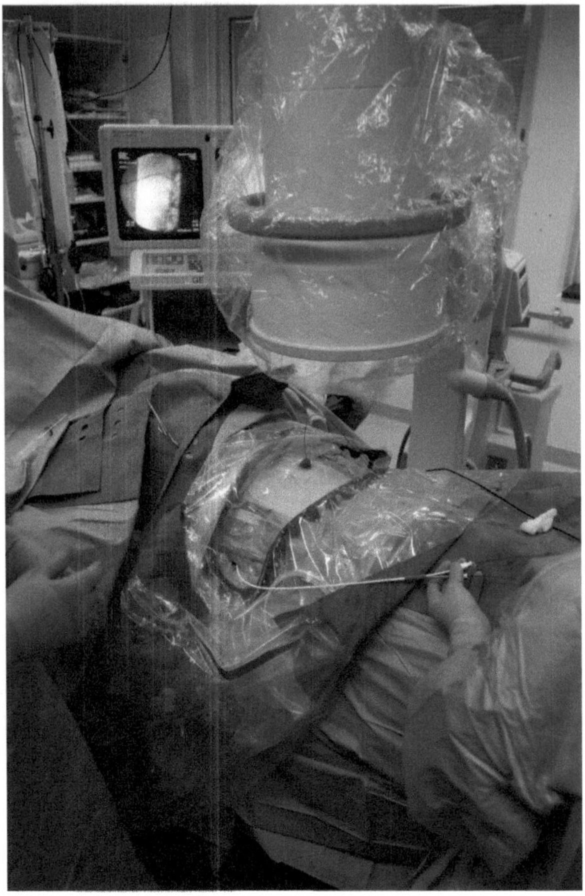

Fig. 18.9 Double-lumen catheter is used to place a second safety guidewire

diverticulum. If no safety guidewire is placed, there is the risk to lose the direction of the incision. However, sometimes the lumen is so small that there is no room for anything else but the laser fibre.

A stenosis of the ureteropelvic junction (UPJ) is incised in a posterolateral direction to avoid cutting into the lower renal pole and to minimize the risk of cutting through any vessel.

Distal strictures are often easier to pass through an antegrade approach than a retrograde one. Sometimes a stenotic orifice is not even possible to identify at cystoscopy but can be passed from above (Fig. 18.14).

A guidewire is passed through the stricture to the bladder or a urinary conduit via antegrade approach. By using a cystoscope, the guidewire is grabbed by biopsy forceps and taken out through the urethra or the stoma (Fig. 18.8). A double-lumen catheter is inserted over the guidewire so that an additional safety guidewire can be placed (Fig. 18.9). With some traction on the working guidewire, a dilation balloon is then placed using an antegrade or a retrograde approach.

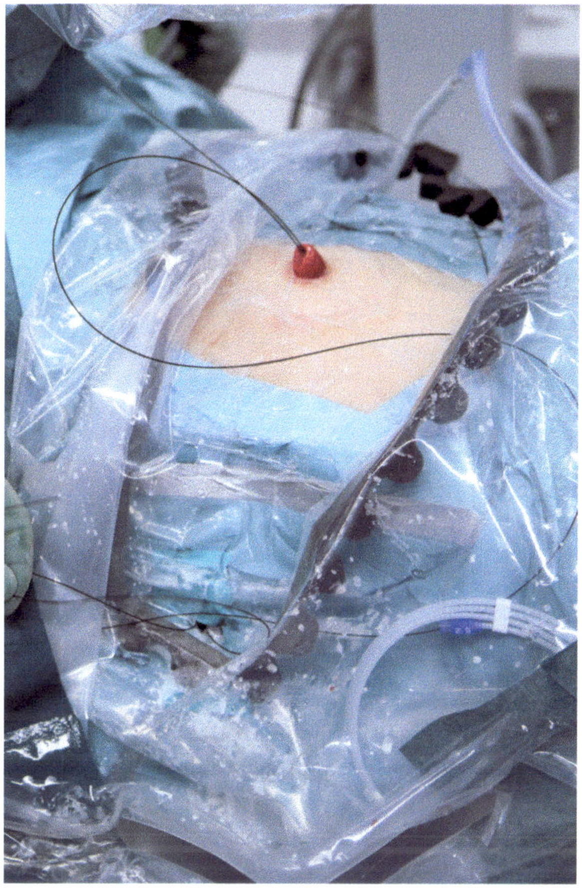

Fig. 18.10 Two guidewires are in place

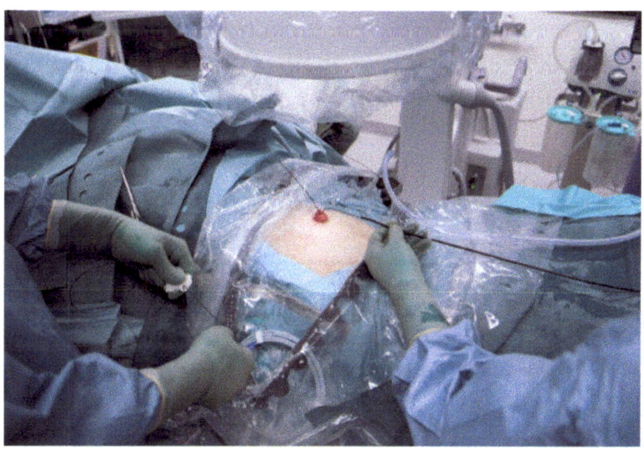

Fig. 18.11 A flexible ureteroscope can be introduced with a retrograde approach over a guidewire that is placed through the nephrostomy channel. Traction is added on the guidewire, facilitating the introduction

Fig. 18.12 A biopsy is taken from a renal pelvic tumour

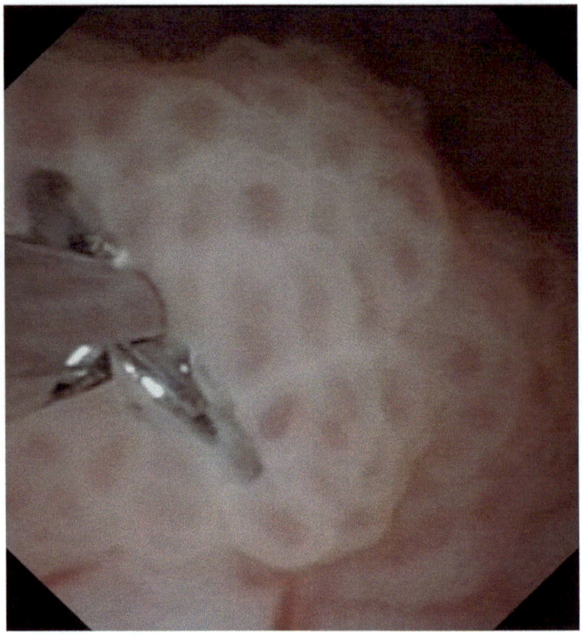

In the ureter, a 15 Ch dilation balloon is usually enough. After dilation, an antegrade pyelography is performed, and the contrast should then pass easily reaching the bladder. Strictures in the ureter or of the ureteral orifice can also be incised by using holmium:YAG laser.

After dilating the stenosis, a double-pigtail stent is placed over the guidewire. Most urologists would leave a stent for 6–8 weeks; however, there is no evidence for this indication. When a stent is in place, the nephrostomy tube may be closed. However, it is advisable to keep the nephrostomy tube in place until the stent is removed. By doing so, the nephrostomy tube will act as a safety route if the stent does not drain sufficiently, and it can also be used for antegrade pyelography when the stent is removed. If contrast does not pass through the ureter to the bladder sufficiently, a second dilation can be performed. However, if the passage is not satisfactory after two procedures, additional dilations are usually not worthwhile.

Fig. 18.13 Balloon dilation of a calyceal diverticulum. (**a**) Opening of a calyceal diverticulum containing a stone. (**b**) Calyceal diverticulum containing a stone, intraoperative fluoroscopic view. (**c**) Dilation balloon introduced through the small opening of the calyceal diverticulum. (**d**) Balloon dilation. (**e**) Ureteroscopic laser treatment of stones after dilation within the calyceal diverticulum

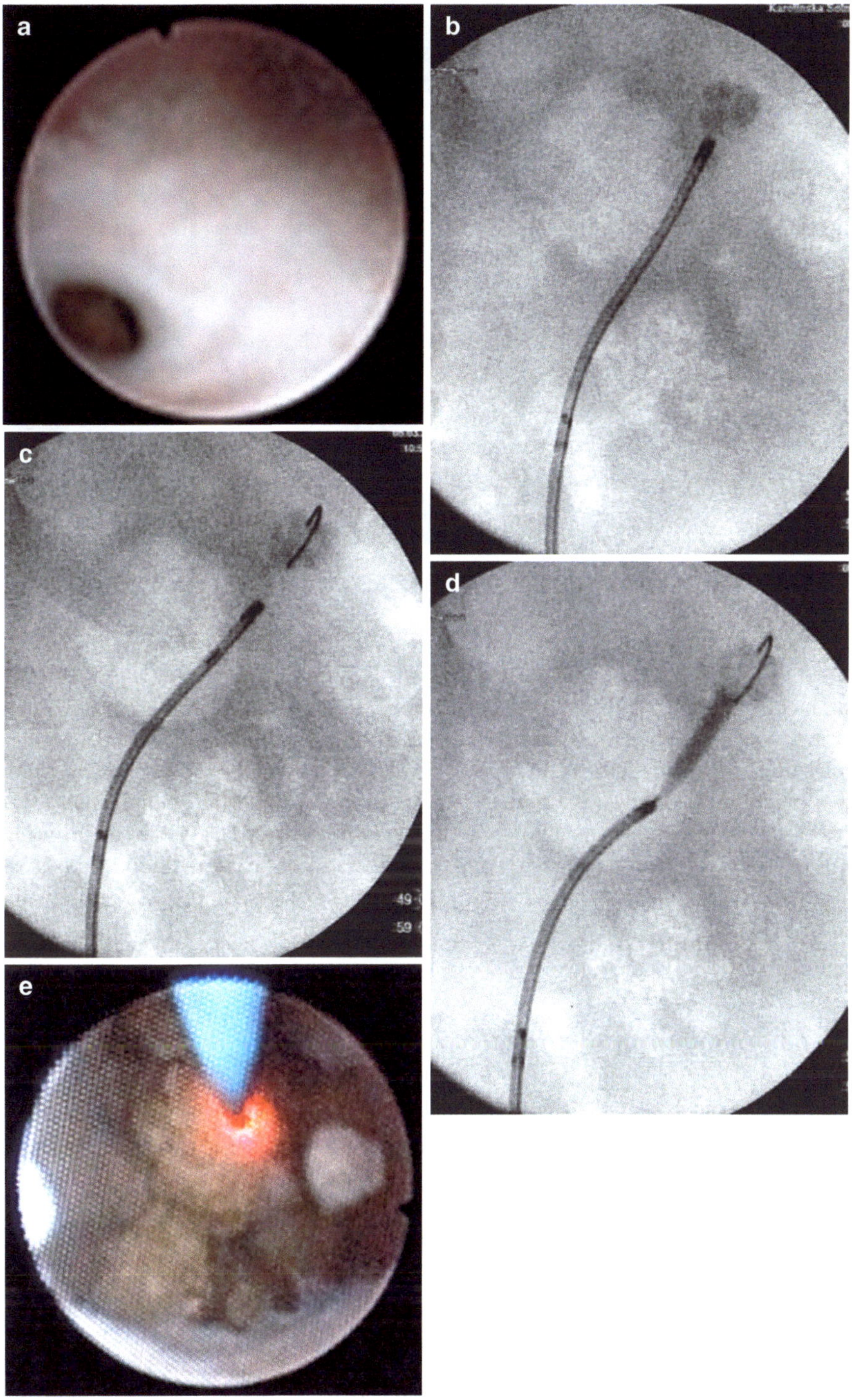
a
b
c
d
e

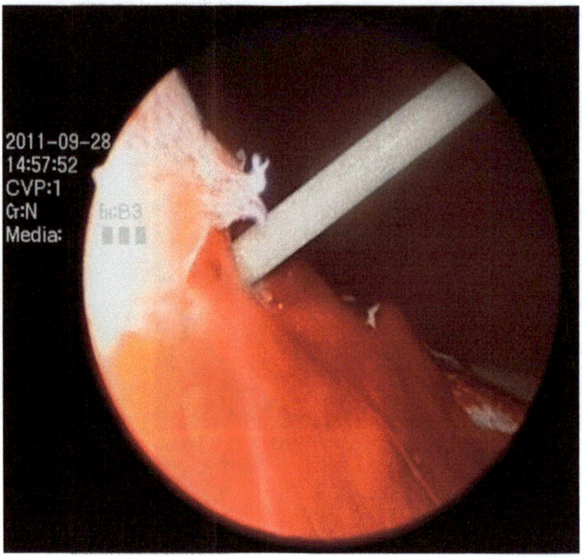

Fig. 18.14 Guidewire through a tight orifice, via antegrade approach

18.4.2 Follow-Up

If antegrade pyelography shows a satisfactory passage of the contrast through the ureter, a radiographic follow-up is performed at 3–6 months. There are no clear rules on how long patients need to be followed. In cases of less severe stenosis and two functioning kidneys, the patient may be followed up at 3–6 months and then released if the result is satisfactory. In other patients with higher risk of recurrence, follow-up for a longer period is recommended. To avoid heavy radiation exposure, an alternative is to follow the patient yearly by means of an isotopic scintigram with forced diuresis.

18.4.3 Tumour in the Renal Pelvis or Ureter

If TCC is confirmed (Fig. 18.15) and organ-sparing treatment is desired, the combination of holmium (Ho):YAG and neodymium (Nd):YAG laser is recommendable for treatment (Fig. 18.16). Nd:YAG is used for coagulation, whereas Ho:YAG is used for ablation. Especially in large tumours, this is very useful. In the UUT, the setting of the Nd:YAG laser may be 30 W and 3 s. For ablative effect of the Ho:YAG laser, one can start using a 6 Hz frequency and then increase energy until the ablative effect is satisfactory. The Nd:YAG and the Ho:YAG lasers are alternated throughout the procedure to minimize the bleeding.

During ablation, the intrarenal pressure should be kept as low as possible to minimize the risk of tumour cell seeding. If the procedure is performed retrogradely,

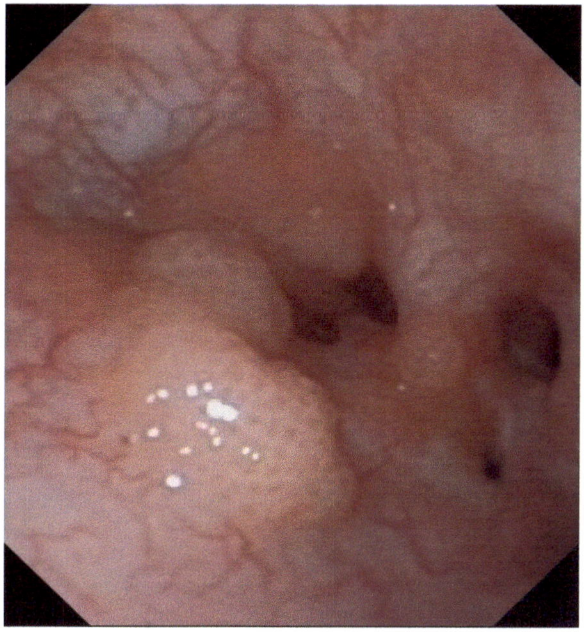

Fig. 18.15 Tumour in the renal pelvis

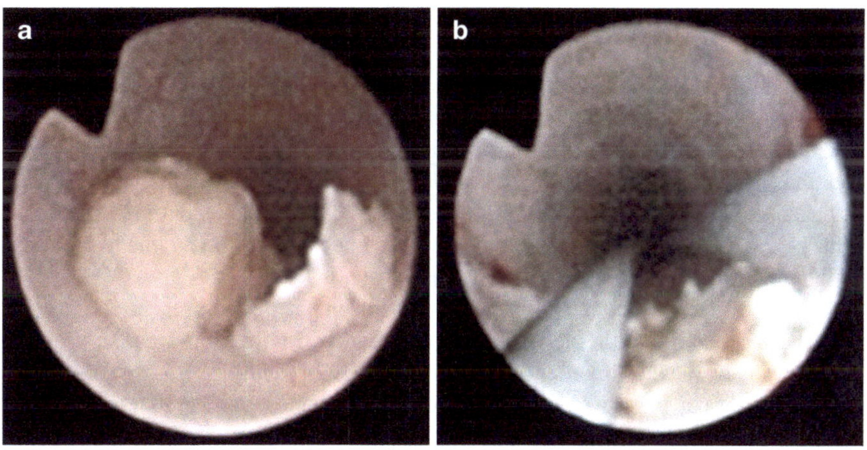

Fig. 18.16 (**a**) Tumour in the ureter. (**b**) Tumour in the ureter after laser ablation

a small catheter (8 Ch with 3 ml in the balloon) in the bladder can usually be put alongside the ureteroscope or a UAS (Fig. 18.17). A UAS may be used if there is a large tumour in the renal pelvis that will take some time to ablate. The use of a UAS will most probably decrease the renal pressure during a long procedure [2, 3]. However, cautiousness should be used not to dilate with force, again to minimize the risk of tumour cell seeding.

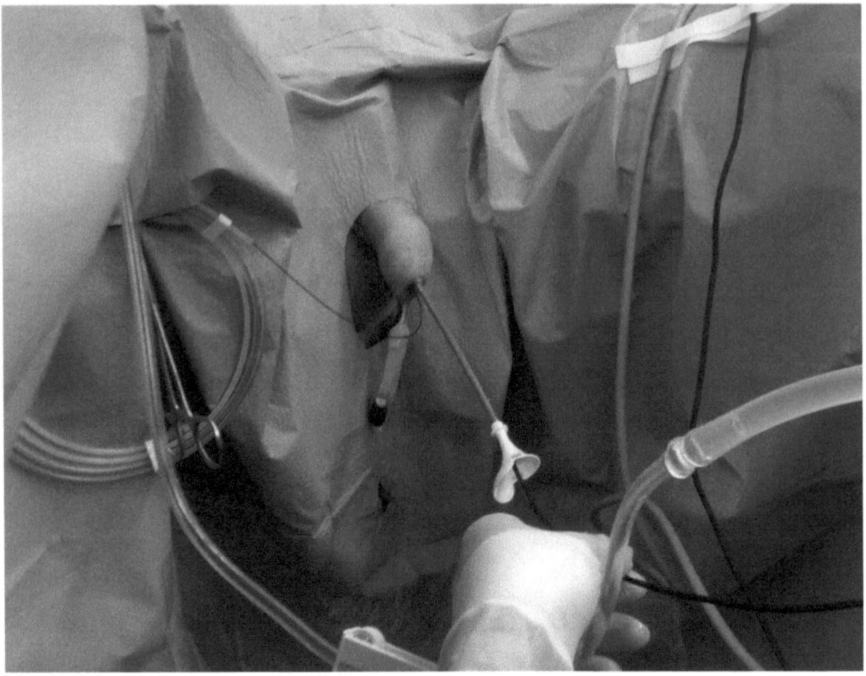

Fig. 18.17 Bladder drainage, using an 8 catheter

If the tumour is large (>15 mm), the treatment may need to be performed in more than one session. A second treatment is then performed after 6 weeks since that will give necrotic tissue the time to pass, which will facilitate the second look. If a JJ stent has been placed after the first procedure, to facilitate passage of necrotic tissue or because a ureteral access sheath has been used, it is advisable to remove the stent after 3–4 weeks. Otherwise, oedema caused by the stent will make the assessment of the mucosa at the second treatment more difficult.

If biopsies have been taken or treatment has been performed in the ureter, a stent must be placed so that the nephrostomy tube can be removed as soon as possible postoperatively, always in order to minimize the risk of tumour seeding in the access tract. After biopsy or laser treatment in the ureter, a stent is left for 10 days or more, depending upon the extent of the laser manipulation.

18.4.4 Follow-Up

It is not clear how often and for how long time patients who have undergone organ-sparing treatment for TCC in the UUT need to be followed. It is clear that radiographic methods are not adequate to detect small recurrences. Therefore, endoscopic follow-up is necessary. Ureteropyeloscopy every 3 months during the first year, every 6 months for the following 1–2 years (depending of the grade of the tumour) and then yearly for at least 5 years. When yearly ureteropyeloscopies are performed, a cystoscopy including urine cytology should be carried out every 6 months.

References

1. Tawfiek E, Bibbo M, Bagley DH (1997) Ureteroscopic biopsy: technique and specimen preparation. Urology 50:117–119
2. Auge BK, Pietrow PK, Lallas CD et al (2004) Ureteral access sheath provides protection against elevated renal pressures during routine flexible ureteroscopic stone manipulation. J Endourol 18:33–36
3. Ng YH, Somani BK, Dennison A et al (2010) Irrigant flow and intrarenal pressure during flexible ureteroscopy: the effect of different access sheaths, working channel instruments, and hydrostatic pressure. J Endourol 24:1915–1920

Chapter 19
The Scrub Nurse's Point of View on ECIRS (Endoscopic Combined IntraRcnal Surgery)

Cristian Demelas, Gianni De Masi, Debora Crepaldi, Elena Bertinaria, Michele Trimboli, Angela Palamuso, Tiziana Girodo, and Debora Coda Zabetta

Abstract ECIRS (Endoscopic Combined IntraRenal Surgery) is an endourologic procedure characterized by a certain degree of complexity under many respects, and the first impression is that the task of the scrub nurse is a very hard one. Since each surgical step is strongly justified and standardized, once understood, their sequence is highly reproducible and easy to teach/easy to learn, so that in the end ECIRS becomes also easy to assist from the point of view of the nursing staff, in spite of the fact that it remains a demanding procedure. All the nursing team is required to have a wide knowledge of all the instruments, devices, and accessories, patient positioning, operating room organization, and ECIRS steps, as well as of a correct post- and preoperative care during the sterilization phase. A phase of "on-the-field" formation is required, and each member of the staff should have defined and well-distributed tasks.

19.1 The Mental Attitude of the Nurse Staff Towards ECIRS

19.1.1 Sharing Understanding and Knowledge of ECIRS Surgical Steps

ECIRS is an endourologic procedure for the treatment of large and/or complex uroli thiasis characterized by a certain degree of complexity under many respects. In fact,

C. Demelas (✉) • G. De Masi
Department of Urology, San Luigi Hospital, University of Torino, Regione Gonzole, 10, 10043 Orbassano (Torino), Italy
e-mail: cristiandemelas@gmail.com; gianni.demasi@gmail.com

D. Crepaldi • E. Bertinaria • M. Trimboli • A. Palamuso • T. Girodo • D. Coda Zabetta
Cottolengo Hospital, Via Cottolengo 9, 10152 Torino, Italy
e-mail: debora.crepaldi@icloud.com; eleninab82@gmail.com; michele.trimboli@yahoo.it; angela.palamuso@virgilio.it; tizialegio@gmail.com; debora.codazabetta@ospedalecottolengo.it

C.M. Scoffone et al. (eds.), *Supine Percutaneous Nephrolithotomy and ECIRS*, DOI 10.1007/978-2-8178-0459-0_19, © Springer-Verlag France 2014 the urologists perform a sequence of surgical steps which may appear very complicated at a first glance, and the first additional impression is that the task of the scrub nurse is a very hard one. Each surgical step is strongly justified and standardized, thus, once comprehended, their sequence becomes highly reproducible and easy to teach/easy to learn. In the end, once the knowledge of ECIRS procedure has been shared and understood, the procedure suddenly becomes rather easy to assist from the point of view of the nursing staff, in spite of the fact that it remains a demanding procedure.

19.1.2 Displaying a Synergic and Versatile Attitude in the Operating Room

From this point of view, the interplay between urologists performing ECIRS and scrub nurse/nurses present in the operating room (OR) is fundamental. Intraoperative synergy and versatility are the keywords for this procedure, which cannot give birth to a successful clinical outcome in the absence of a careful and interactive cooperation among all the members of the team participating to ECIRS.

In particular, definite tasks have to be fulfilled by a prepared scrub nurse during the procedure [1]:

- To know perfectly all the surgical steps of ECIRS, as we said before.
- To know the functioning of all instruments, accessories, and devices, their sequence of use, and their fundamental or optional roles.
- To be able to control and correctly assist the various steps of ECIRS, actively proposing adequate solutions to aid the surgeon.
- To know how to manage during unforeseen events or complications.

This kind of contribution can reduce the risk of complications, shorten the operating times, and improve the quality of the work and the clinical results, making the difference between a common PNL and an optimal PNL.

Other relevant synergies are those among urologists, scrub nurse, the radiology technician, anesthesiologist, and supporting OR nurse team.

19.1.3 Learning Pre-, Intra-, and Postoperative Preparation and Management of All the Endourologic Armamentarium

Additionally, a wide knowledge of all the instruments, devices, and accessories is required not only to the surgeon but also to the nurses, as well as a correct post- and preoperative care during the sterilization phase. Before starting ECIRS, everything must be ready to use, sterile, and perfectly functioning, according to the internal checklists.

All our team (scrub nurses and OR nurses) has undergone a phase of "on-the-field" formation, a number of ECIRS (at least 15) have been needed to complete the training, and subsequently some tools have been produced (as the list of all instruments required for antegrade and retrograde endoscopy or sterilization protocols for flexible endoscopes).

Each member of the staff behaves according to previously defined and well-distributed tasks, without standing in the way of each other. Setup of frequency and energy of the laser (Fig. 19.1a) and regulation of the LithoClast Master (Fig. 19.1b); switch between the ready and pause status; functioning of the C-arm; memorization of the fluoroscopic and ultrasound images; setup of the video system in terms of white balance, brightness, contrast, zoom, and double focus; and management of the AIDA Storz system with the possibility of storing video and images are some of the tasks to share among each other, according to organizational and management internal protocols.

19.2 Operating Room Preparation

Care should be taken to prepare the operating room according to the local requirements. For instance, our present OR being a rectangle, the surgical bed has to be put oblique towards the right or the left in order to create enough space for all the devices. Usually, we prepare the floor with adequate absorbing coverings, to afford possible fluid spilling during the procedure. The operating bed must be adaptable for the lithotomic position, radiotransparent, and movable to obtain enough space underneath for the C-arm (Fig. 19.2).

The OR, after standard cleaning, has to be filled with all the devices ready for use: anaesthesiologist's respirator, ultrasound, fluoroscopy screen and C-arm, laser and LithoClast Master with the related pedals, video tower with two monitors (or a single one with the possibility of splitting the two images from antegrade and retrograde endoscopy) and two video cameras, chair with wheels for the surgeon, heating/irrigation devices, 50 liters fluid aspirator, and operating trays (Fig. 19.3).

Everything must have been preliminarily checked for efficient functioning. The disposition of each element we mentioned is not casual but arranged according to standardized schemes, different for the right and the left side (see Chap. 11). One of the most important things is that the surgeons must always be able to look at the monitor and at the fluoroscopy screen at the same time without problems.

Before the patient enters the OR, also the three sterile operating trays must be almost ready, with all the instruments and accessories sterile and ready to be opened within the room on a dedicated table. Also lead aprons and collars with the related dosimeters must be readily worn by all the personnel in the OR, to prevent radiation exposure (Fig. 19.4) [2, 3].

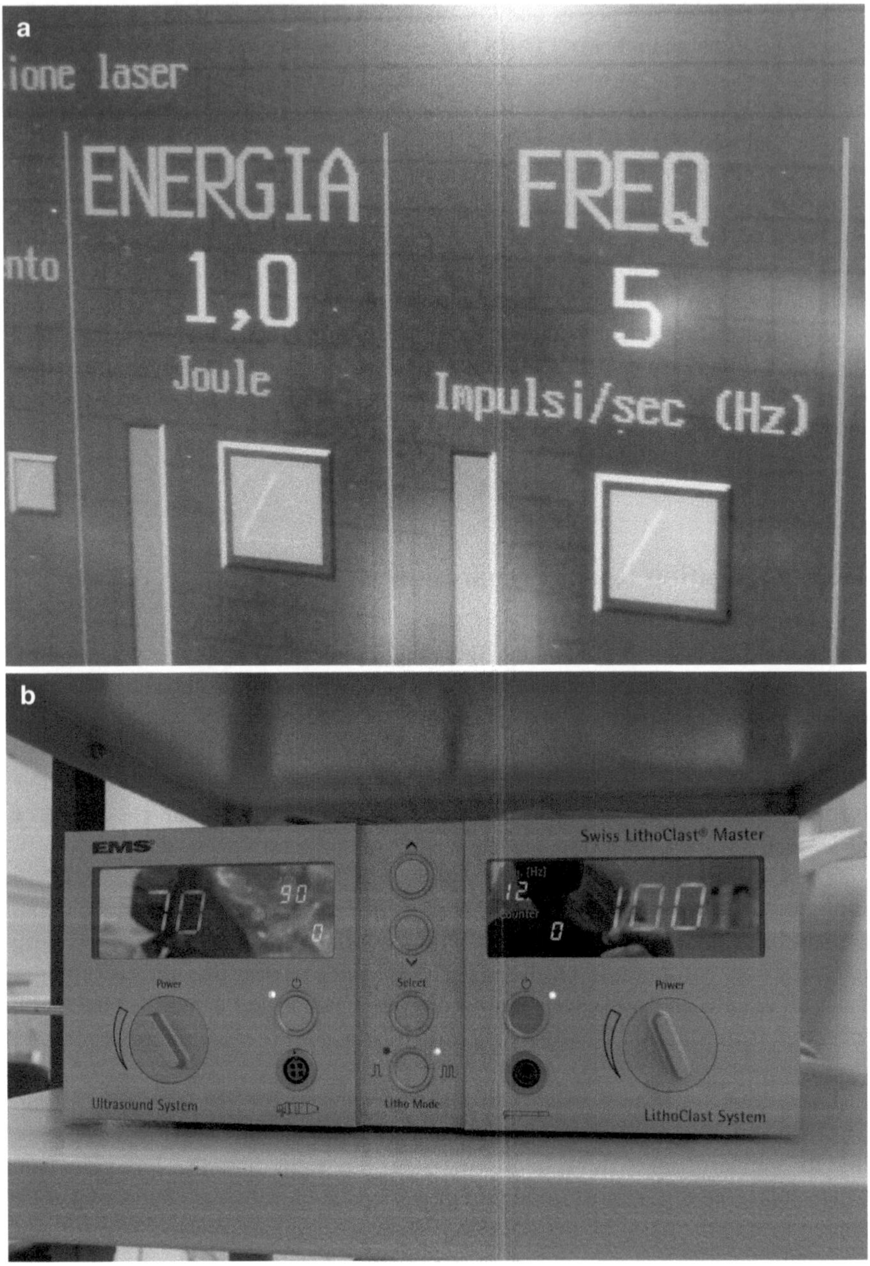

Fig. 19.1 Setup of laser frequency and energy (**a**) and of the combined ballistic/ultrasound lithotripsy device (**b**)

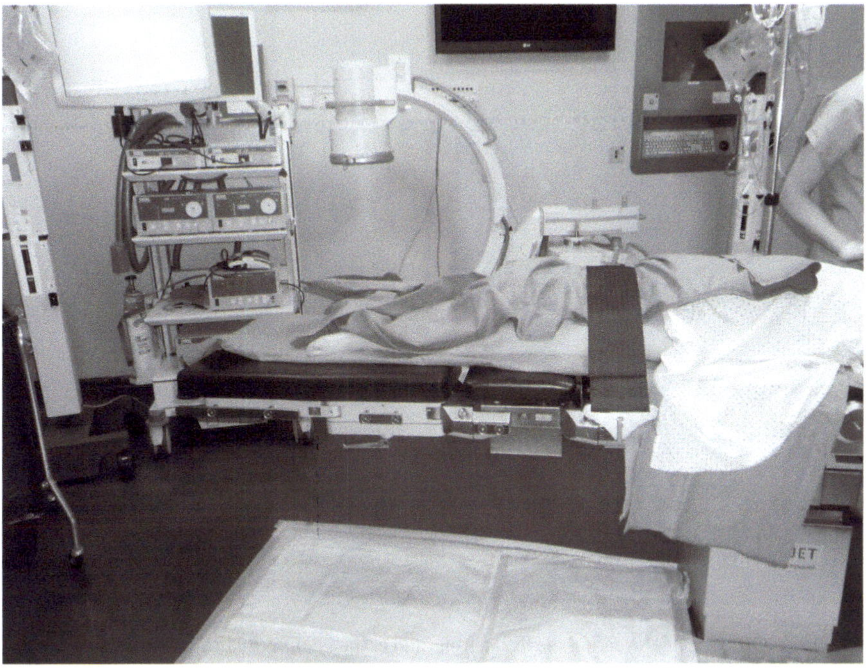

Fig. 19.2 Floor absorbent covering and oblique surgical bed, translated to create the space for the C-arm

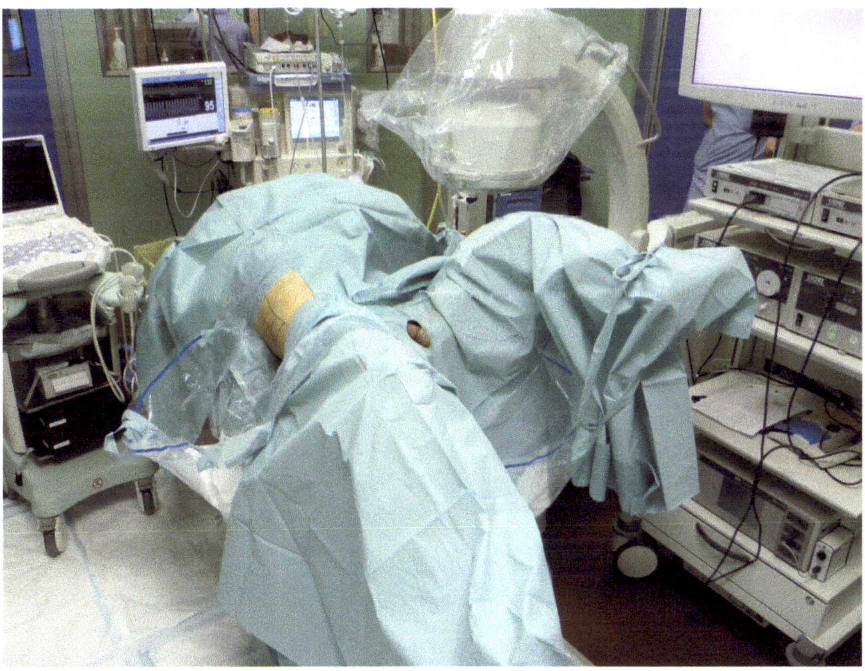

Fig. 19.3 Overview of the full OR ready to start ECIRS

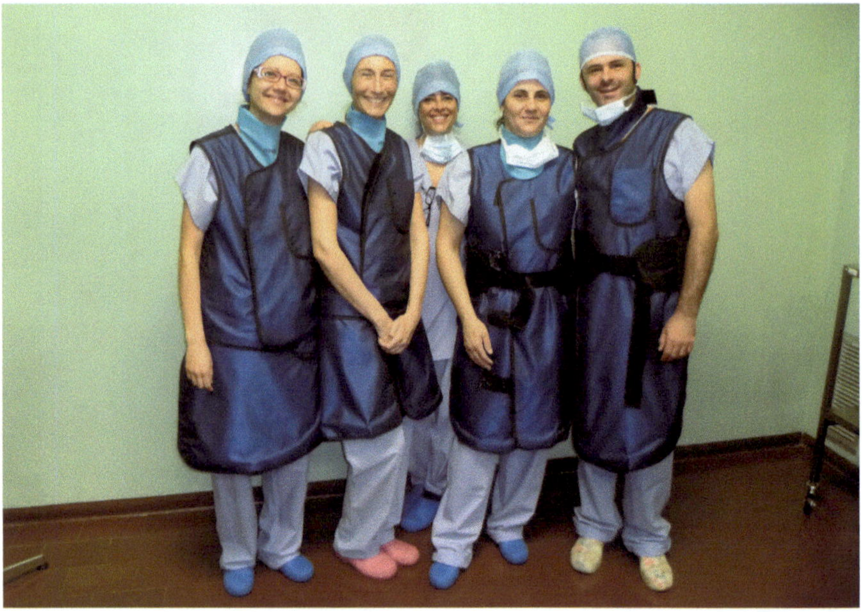

Fig. 19.4 OR personnel wearing the lead aprons and collars before ECIRS

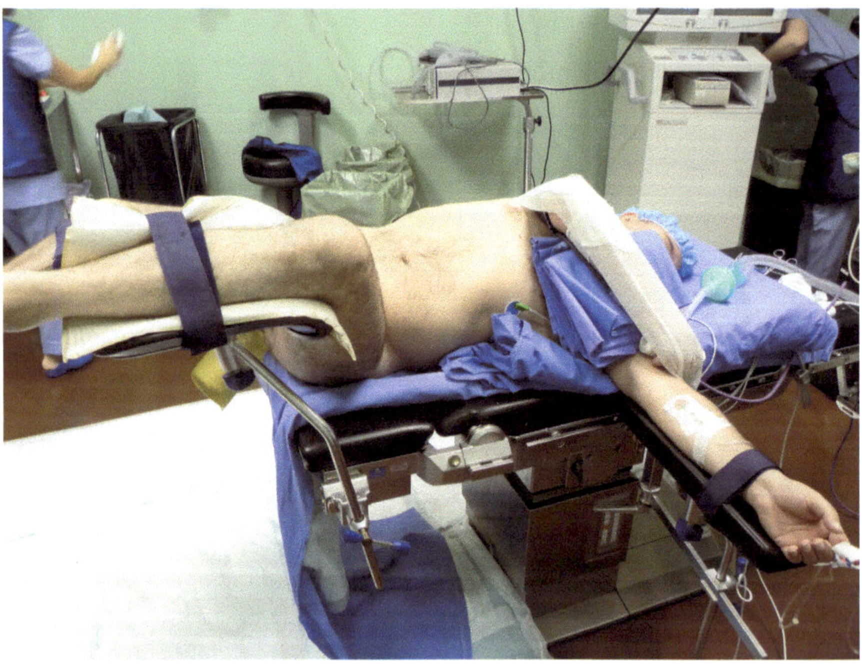

Fig. 19.5 Patient in the final Galdakao-modified supine Valdivia position

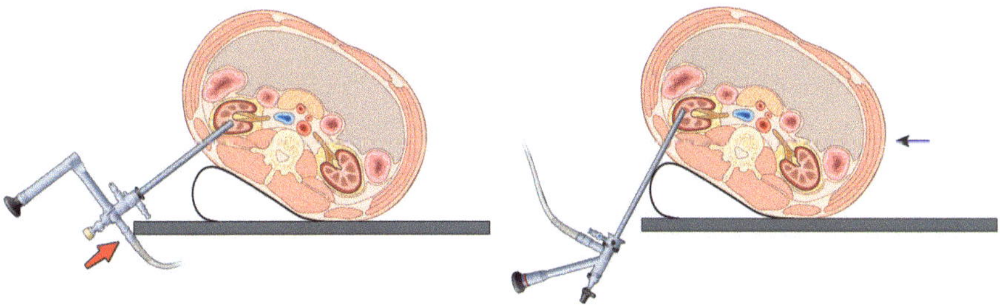

Fig. 19.6 There has to be enough space for nephroscopic manipulation under the area of the percutaneous access, without being hindered by the border of the surgical table (arrow = direction in which the patient has to be moved) (© Carole Fumat)

19.3 Patient Positioning

Patient positioning is a task implying serious responsibilities, thus to be shared among nursing staff, surgeon, and anaesthesiologist, since if incorrect, it may cause a variety of lesions, sometimes transient but sometimes irreversible.

The Galdakao-modified supine Valdivia positioning of the patient [4] is less tiring than the alternative traditional position, requiring to turn the anaesthetized patient from the dorsal lithotomic initial position to the prone one. Adequate paddings should be placed, and the patient should be correctly fixed in the final position, with self-adhesive bandages such as peha-haft (Fig. 19.5). Care to avoid excessive abduction of the limbs or tracheal tube/vascular accesses displacement should be taken while moving the patient.

Also ECIRS requirements have to be kept in mind, for instance, the contralateral leg should not hinder retrograde access with the semirigid ureteroscope, or enough space should be left under the flank for nephroscopic manipulation (Fig. 19.6).

19.4 Sterile Draping

After skin disinfection of both antegrade (Fig. 19.7a) and retrograde surgical fields (Fig. 19.7b), sterile drapings can be applied for ECIRS, consisting in one original endourologic draping for TURB/TURP with the bags for draining fluids and another one arranged for the percutaneous zone according to a personal solution (Fig. 19.3), trying to avoid irrigation liquid spilling on the floor or on the surgeon during the whole procedure. We established a sort of sequence in the application of all the sterile drapings (Fig. 19.8), starting from the legs, going on with the thorax, and finishing with the abdomen, sealing all the field with adhesive stripes.

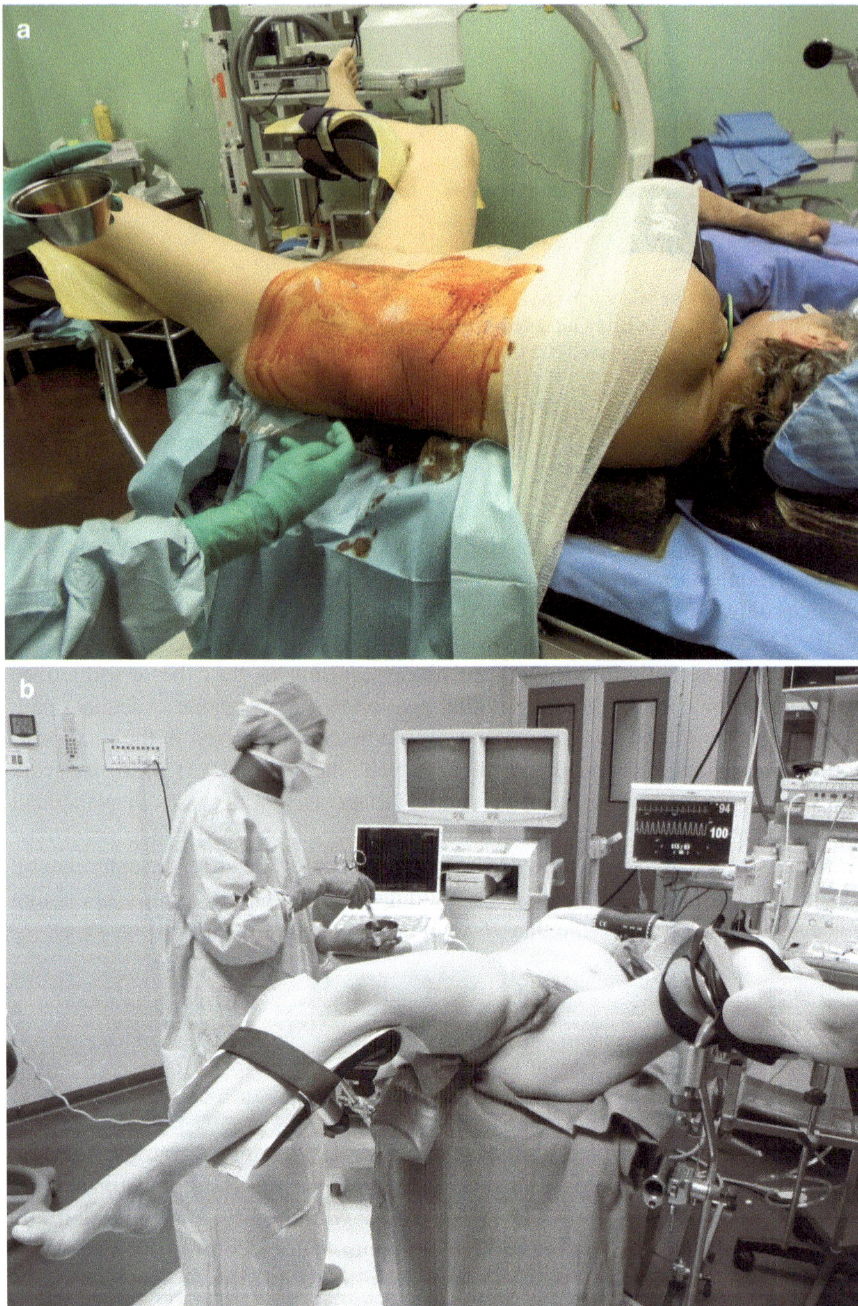

Fig. 19.7 Skin disinfection of both antegrade (**a**) and retrograde (**b**) surgical fields

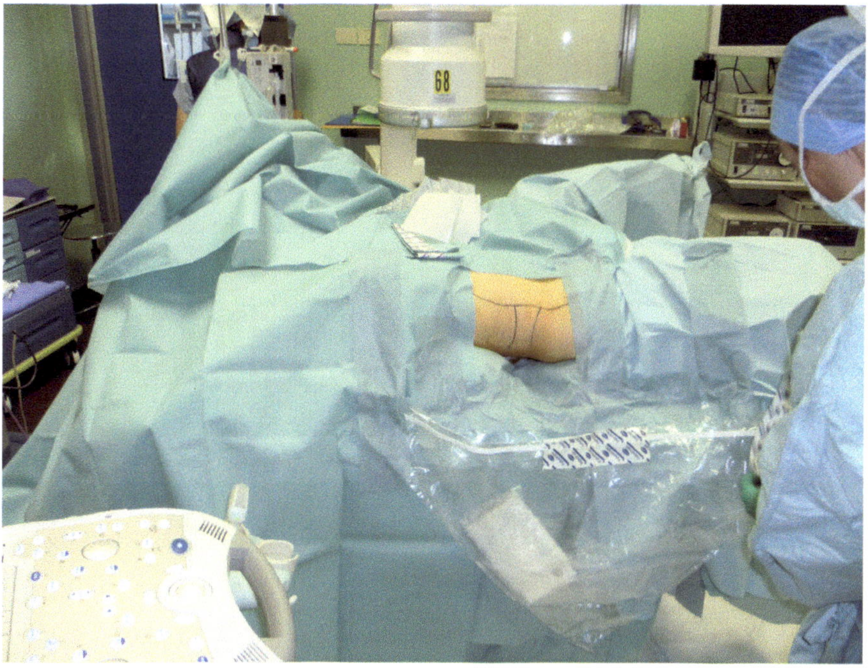

Fig. 19.8 Final sterile draping of the patient, first the legs, then the thorax, and finally the abdomen, sealed on every side

19.5 Preparation of the Surgical Tables

1. One surgical sterile tray is for all the surgical drapings and the sterile gowns and gloves. Sterile coverings are prepared also for the ultrasound probe, the head of the C-arm, and the surgeon's chair with wheels (Fig. 19.9).
2. Another surgical sterile tray is for the retrograde access, carrying semirigid 6–7.5 Ch and flexible ureteroscopes, the digital flexible ureteroscope being always ready although still sealed; cystoscope with 30° optics and forceps for stent removal; optic cable; guidewires; 20 cc syringes (one empty, one with saline, one with contrast); lubricant; ureteral access sheath when required; ureteral catheter/stent; urethral catheter; water cable for heated irrigation; and laser fibers (Fig. 19.10).
3. Another surgical sterile tray is for the percutaneous procedure, carrying rigid and flexible nephroscopes, the digital one being always at disposal although still sealed; probes of LithoClast Master; optic cable; water cable for heated irrigation; three cups (one empty, one with saline, and one with contrast); 20 cc syringes; lubricant; 18G Chiba needle; Alken dilators; Amplatz dilators; balloon dilators; 0.038″ hydrophilic guidewire; extraction basket like N-Perc; and pyelostomy (Fig. 19.11).

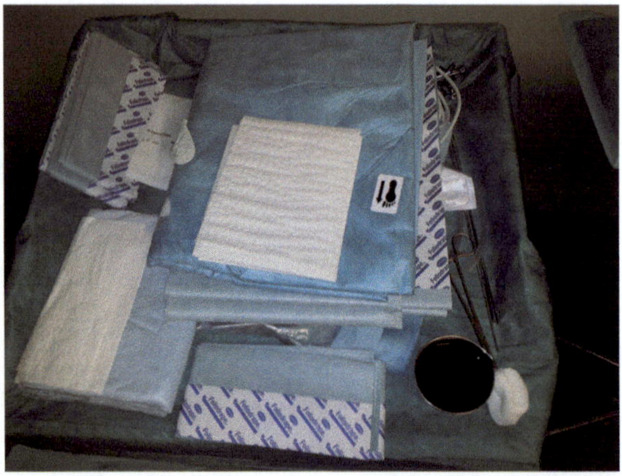

Fig. 19.9 Table for sterile drapings

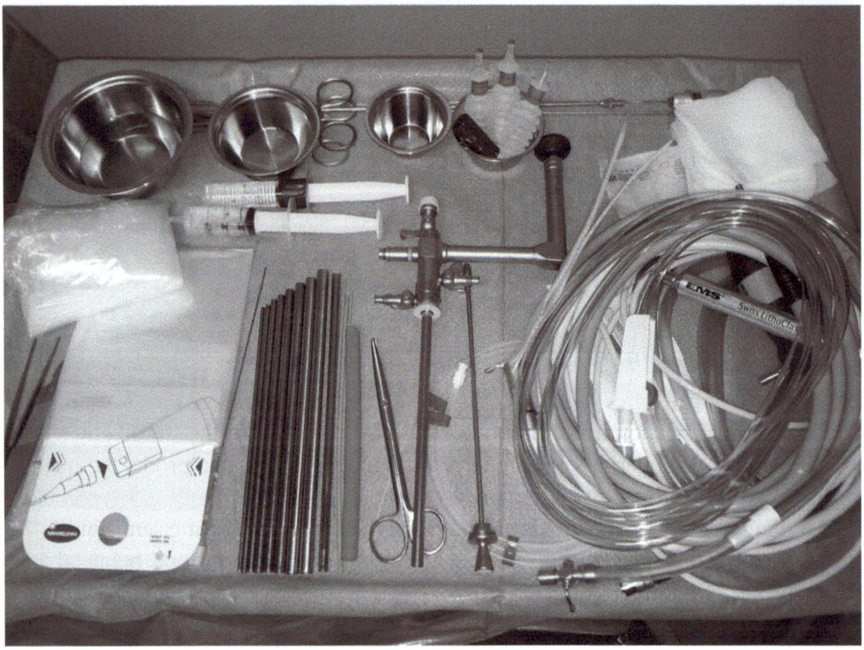

Fig. 19.10 Table for antegrade access

The correct preparation of the surgical trays requires the preliminary briefing on the clinical case with the surgeon (adult patient or child, previous surgeries meaning more likely Alken than balloon for tract dilation, morbidly obese patient needing the extra long 25 cm nephroscope, etc.) in order to foresee the intraoperative needs and to plan together the strategy in terms of dilation system and size of the access.

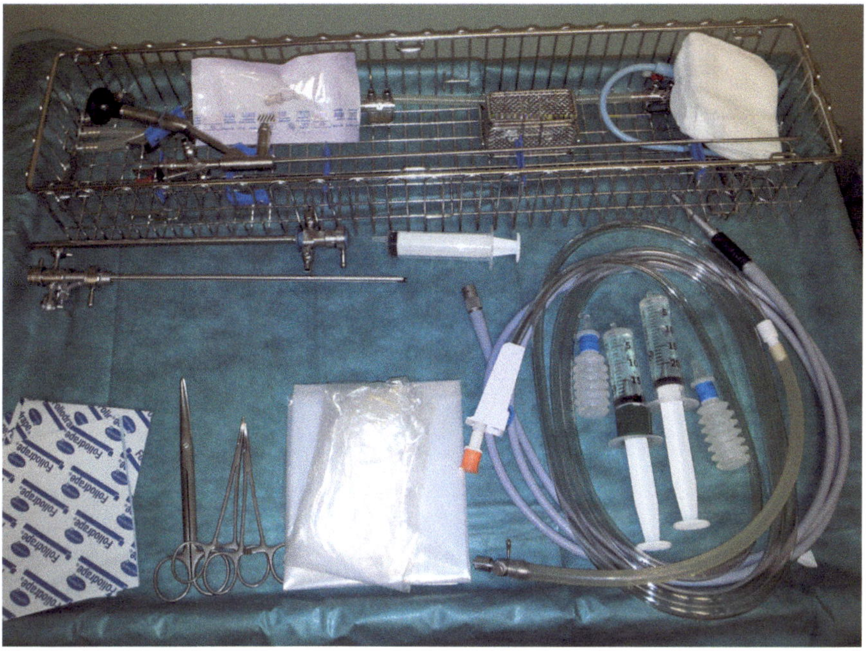

Fig. 19.11 Table for retrograde access

Fig. 19.12 Check the presence of all the coaxial Alken dilators and their correct insertion one over the other

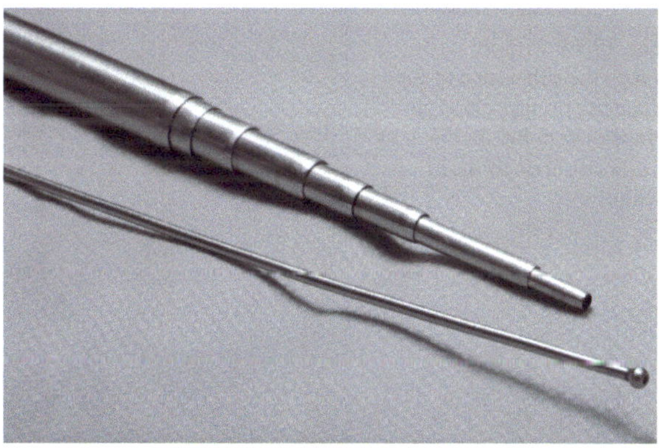

19.6 Some Tips and Tricks

Here is a short list of "tips and tricks" which may be obvious for many but which we have learned with the experience to pay attention to:

- Preliminarily check that all the coaxial telescopic metallic dilators of Alken are present and easily roll one over the other (this does not happen if they have not been adequately cleaned) (Fig. 19.12).

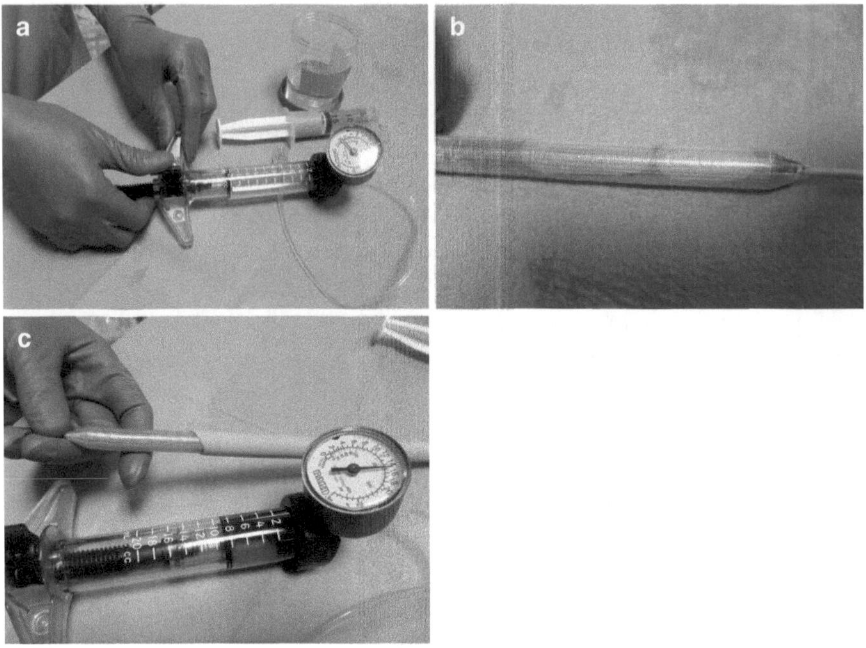

Fig. 19.13 Correctly prepare the balloon injecting contrast (**a**), avoiding to produce air bubbles (**b**) and never forgetting to pass the balloon within the Amplatz sheath before inflating it (**c**)

Fig. 19.14 Preliminarily verify the coherence of the diameter of the operating channel with the diameter of the accessories to insert within

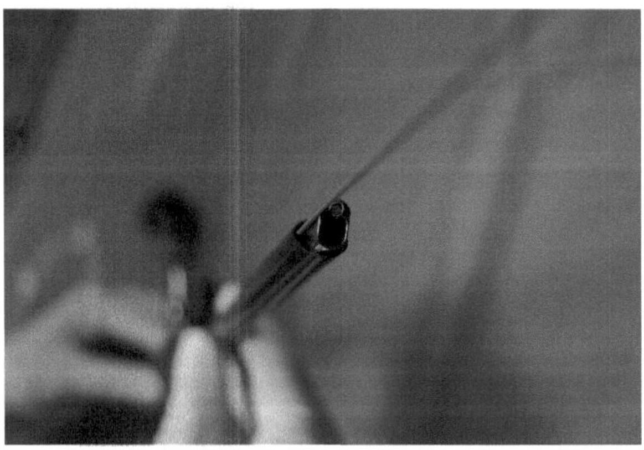

- Correctly prepare the balloon injecting contrast (Fig. 19.13a), avoiding to produce air bubbles (Fig. 19.3b); attention to the side with the diagonal cut of the Amplatz sheath, which, should be positioned toward the tip of the dilated balloon (Fig. 19.13c).
- Always verify the coherence of the diameter of the operating channel of all the semirigid and flexible instruments with the accessories to insert within (like baskets or forceps). This avoids to open too large accessories, not able to pass within, and to waste them (Fig. 19.14).

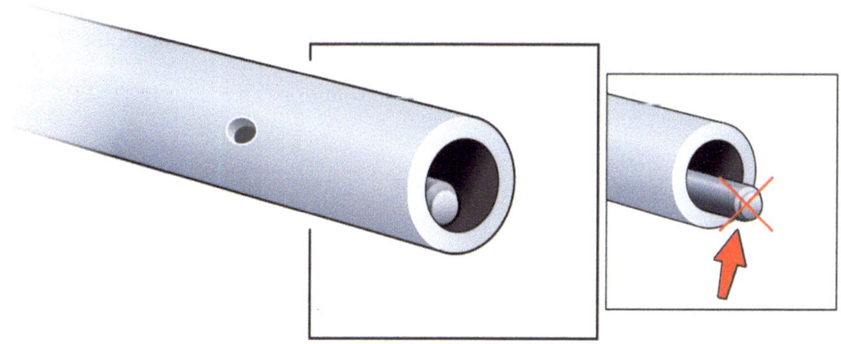

Fig. 19.15 Correctly mounted ballistic probe of the LithoClast Master (arrow = wrong position of the ballistic probe) (© Carole Fumat)

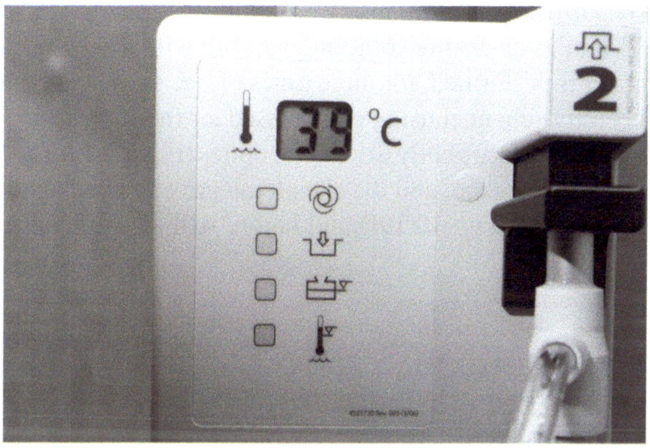

Fig. 19.16 Setup of the heating of the irrigation fluids (the device also avoids air bubble formation)

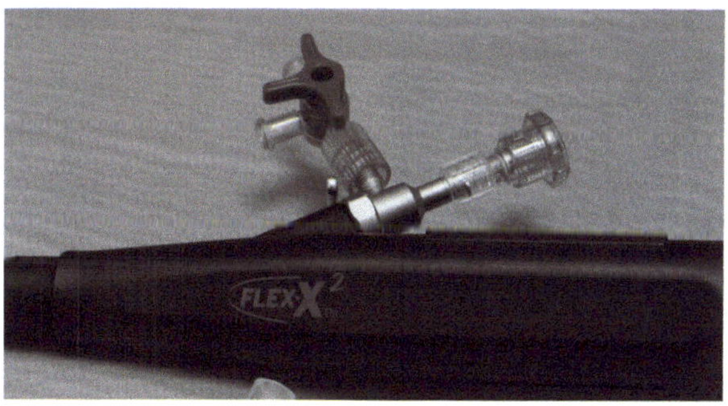

Fig. 19.17 Port Seal and three-branched tap for flexible ureteroscope

- Mount correctly the LithoClast Master, with particular reference to the ballistic probe that has not to protrude (no more than in the drawing because otherwise it hinders ultrasound functioning, not less because otherwise it does not work) (Fig. 19.15).
- Switch off the heating of the irrigation fluids during ultrasound lithotripsy, to avoid overheating (this is not necessary during ballistic only or stone laser lithotripsy) (Fig. 19.16).

- Always prepare in advance the Port Seal and the three-branched tap for the flexible ureteroscope, to avoid bad vision due to the pouring out of all the irrigation fluid (Fig. 19.17).

19.7 In the Sterilization Central

At the end of surgery, the work of the nursing team is not over. In fact, the correct management of all the endourologic armamentarium and the application of standardized protocols of sterilization have to be followed. For instance, the laser fibers have to be washed, cut, peeled, and checked with the dedicated inspecting device controlling its integrity before sterilization processing (Fig. 19.18).

For the flexible endoscopes, a first test of capacity verifies the integrity of the sheath (pressure progressively diminishes in case of damage, Fig. 19.19a). After 15 min in cleansing solution, washing with a pressurized pistol and demineralized water is performed, for three times of one minute each. Water is eliminated from the operative channel using compressed air (no more than 50 kPa, Fig. 19.19b) and the outside surface gently dried. The optics (Fig. 19.19c) and the flexibility (Fig. 19.19d) are then checked, and the sheath integrity verified again (Fig. 19.19e), after putting all the taps (Fig. 19.19f) and before sealing the final product in Sterrad. Attention

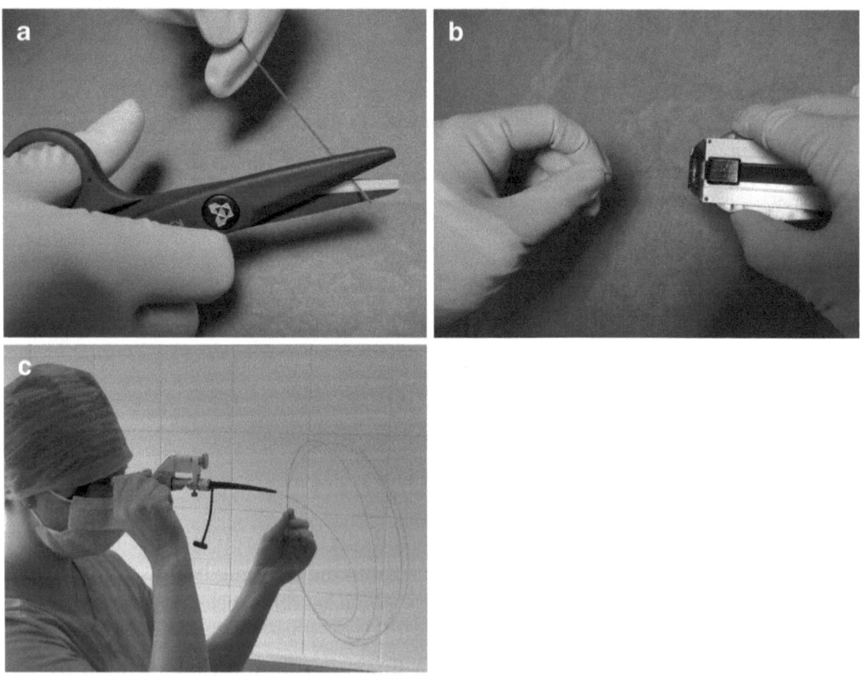

Fig. 19.18 Preparation of the laser fiber after its use: (**a**) cutting, (**b**) peeling, (**c**) visual checking of the laser fiber

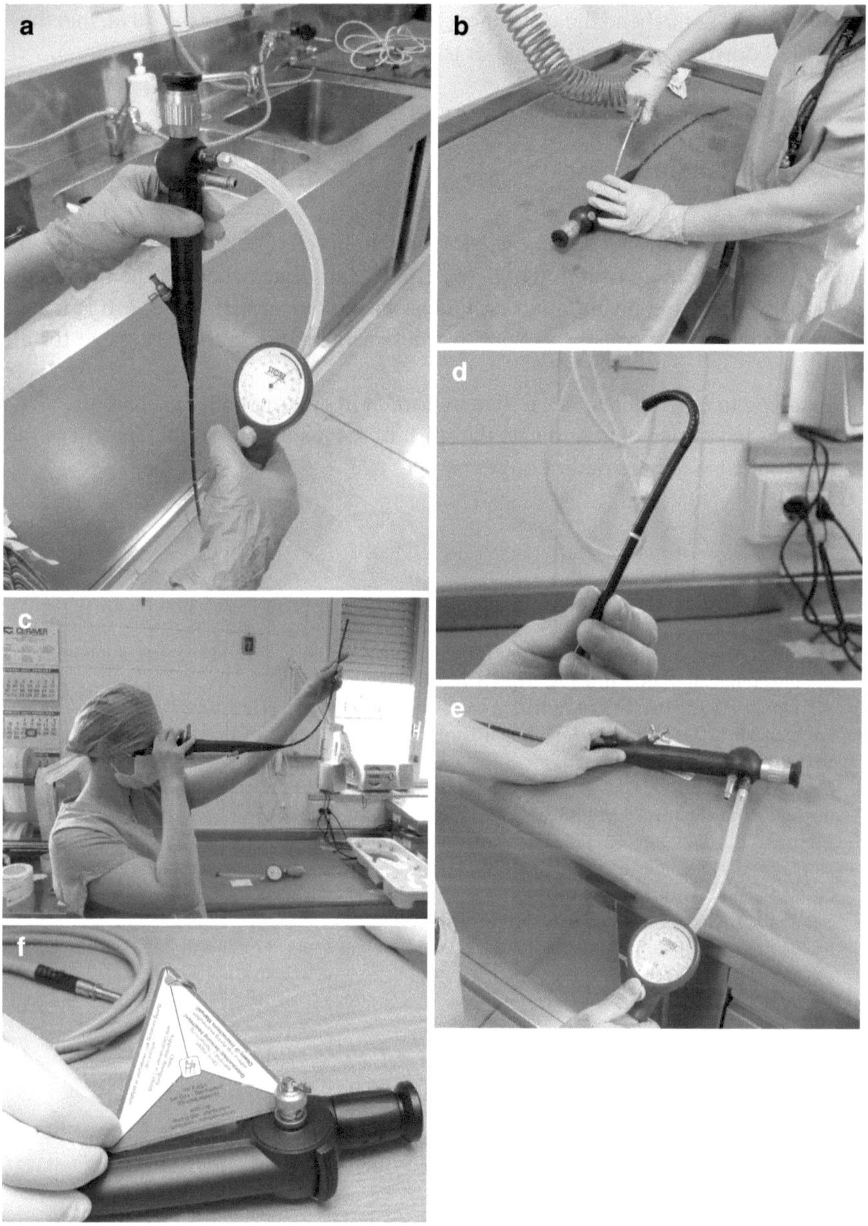

Fig. 19.19 Various steps of flexible ureteroscope care in the sterilization central : sheath integrity control (**a**), drying of the working channel (**b**), check of the optics (**c**) and of the flexibility (**d**), second sheath integrity control (**e**), after putting all taps (**f**)

should be paid not to bend the instruments too much, overloading the guys, that they do not fall down or receive any kind of trauma [5, 6].

19.8 Conclusions

Nursing assistance to ECIRS requires for sure an initial effort, largely rewarded by the satisfaction coming from the final results. The absolute benefit of the patient (in terms of comfortable positioning, easy anaesthesiological assistance, efficacy and safety of the percutaneous procedure, painless awakening) is the best prize for all our work.

Teaching to other colleagues is also important in order not only to share the technical notes but also to communicate the spirit of the team, for the final benefit of the patients and also to be proud of our expertise.

References

1. Bush WH, Jones D, Brannen GE (1985) Radiation dose to personnel during percutaneous renal calculus removal. AJR Am J Roentgenol 145:1261–1264
2. Majidpour HS (2010) Risk of radiation exposure during PCNL. Urol J 7:87–89
3. Laureano F (2001) Percutaneous nephrostolithotomy: a means of managing urinary calculi. Semin Perioper Nurs 10:54–59
4. Cracco CM, Scoffone CM, Poggio M, Scarpa RM (2010) The patient position for PNL: does it matter? Arch It Urol Androl 82:30–31
5. Clemens JQ, Dowling R, Foley F, American Urological Association, Society of Urologic Nurses and Associates et al (2010) Joint AUA/SUNA white paper on reprocessing of flexible cystoscopies. J Urol 184:2241–2245
6. Semins MJ, George S, Allaf ME, Matlaga BR (2009) Ureteroscope cleaning and sterilization by the urology operating room team: the effect on repair costs. J Endourol 23:903–905

Chapter 20
Intraoperative Complications: How to Avoid Them?

Francisco Pedro Juan Daels and Mariano Sebastian Gonzalez

Abstract At present, PNL is the minimally invasive technique of choice to treat complex renal stones. Despite being a safe surgical intervention, PNL is not exempt from potential complications, which can arise at any stage of the procedure: patient positioning, renal puncture, tract dilation, intraoperative manipulation, stone fragmentation and postoperative management. Besides being the majority of them minor, they can be kept to a minimum in experienced hands with the development of new techniques and improved technologies. However, patient positioning-related complications are not considered in any classification, as well as those related to anaesthesiological problems, which are the ones minimised adopting ECIRS in the Galdakao-modified supine Valdivia position. In particular, with regard to the potential complications due to decubitus, haemodynamic conditions, management of the respiratory tract and the relative location of the colon with respect to the puncture site, PNL performed in supine decubitus or in any of its variations proves to be safer than in prone decubitus.

20.1 Introduction

At present, percutaneous nephrolithotomy (PNL) is the minimally invasive technique of choice to treat complex renal stones. Despite being a safe surgical intervention, PNL is not exempt from potential complications, which can arise at any stage of the procedure: patient positioning, renal puncture, tract dilation, intraoperative manipulation, stone fragmentation and postoperative management.

F.P.J. Daels, MD (✉) • M.S. Gonzalez, MD
Department of Urology, Instituto Universitario del Hospital Italiano de Buenos Aires, Buenos Aires, Argentina
e-mail: pedro.daels@hospitalitaliano.org.ar; mariano.gonzalez@hospitalitaliano.org.ar

C.M. Scoffone et al. (eds.), *Supine Percutaneous Nephrolithotomy and ECIRS*,
DOI 10.1007/978-2-8178-0459-0_20, © Springer-Verlag France 2014

20.2 Positioning-Related Complications

Placing a relaxed, anaesthetised patient from supine to prone decubitus is not an easy task. It implies great maneuvring and requires to be performed with great care and coordination to avoid extreme extensions and flexions that may hurt neck and shoulders.

Neurological lesions have been described as a consequence of the extreme rotation of the head, such as hemiparesis, quadriparesis, quadriplegia, cerebrovascular accidents and brachial plexus injury [1–4]. Fortunately, however, all these severe lesions are extremely infrequent.

The probability of these complications diminishes considerably when the patient's final position is supine decubitus or any of its variations [5–9], as its manoeuvring is much less or virtually nil (see also Chap. 8).

20.2.1 Pressure-Point-Area-Related Complications

Prone decubitus requires the surfaces of the body that are in contact with the operating table to be thoroughly padded. A wide variety of lesions have been described as a result of prone decubitus: skin necrosis of the forehead, nose, malar region, chin, eyebrows, ears, iliac crests and genitals [10–13]; dermatitis [14]; tracheal compression [15]; macroglossia; oropharyngeal congestion; oedema of the superior respiratory tract [16]; visceral ischemia; peripheral neuropathies in elbows, knees and toes; and amaurosis [17].

Postoperative blindness after a non-ophthalmological surgery is a rare phenomenon, but in two out of three cases, it occurs after surgery with the patient in prone decubitus [18]. The mechanism could be the direct external compression of the ocular globe, causing an increase in the intraocular pressure, the consequent ischemia on the retina and the loss of sight (Hollenhorst syndrome) [19]. Another factor could be that the prone position itself increases the intraocular pressure, and if this pressure is the same as the mean arterial pressure, which is reduced by the anaesthetic, a relative ischemia of the optic nerve might take place [20]. Amaurosis occurs in 0.2 % of the surgeries in prone decubitus [21].

None of these complications has been reported in supine decubitus, presenting much less opportunity for injury to the patient, since the above-mentioned structures do not come into contact with the operating table. As to the Galdakao-modified supine Valdivia position, care must be taken here to avoid with adequate paddings localised pressures of upper and lower limbs and to tilt the pelvis and thorax equally to avoid stress on the lumbar spine.

20.2.2 Haemodynamic Disorders

The prone decubitus produces significant changes in the blood distribution, breathing movements and lung perfusion. The fact that the thorax is lying on the surface of the operating table restricts respiratory movements. Owing to this, intermittent positive pressure ventilation is necessary to bear the weight of the chest [22]. This results in an increased intrathoracic pressure, which leads to a reduction in venous back flow, both cephalic and caudal [23]. This circulatory disorder is particularly relevant in obese, elderly and hypovolaemic patients.

In the supine decubitus and its variations, the rib cage moves freely, avoiding such haemodynamic disorders.

20.2.3 Management of the Respiratory Tract

Air tract control and resuscitation maneuvers are difficult in the prone position. Any complication (involuntary disintubation, the need for cardiopulmonary resuscitation, etc.) means the need to move the patient immediately into supine decubitus, which is extremely difficult to do in the middle of a surgical procedure [24].

However, if the patient is treated in supine decubitus, in the event of an emergency, the anaesthesiologist is comfortable and free to work.

20.3 Puncture-Related Complications

An ideal renal puncture should fulfil three conditions:

1. It should avoid lesion of any neighbouring organ. If the kidney is in normal position (as shown by the preoperative computed tomography), the puncture should be performed in the safe area for lumbar puncture as described in Chap. 13.
2. The needle, having passed through the renal parenchyma, should penetrate the urinary tract through the papilla of the selected calyx.
3. The needle should follow the same direction of the axis of the neck of the calyx.

20.3.1 Colon Lesions

Even if a correct puncture is independent from the decubitus of the patient, it is worth noting that in supine decubitus (or in its variations), the colon moves away from the puncture area by an average of 2.5 cm, therefore decreasing the risk of its perforation. This has been shown by a work carried out at our department at the Hospital Italiano of Buenos Aires, where we compared 20 computed tomography scans of the abdomen and pelvis of patients positioned in prone and intermediate supine decubitus, respectively [25]. There is also the research by Hopper, which has become a classic, which compares the frequency of occurrence of retrorenal colon in prone and supine decubitus, 1.9 % in supine decubitus and 4.7 % in prone position, respectively [26]. This is the reason why pre operative tomography is of vital importance as a safety precaution for the percutaneous procedure as any anatomic alteration would be revealed [27].

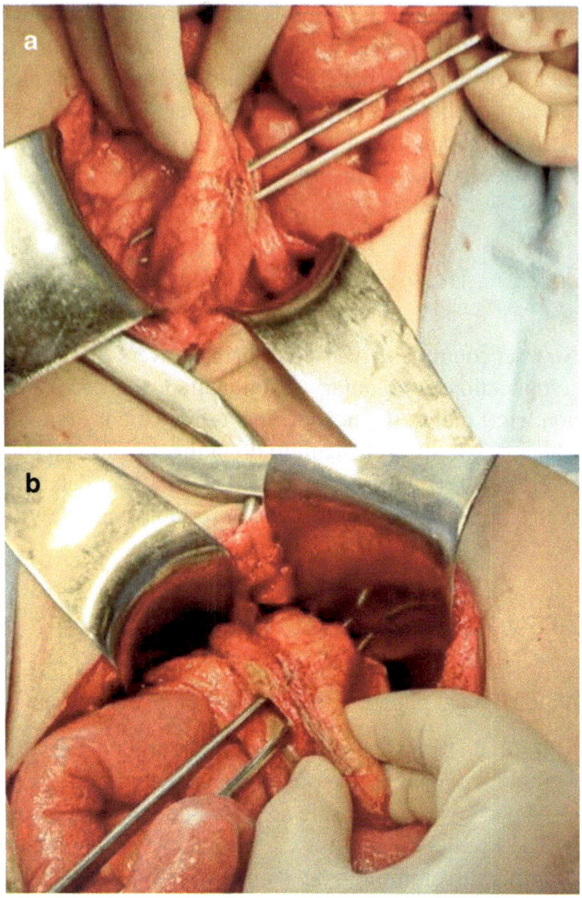

Fig. 20.1 (**a**) Intraperitoneal bowel perforation (**b**) Intraperitoneal bowel lesion, surgical repair

The diagnosis of colonic perforation could be intraoperative, but it tends to be immediately postoperative. The damage can be either retroperitoneal or intraperitoneal (Fig. 20.1a, b). The clinical manifestations of peritonitis indicate intraperitoneal lesion, which can be confirmed radiologically by a nephrostomy control with contrast medium. A retroperitoneal lesion can often clear itself up spontaneously without the need of active maneuvers except for corresponding ones of support. On the other hand, an intraperitoneal lesion must be repaired immediately. Sometimes a complementary derivative transitory colostomy is required. The longer it takes to resolve, the greater the risk of patient mortality. Every hour counts.

20.3.2 Pleural Lesions

Any intercostal puncture passes through the diaphragm and increases the risk of pneumothorax, hydrothorax and/or haemothorax. The incidence of liquid accumulating in the pleura varies between 3 and 38 % when the puncture is performed

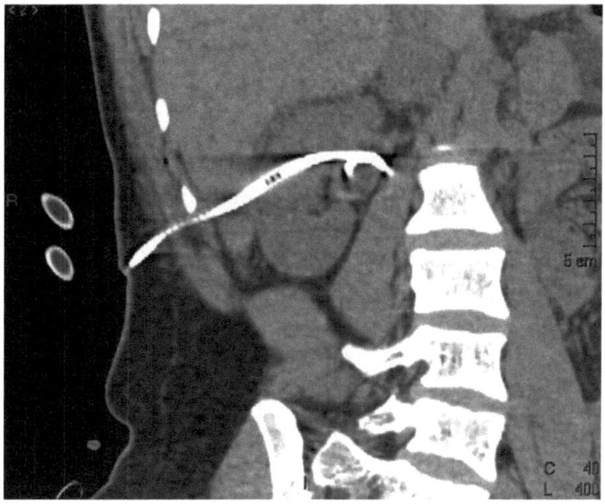

Fig. 20.2 CT scan demonstrating the transhepatic passage of the nephrostomy tube (Courtesy of A. Hoznek)

above the 11th rib [28, 29]. The lung and pleura can be damaged when the decision is made to reach the kidney by a puncture above the 11th rib [30]. Hopper states that these cases reach 86 % in the right pleura and 29 % in the right lung and on the side 79 % in the left pleura and 14 % in the left lung.

These lesions often clear up by themselves spontaneously. Only in cases of extensive pneumothorax or haemopneumothorax is it necessary to place underwater seal thoracic drainage. Open surgery is seldom required.

20.3.3 Hepatic Lesions

Hepatic lesions are unusual (Fig. 20.2). They are found to be associated with hepatomegaly or right punctures above the eleventh rib. They do not often require an active resolution.

20.3.4 Splenic Lesions

Splenic lesions are also unusual. They are associated with splenomegaly or left punctures above the 11th rib. They often bleed in an unconstrained manner and may require splenectomy. Although a recent paper has shown the possibility of a conservative form of treatment, this seems to be only an exceptional option [31].

20.3.5 Other Visceral Injuries

Other unusual lesions which have been described, such as biliary, duodenal and intestinal mesenteric ones, are generally caused by the perforation of the renal pelvis by exaggerated progression of a dilator or needle.

20.3.6 Vascular Lesions

The second objective of the needle, as well as avoiding a lesion of a neighbouring organ, is to reach the urinary tract passing through the renal parenchyma without causing arterial bleeding. In order to reduce this risk to the upmost, it is necessary to know the arrangement of the renal artery and its branches in relation to the pelvis and the calyces. The vascularisation of the kidney is detailed in Chap. 6.

The safest area for the puncture is normally the dorsal calyx of the lower pole. It is especially important to bear in mind the pathway of the infundibular arteries, and thus the safest way to access the urinary system percutaneously is frontally through the papilla of a calyx, following the axis of the infundibulum [32–34]. A vascular lesion may occur as the consequence of an intrarenal puncture through the infundibulum. In fact, the puncture of the kidney through the infundibulum of an upper pole calyx is very dangerous, as this zone is completely surrounded by large blood vessels, both venous and arterial. In the casts, when the puncture was via the neck, 67 % of the cases presented vascular lesion, of which 26 % presented arterial lesion. When the puncture is through a mid-renal infundibulum, 23 % of the cases present lesion to blood vessels. When the puncture is through a lower pole infundibulum, 13 % of cases present a vascular lesion.

These findings clearly show that the puncture through the infundibulum is not a safe access, since there is a high risk of lesion to an arterial blood vessel [35]. On the other hand, access through the papilla showed venous lesion in 8 % of the cases (regardless to the selected calyx) and no arterial lesions.

Additionally, following the same criterion of intending to avoid lesions to infundibular blood vessels that run parallel to the calyceal necks, not only should the tip of the papilla be punctured but the needle should also follow the direction of the axis of the calyceal neck (a further condition for an ideal puncture). This way, the needle, once inside the calyx, has a long endoluminal pathway towards the pelvis, decreasing the risk of coming out and causing arterial lesions.

Unfortunately, the projection of a straight line that follows the axis of the inferior calyx and passes through the centre of the papilla generally enters the skin at a point outside the safe area for lumbar puncture. This means that an ideal puncture is very rarely feasible. Therefore, the precaution should always be taken of advancing the needle just a few millimetres, once the papilla is punctured, and removing its mandrel by introducing a guide wire towards the renal pelvis in order to maintain the way.

20.4 Dilation-Related Complications

Once the guide wire is inserted, the access tract is dilated. Throughout this step, the main concern is to avoid an exaggerated progression of the dilators inside the urinary tract. It is also opportune to remember that the punctured calyx tends to be occupied by stones, and untimely dilation can cause damage to the mucosa. These complications during the dilation are avoided by making precise, gentle and controlled movements.

A current controversy is what calibre to use in order to dilate. It is accepted that the greater the calibre of the Amplatz sheath inserted, the greater the risk of lacerations on the one hand but, on the other hand, the shorter the operating time (as it enables the extraction of larger-sized fragments) and a guarantee of lower intrarenal pressures, decreasing the risk of sepsis.

The dilation usually makes any mistake made during the puncture evident. Thus, a peripheral papillary puncture can lead to bleeding due to parenchymal laceration during the dilation.

When bleeding is present, it must be determined whether it is venous or arterial (Fig. 20.3a–c). Venous bleeding is easy to solve. A simple occlusion of the venous flow for a few minutes triggers the quick clot formation and allows the procedure to continue without major frights. However, arterial bleeding, fortunately far less common, is a urological emergency which requires an immediate solution by means of a superselective embolisation (Fig. 20.3d–g).

20.5 Manipulation-Related Complications

Although there are various potential complications at this stage, all of them can be easily prevented or limited. The first is the loss of the nephrostomy tract due to the slipping out of the Amplatz sheath. This is prevented by means of a previous safety guide wire insertion, especially the “through and through” (kebab) guide wire. In case the access tract is lost, it may be quickly regained with a safety guide wire in place. The nephroscope follows the guide wire and the sheath is reinserted.

With no safety guide wire in place, the same situation becomes more complex. It may be of help to retrogradely inject contrast medium mixed with indigo carmine or a little air into the ureteral catheter; the dye or the bubbles will come out through the fistulous tract, observed by the nephroscope and under radioscopic control. During these manoeuvres, it is important to use the smallest amount of fluids possible, for the shortest length of time possible (especially if it is not saline), to avoid an absorption syndrome [36–38]. The absorption syndrome is a rarity when the sheath is adequately placed within the urinary tract but proves to be a potentially severe complication when the fluids are dispersed in the retroperitoneum, requiring clinical and nephrological management and high complexity support and control.

If the attempt of regaining the lost access tract is not successful, an alternative correct decision could be to create a new access tract re-puncturing the patient or to suspend the procedure (possibly inserting a double-J stent) programming a further surgery later on.

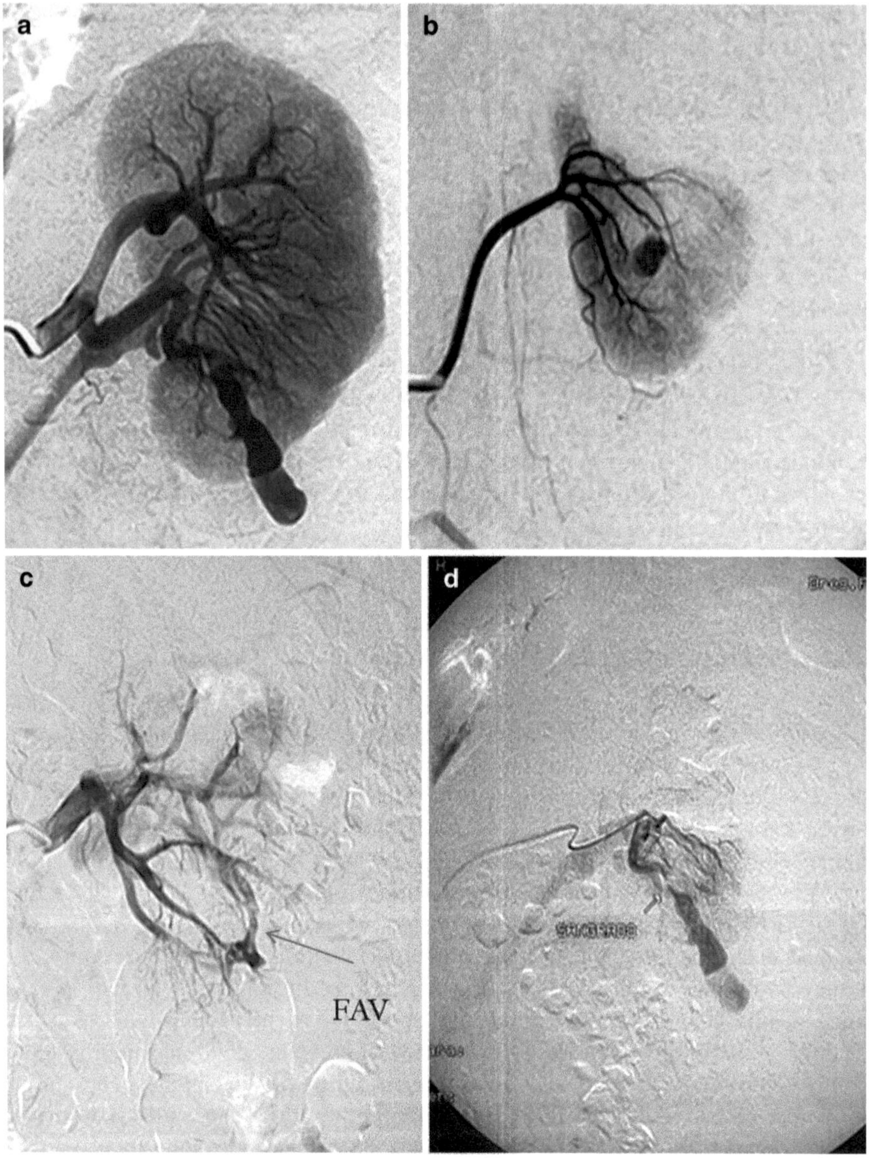

Fig. 20.3 (**a**) Arteriographic evidence of renal active bleeding (**b**) Arteriographic evidence of a pseudoaneurysm (**c**) Arteriographic evidence of an *arrow*: arteriovenous fistula (**d**) Selective arteriographic catheterisation of the vascular lesion (**e**) Superselective embolisation of the vascular lesion (**f**) Postembolisation control: arterial phase (**g**) Postembolisation control: nephrographic phase: ischemic area

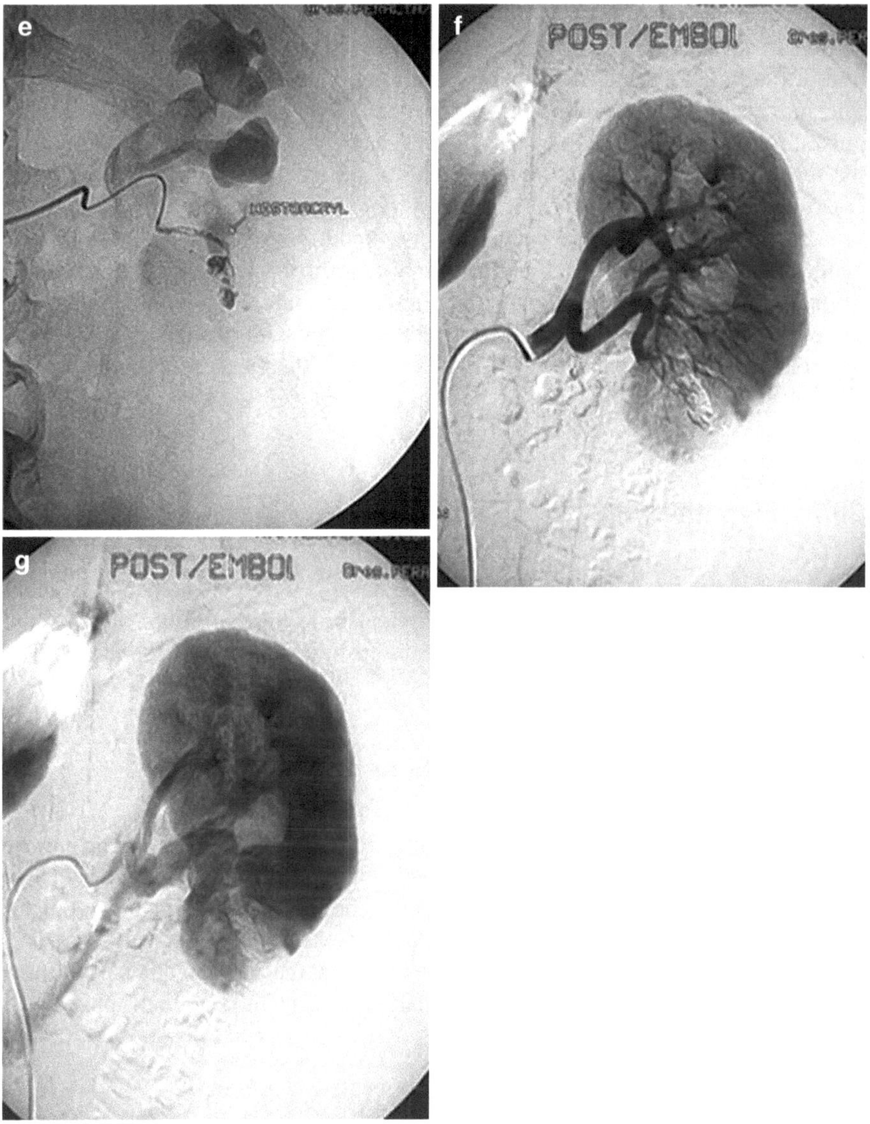

Fig. 20.3 (continued)

20.6 Fragmentation-Related Complications

Usually, complex calculi need to be fragmented in order to make their extraction possible via the Amplatz sheath. Any available energy can be used, whether ultrasonic, pneumatic, electrohydraulic or laser. Each one has different physical features as well as potential harmful mechanisms causing lesion to the surrounding mucosa.

For instance, the obstruction of the probe of the sonotrode during ultrasonic lithotripsy can cause thermal lesions. The expansive features of the explosive evaporation of the liquid around the electrohydraulic fibre can cause mucosal laceration. The movement of the probe being propelled by pneumatic or electromagnetic pulses, following the principles of ballistics, can cause mechanical perforation of the renal cavities. The hyperthermia of the tip of the laser fibre, if inadequately controlled, can cut through tissues as if they were butter.

In principle, none of these complications should force the procedure to be suspended, and they can be solved spontaneously by inserting a nephrostomy at the end of the procedure to guarantee a low intraluminal pressure. It is possible to prevent these problems by using any of these energy sources with gentleness and always working under permanent endoscopic vision on the calculus, keeping as far as possible from the mucosa.

20.7 Hypothermia

It may be unusual, but hypothermia has been described as a phenomenon possibly and inadvertently occurring when any surgical procedure is prolonged in time. Therefore, in such cases, it is advisable to administer tepid irrigation solutions [39].

20.8 Exiting-Related Complications

Once the procedure is finished, a nephrostomy drain is usually left in, which may be somehow painful. Nevertheless, increasingly more and more research seems to show an advantage of leaving the patient at the end of the procedure without nephrostomy drainage, in other words, tubeless [40, 41]. The nephrostomy aims at guaranteeing low pressure inside the urinary tract. For that reason, it is indicated in cases of persistent lithiasic remains, bleeding that can result in potentially obstructive blood clots and previous urinary infections.

20.9 Conclusions

Complications occurring during or after PNL may occur with a rate of up to 83 % and have been stratified according to their severity [42–48]. It is important to realise that, besides being the majority of them minor, they can be kept to a minimum in experienced hands with the development of new techniques and improved technologies. However, patient positioning-related complications are not considered in any classification of PNL complications, as well as those related to anaesthesiological problems.

In spite of all the above-mentioned potential complications, PNL is still a procedure that is minimally invasive, very therapeutic (whether or not in combination with endoscopic or laparoscopic procedures) and scarcely painful. It implies a short hospitalisation time and convalescence and has virtually no after-effects. Thus, PNL is definitely a useful and safe tool to treat complex calculi.

With regard to the potential complications due to decubitus, haemodynamic conditions, management of the respiratory tract and the relative location of the colon with respect to the puncture site, PNL performed in supine decubitus or in any of its variations proves to be safer than in prone decubitus.

To conclude, there are ten points to bear in mind when carrying out a PNL:

1. Put together a stable surgical team defining the precise role of each of its members.
2. Be knowledgeable of and have available a complete set of endoscopic instrumentation.
3. Work in a relaxed environment.
4. Perform a thorough preoperative assessment of the patient, with negative urine culture.
5. Perform a preoperative computed tomography of the abdomen and pelvis.
6. Carry out the puncture in the safe area for lumbar puncture: below the eleventh rib, outside the paravertebral muscles, above the iliac crest and inside the free end of the 12th rib.
7. Puncture the tip of the papilla of the selected calyx, following the axis of the calyceal neck as much as possible.
8. Penetrate the urinary tract by a few millimetres and insert a safety guide wire.
9. Fragment and extract the stones delicately under direct vision.
10. Never be in a hurry and never underestimate the procedure you are performing.

References

1. Langmayr J, Ortler M, Obwegeser A, Felber S (1996) Quadriplegia after lumbar disc surgery. A case report. Spine 21:1932–1935
2. Anderton J, Schady W, Markham D (1994) An unusual cause of postoperative brachial plexus palsy. J Anaesth 72:605–607
3. Schwartz D, Drummond D, Hahn M et al (2000) Prevention of positional brachial plexopathy during surgical correction of scoliosis. Spinal Disord 13:178–182
4. Winfree C, Kline D (2005) Intraoperative positioning nerve injuries. Surg Neurol 63:5–18
5. Valdivia Uria J, Valle J, Villarroya S et al (1990) Why is percutaneous nephrostomy still performed with patient prone? J Endourol 4:269–272
6. De Sio M, Autorino R, Quarto G et al (2008) Modified supine versus prone position in percutaneous nephrolithotomy for renal stones treatable with a single percutaneous access. a prospective randomized trial. Eur Urol 54:196–202
7. Ibarluzea G, Scoffone C, Cracco C et al (2007) Supine Valdivia and modified lithotomy position for simultaneous anterograde and retrograde endourological access. BJU Int 100: 233–236

8. Daels F, Gonzalez M, Garcia Freire F et al (2009) Percutaneous lithotripsy in Valdivia-Galdakao decubitus position: our experience. J Endourol 23:1615–1620
9. Valdivia Uría JG, Valle Gerhol J, López López JA (1999) Percutaneous nephroscopy technique in supine position. Braz J Urol 25:263–267
10. Anderton J (1991) The prone position for the surgical patient: a historical review of the principles and hazards. Br J Anaesth 67:452–463
11. Jain Y, Bithal P, Rath J (2007) Pressure score on malar prominences by horseshoe headrest in prone position. Anaesth Int Care 35:304–305
12. Moore D, Edmunds L (1950) Prone position frame. Surgery 27:276–279
13. Ray C (1987) New kneeling attachment and cushioned face rest for spinal surgery. Neurosurgery 20:266–269
14. Jericho B, Scaria G (2003) Contact dermatitis after use of the prone positioned. Br Anesth Analg 19:1–4
15. Kai Y, Yamaoka A, Irita K, Zaitsu A, Takahashi S (1995) Transient tracheal obstruction during surgical correction of scoliosis in a patient with Marfan's syndrome. Masui 44:868–873
16. Szabo M, Denman W, Marota J, Roberts J (1997) Evaluation of airway edema in patients operated on in the prone position. J Neurosurg Anaesthesiol 9:380
17. Cheng M, Todorov A, Templehoff R et al (2001) The effect of prone positioning on intraocular pressure in anesthetized patients. Anaesthesiology 95:1351–1355
18. Lee L (2003) Postoperative visual loss registry: preliminary analysis of factors associated with spine operations. ASA Newsl 67:7–8
19. Roth S, Tung A, Ksiazek S (2007) Visual loss in a prone-positioned spine surgery patient with the head on a foam headrest and goggles covering the eyes: an old complication with a new mechanism. Anesth Analg 104:1185–1187
20. Lee L, Posner K (2006) The American Society of Anaesthesiologists Postoperative visual loss registry: analysis of 93 spine surgery cases with postoperative visual loss. Anaesthesiology 105:652–659
21. Stevens W, Glazer P, Kelley S et al (1997) Ophthalmic complications after spinal surgery. Spine 22:1319–1322
22. Palmon S, Kirsch J, Deppe J, Toung T (1998) The effect of the prone position on pulmonary mechanics is frame dependent. Anesth Analg 87:1175–1180
23. Lee T, Yamg L, Chen H (1998) Effect of patient position and hypotensive anesthesia on inferior vena cava pressure. Spine 23:941–948
24. Tobias D, Mencio G, Atwood R, Gurwitz G (1994) Intraoperative cardiopulmonary resuscitation in the prone position. J Pediatr Surg 29:1537–1538
25. Gonzalez MS, Billordo Peres N, Garcia Marchibena P et al (2009) Colon position in ventral and intermediate dorsal decubitus (Valdivia). J Endourol 23(Suppl 1):A49, World Congress of Endourology 2009, abstract MP4-19
26. Hopper K, Sherman J, Luethke J, Ghaed N (1987) The retrorenal colon in the supine and prone patient. Radiology 162:443–446
27. LeRoy A, Williams H Jr, Bender C (1985) Colonic perforation following percutaneous nephrostomy and renal calculus removal. Radiology 155:83–85
28. Gupta R, Kumar A, Kapoor R et al (2002) Prospective evaluation of safety and efficacy of the supracostal approach for percutaneous nephrolithotomy. BJU Int 90:809–813
29. Munver R, Delvecchio FC, Newman GE, Preminger GM (2001) Critical analysis of supracostal access for percutaneous renal surgery. J Urol 166:1242–1246
30. Robert M, Maubon A, Roux JO et al (1999) Direct percutaneous approach to the upper pole of the kidney: MRI anatomy with assessment of the visceral risk. J Endourol 13:17–20
31. Desai A, Jain S, Benway B et al (2010) Spleen injury during percutaneous nephrolithotomy: a case report with a novel management technique. J Endourol 24:541–545
32. Valer Algarabel J, Valdivia Uria J, Orozco J et al (1992) Anatomia renal aplicada a la cirugia percutánea, Cuadernos de Endourologia. Hospital Clinico Universitario, Zaragoza

33. Sampaio F (1992) Anatomic background for intrarenal endourologic surgery. J Endourol 6:301–304
34. Sampaio F, Zanier J, Aragao A (1992) Intrarenal access: three dimensional anatomical study. J Urol 148:1769–1773
35. Sampaio F, Aragao A (1990) Anatomical relationship between the intrarenal arteries and the kidney collecting system. J Urol 143:679–681
36. Koroglu A, Toga T, Cicek M et al (2003) The effects of irrigation fluid volume and irrigation time on fluid electrolyte balance and hemodynamics in percutaneous nephrolithotripsy. Int Urol Nephrol 35:1–6
37. Rozentsveig V, Neulander E, Roussabrov E et al (2007) Anesthetic considerations during percutaneous nephrolithotomy. J Clin Anesth 19:351–355
38. Gehring H, Nahm W, Zimmermann K et al (1999) Irrigation fluid absorption during percutaneous nephrolithotripsy. Acta Anaesthesiol Scand 43:316–321
39. Roberts S, Bolton D, Stoller M (1994) Hypothermia associated with percutaneous nephrolithotomy. Urology 44:832–835
40. Tefekli A, Altunrende F, Tepeler K et al (2007) Tubeless percutaneous nephrolithotomy in selected patients: a prospective randomized comparison. Int Urol Nephrol 39:57–63
41. Shah H, Khandar A, Sodha H et al (2009) Tubeless percutaneous nephrolithotomy: 3 years of experience with 454 patients. BJU Int 104:840–846
42. De La Rosette JJ, Zuazu JR, Tsakiris P et al (2008) Prognostic factors and per cutaneous nephrolithotomy morbidity: a multivariate analysis of a contemporary series using the Clavien classification. J Urol 180:2489–2493
43. Tefekli A, Ali Karadag M, Tepeler K et al (2008) Classification of percutaneous nephrolithotomy complications using the modified Clavien grading system: looking for a standard. Eur Urol 53:184–190
44. Zuazu JR, Hruza M, Rassweiler JJ, De Rosette JJ (2010) The Clavien classification system to optimize documentation of PCNL morbidity. Arch Ital Urol Androl 82:20–22
45. De La Rosette J, Assimos D, Desai M, CROES PCNL Study Group (2011) The Clinical Research Office of the Endourological Society percutaneous nephrolithotomy global study: indications, complications and outcomes in 5,803 patients. J Endourol 25:11–17
46. Ozden E, Mercimek MN, Yakupoglu YK et al (2011) Modified Clavien classification in percutaneous nephrolithotomy: assessment of complications in children. J Urol 185:264–268
47. Labate G, Modi P, Timoney A et al (2011) The percutaneous nephrolithotomy global study: classification of complications. J Endourol 25:1275–1280
48. Seitz C, Desai M, Haecker A et al (2012) Incidence, prevention, and management of complications following percutaneous nephrolitholapaxy. Eur Urol 61:146–158

Chapter 21
Antibiotic Prophylaxis and Infectious Complications in PNL

Oscar R. Negrete-Pulido and Jorge Gutiérrez-Aceves

Abstract Postoperative infection in PNL represents one of the most feared and life-threatening complications in current urologic practice. In this chapter the importance of a correct preoperative evaluation of the patient and of the related risk factors is described; adequate antibiotic prophylaxis and intraoperative measures to prevent the development of infectious adverse events are indicated; early postoperative signs that could anticipate the development of a sepsis, in order to achieve a timely diagnosis and establish early measures that consequently will reduce morbidity and mortality, are identified. These are the basic principles and key points that will help us to perform a secure PNL, limiting intraoperative risk.

21.1 Introduction

Postoperative infection in percutaneous nephrolithotomy (PNL) represents one of the most feared and life-threatening complications in current urologic practice. In this chapter we will:

1. Describe the importance of a correct preoperative evaluation of the patient and of the related risk factors.
2. Indicate adequate antibiotic prophylaxis and intraoperative measures to prevent the development of infectious adverse events.

O.R. Negrete-Pulido, MD (✉)
Department of Urology, Lithiasis and Endourology Clinic, Urology,
Hospital Ángeles LEÓN, Hospital Regional de Alta Especialidad del Bajío,
Blvd. Milenio 130 San Carlos la Roncha C.P. 37670, León, Guanajuato, Mexico
e-mail: ornegrete@hotmail.com

J. Gutiérrez-Aceves, MD
Department of Urology, Wake Forest School of Medicine, Medical Center Boulevard,
Winston-Salem, NC 27157, USA
e-mail: jgutierr@wakehealth.edu

C.M. Scoffone et al. (eds.), *Supine Percutaneous Nephrolithotomy and ECIRS*,
DOI 10.1007/978-2-8178-0459-0_21, © Springer-Verlag France 2014

3. Identify early postoperative signs that could anticipate the development of a sepsis, in order to achieve a timely diagnosis and establish early measures that consequently will reduce morbidity and mortality.

PNL is considered a safe procedure for the management of renal stones [1]. It is an invasive procedure with a wide reported complication rate that ranges from 3 to 83 % according to different authors [2, 3]. Indeed, urosepsis and urinary tract infections in PNL represent a dangerous situation when postoperative septicemia or severe sepsis develops. Urinary sepsis has a low reported incidence that ranges from 0.3 to 1 % but a very high (66–80 %) mortality rate [2, 4, 5].

Postoperative fever is a common and usually not exceptional adverse event, with a reported incidence from 10.4 up to 38.9 % [2, 6, 7]. It is well known that it is not always secondary to an infectious process, but the related literature frequently considers it in any case an infectious complication. In spite of its benign clinical course, postoperative fever deserves close observation and the maintenance of a high index of suspicion, because 0.3–9.3 % of patients can develop potentially life-threatening sepsis [6].

21.2 Pathogenesis of Urosepsis/Septic Shock

Most of the stones that are managed today by PNL are infected stones (magnesium ammonium phosphate or calcium carbonate) derived from persistent infection caused by urease-producing bacteria; in industrialized countries these represent up to 15 % of urinary calculi [8]. Noninfected stones (calcium oxalate or uric acid stones) are also frequently associated with bacterial colonization or active infections caused by associated factors like urinary flow obstruction and urine stasis.

The bacteria are incorporated into the interstices of the stone, establishing their own biofilm environment and becoming difficult or impossible to eradicate without removal of the calculus. Stones can also injure the urinary tract, and this damage can further facilitate bacterial colonization [9].

An infectious complication is triggered when during PNL urinary bacteria and their products enter the bloodstream via pyelovenous, pyelolymphatic, and pyelotubular backflow and forniceal rupture, caused by a mixture of events related to the surgery per se (such as vascular, lymphatic, and urothelial disruption secondary to renal access; increased pressure into the collecting system during nephroscopy; stone manipulation producing an intense release of bacteria and endotoxins), triggering a systemic inflammatory response.

A generalized neurohumoral pro- and anti-inflammatory response takes place. This begins with cellular activation of monocytes, macrophages, and neutrophils that interact with endothelial cells through numerous pathogen recognition receptors [10]. A further host response includes the mobilization of plasma substances, such as tumor necrosis factor (TNF), interleukins (ILs), caspases, proteases, leukotrienes, kinins, reactive oxygen species, nitric oxide (NO), arachidonic acid, platelet activating factor (PAF), and eicosanoids. TNF-α and IL-1 are the most important pro-inflammatory cytokines and exhibit similar biologic properties. They influence the temperature regulatory centers in the hypothalamus, resulting in fever. They also have an effect on the reticular formation in the brain stem, which renders the patient somnolent and comatose. Release of adrenocorticotropic hormone (ACTH) in the pituitary gland is increased; therefore, the adrenal gland is stimulated. These factors also stimulate hematopoietic growth factors, which leads to the formation of new neutrophils and the release of stored ones. The neutrophils are additionally activated and produce bactericidal substances, such as proteases and oxygen radicals. B and T lymphocytes are stimulated for the synthesis of antibodies and cellular immune reaction. In the continuing septic process, however, apoptosis of B cells, CD4 helper cells, and follicular dendritic cells causes an anti-inflammatory immune suppression, called transient immune paralysis [11]. Activation of complement and coagulation cascades further amplifies this chain of events. Microvascular injury, thrombosis, and loss of endothelial integrity (capillary leak) take place and result in tissue ischemia. This diffuse endothelial disruption is responsible for the multiple organ failure (MOF) and the global tissue hypoxia accompanying severe sepsis/ septic shock [12].

21.3 Bacteriology

Pathogens associated with urinary tract infections (UTIs) and urosepsis have not varied greatly over the last decades except for the considerable changes in their resistance patterns [13, 14]. A continuous assessment of local patterns is important in order to establish the most appropriate and effective antibiotic regimens to prevent infectious complications.

Escherichia coli remains the single most common microorganism to cause UTIs. This is followed by Klebsiella and Proteus spp., frequently associated with stone disease. Furthermore, the increasing presence of Gram-positive bacteria such as Enterococcus and Staphylococcus should be noted.

DasGupta et al. reported that 40 % of urology inpatients had Gram-positive organisms, Enterococcus accounting for 27 % [15]. Several reports have shown that other organisms have increased not only their incidence but also their resistance to antibiotics commonly used in urology, including trimethoprim, quinolones, cephalosporins, and aminoglycosides, such as gentamicin; this is the case for Pseudomonas aeruginosa, methicillin-resistant Staphylococcus aureus, Serratia spp., and Clostridium difficile [16]. Resistance of Pseudomonas to quinolones is reported in up to 20 % of urology inpatients, with multiresistant Pseudomonas outbreaks encountered in endourologic units [17]. Kashanian et al. [18] recently reported in a retrospective analysis 25 % resistance of *E. coli* to ciprofloxacin. This rise in resistance of urinary pathogens towards quinolones has been reported worldwide and might be the consequence of its overuse due to its efficacy in treating other infections and uncomplicated UTIs, as well as its misuse as prophylaxis in some urologic diagnostic procedures.

21.4 Preoperative Evaluation

21.4.1 Identifying Risks for Infectious Complications

All patients who are being considered for PNL should be strictly evaluated with a complete medical history, physical examination, and laboratory tests, including an obligatory urine culture. This will help identifying those patients with a high risk for the development of an infectious complication [19]. There are well-recognized risk factors that can be categorized under the following headings.

21.4.1.1 Related to the Patient

There are several patient characteristics known to increase the risk of infectious complications after surgery. Patients who are immunosuppressed for different causes, among others those with malignant or autoimmune diseases receiving chemotherapy or chronic use of corticosteroids, usually have impaired infection resistance. Also patients of advanced age or poor nutritional status, with diabetes, obesity, and significant kidney or liver diseases, and female patients have a higher risk [20].

Other risk factors that occasionally are present in stone disease patients are anatomic anomalies, voiding dysfunctions, and urinary diversions. Many of these patients will have a positive urine culture and must receive preoperative antibiotics appropriately tailored to culture-specific organisms; at the end of treatment, urinary cultures must be repeated.

21.4.1.2 Related to the Stone Disease

Any procedure performed in patients with urolithiasis represents a high risk of developing infectious complications because of factors related to the stones (obstruction or hydronephrosis, active infection) and their management (frequent use of antibiotics and instrumentation, indwelling catheters, and ureteral stents), both increasing the possibility of colonization and chronic bacteriuria.

Rao et al. reported that bacteriuria and pyuria are risk factors for bacteremia; they also found that preoperative bacteriuria had a positive predictive value (PPV) of 0.53 for detection of endotoxemia, another important risk factor for the development of urosepsis [20]. The Clinical Research Office of the Endourological Society (CROES) PCNL global study, a prospective global database of indications and outcomes of PNL, included 5,803 patients and found that a positive culture is associated with a twofold risk of fever in the postoperative period. Also the presence of staghorn calculi and the use of a prior nephrostomy tube were shown to independently increase the risk of fever by approximately 60 % [6].

21.5 Intraoperative Management and Risk Factors: Reducing Risks

21.5.1 Prophylactic Antibiotic Therapy

Prophylaxis means a brief course of antibiotics administered before or at the start of an intervention and is used to minimize the infectious complications resulting from diagnostic and therapeutic interventions. While the rationale for the use of antibiotics is well accepted, possible side effects and development of antimicrobial resistance patterns are potential risks. Therefore, an antibiotic prophylaxis policy should be well considered and based on high levels of evidence [21].

For prophylactic antimicrobial administration to be optimally effective, timing and dosing are critical. Infusion of the first dose should begin within 60 min of the surgical incision (with the exception of 120 min for intravenous fluoroquinolones and vancomycin). Correct dosing is equally important. Some drugs should be adjusted to the patient's body weight. Oral administration is as effective as the intravenous route for antibiotics with sufficient bioavailability. Additional doses are required intraoperatively if the procedure extends beyond two half-lives of the initial dose [22].

It is generally agreed that patients who are scheduled for PNL must have a negative urine culture before surgery. Unfortunately, this is not always possible to adhere to because of stone or urinary tract colonization; in these patients, appropriate antibiotic therapy should start at least 1 week before the planned procedure. Results of urine cultures from patients with stones are not predictive of stone bacteriology, especially in those with struvite stones. Therefore, this group should receive broad-spectrum antibiotic therapy, specific to the cultured bacteria but also likely to be effective against urease-producing organisms residing in the stone.

In the last three decades, several studies have been published demonstrating the benefit of prophylactic antibiotics in PNL independently of the drug and scheme studied.

Charton and coworkers [23] found in patients who had negative cultures and who did not receive antibiotics an incidence of 35 and 10 % of post-PNL bacteriuria and fever without sepsis or bacteremia, respectively.

Later, Darenkov and associates [24] demonstrated that patients who received preoperative intravenous or oral ciprofloxacin to reduce the risk of postoperative urinary infection compared with a nontreatment group showed an incidence of 0 and 17 %, respectively, versus 40 % in the arm without therapy.

Lately, Mariappan and colleagues [25] compared a historical cohort as a control arm that received gentamicin as a unique preoperative dosage [26] with a treatment group that received 1 week of ciprofloxacin 500 mg/day preoperatively and showed that in patients with stones >20 mm or dilated pelvicalyceal systems, the risk of postoperative urosepsis development diminished significantly up to three times (relative risk (RR) = 3.4) as well as systemic inflammatory response syndrome (SIRS) (RR = 2.9) in patients who received ciprofloxacin.

Recently, Seyrek et al. [27] showed that ampicillin–sulbactam and cefuroxime are equally effective in terms of prevention of inflammatory response syndrome and did not find any difference between different schemes of duration of antibiotic maintenance, concluding that a single dose administration is sufficient.

Also, Dogan and coworkers [28] in a prospective comparative study on 81 patients with preoperative sterile urine found that a single dose of ofloxacin given during anesthetic induction was associated with the same incidence of fever, bacteriuria, and bacteremia as ofloxacin administered until the time of nephrostomy tube removal.

Komar and colleagues [29] analyzed various risk factors for urosepsis following PNL and studied the role of 1-week nitrofurantoin before surgery in reducing the risk of urosepsis. They found that nitrofurantoin prophylaxis resulted in decreased risk factors as culture positivity (30.2 % vs. 8.3 %, odds ratio 0.36, $p=0.087$), endotoxemia (41.9 % vs. 17.5 %, odds ratio 0.22, $p=0.001$), and consequently SIRS (49 % vs. 19 %, odds ratio 0.31, $p=0.01$).

Published literature suggests that antimicrobial prophylaxis is unnecessary after wound closure or on termination of an endoscopic procedure, but considering that PNL could be associated with a preexisting infection, infectious stone, or manipulation of an indwelling catheter, the subsequent course of antimicrobials (therapeutic rather than prophylactic) might include a period extending beyond 24 h from the conclusion of the procedure. In the absence of preexisting bacterial colonization, there is no evidence that prophylaxis should extend beyond 24 h. In cases where prolonged catheterization follows the procedure (i.e., nephrostomy tube and/or double J stent), antimicrobial therapy at the time of catheter removal may be therapeutic rather than prophylactic, because colonization likely has occurred [30].

Recently, both the European and American Urological Associations published guidelines and recommendations for best practice in antibiotic prophylaxis in urologic surgery [21, 30, 31] (Fig. 21.1). These guidelines are extremely helpful to standardize the administration of antibiotics prior to surgery. However, local practice should be based on or adjusted according to local or even hospital microbiologic patterns and requirements, so it is crucial that each center and department reviews regularly its infection patterns and antibiotic resistance.

21.5.2 Urine and Stone Bacteriology

Mariappan et al. demonstrated that stone and pelvic urine cultures obtained during surgery are better predictors of potential urosepsis than bladder cultures [28]; they found that bladder urine cultures were positive in 11.1 % of cases versus 35.2 and 20.4 % of stone and pelvic urine cultures, respectively. Stone culture showed the

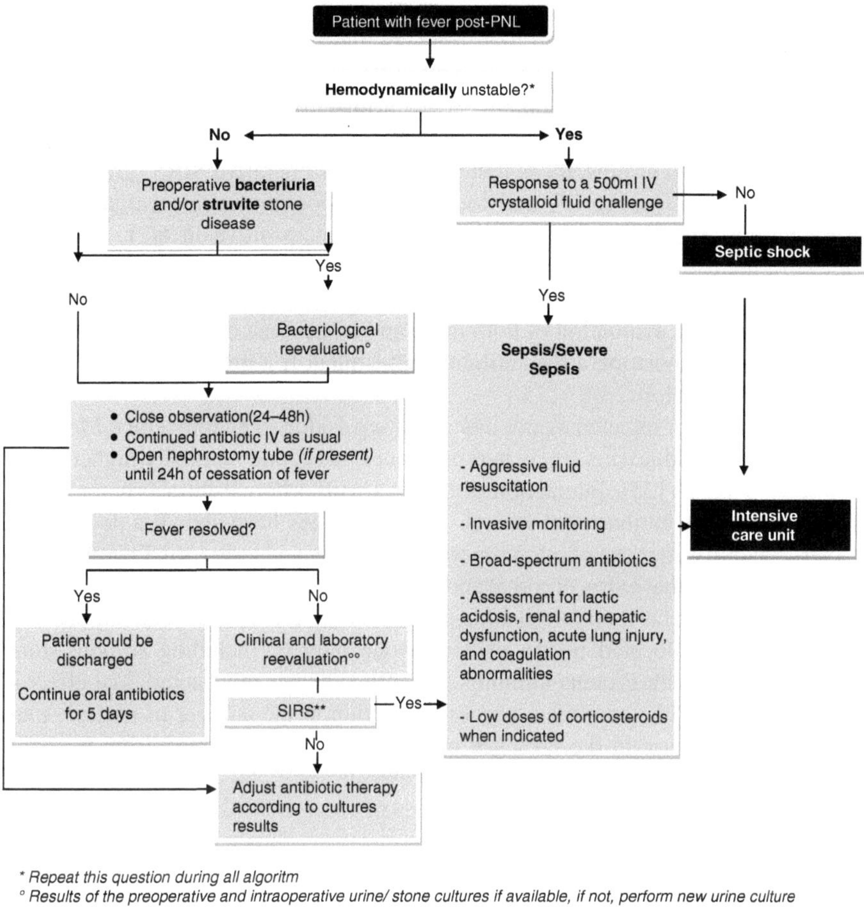

Fig. 21.1 Management algorithm in patients with infectious complications after PNL (Modified from Ref. [50])

greatest PPV (0.7). Infected bladder urine did not always carry identical bacteria to those found in the upper tract. Patients with pelvic- or stone-positive cultures showed a relative risk for urosepsis at least four times greater than the rest of the cohort. In this study, bladder urine did not predict SIRS. Also, they found that pre-operative hydronephrosis and stones larger than 20 mm correlated with positive stone and pelvic urine cultures.

Margel and associates [32] obtained similar results. They found different pathogens between bladder urine and stones in 35 % of cases; colonized stones were associated with sterile urine culture in 25 % of patients. The relative risk (RR) of SIRS when the stone culture was positive was 3.6. Dogan and associates [33] also found an increased risk of postoperative fever and sepsis in the group of patients with positive stone and first urine obtained after puncture cultures. They found 35 % of positive stone cultures and 10 % of upper tract urine positive cultures in patients with negative preoperative urine cultures or those who received appropriate antibiotic therapy before surgery. Recently, Lojanapiwat [34] divided 200 patients in two groups, those that presented postoperative SIRS (group I) and those that did not (group II), and found that preoperative urine culture, pelvic urine culture, and stone culture, respectively, were positive in 66.1, 46.4, and 48.2 % of the patients in group I, but only 10.4, 3.5, and 3.5 % for the corresponding specimens in group II. These findings underline the importance of intraoperative microbiologic evaluation of both urine and stones; the obtained cultures may be a guide in the postoperative antibiotic adjustment if a more serious infectious complication develops.

Manipulation of infected stones can cause sepsis due to endotoxemia. McAleer, et al. measured endotoxins levels in renal stones and found markedly higher levels in infection stones [35]. Interaction of bacteria with different intracorporeal lithotripters may have antibacterial effects. In vitro studies have shown a decrease of bacteria viability after use of intracorporeal lithotripsy and laser [36]. Our group has reported recently that extracorporeal shock wave or intracorporeal lithotripsy, using all the alternatives currently available, is significantly effective at reducing the viability of bacteria located inside artificial stone models, including struvite stone models infected with Proteus mirabilis [37–39]. Whether this bactericidal effect is desirable is still to be answered, because reduction in the number of bacteria may represent an increase in the presence of proteins/endotoxins freed from bacterial cell lysis, therefore increasing the risk of urosepsis.

21.5.3 Renal Pelvic Pressure During Surgery

Renal pelvic pressure (RPP) greater than 30 mmHg has been shown to result in pyelovenous and pyelolymphatic backflow. Troxel and Low, in a prospective study that included 31 patients, found that RPP greater than 30 mmHg was recorded only in eight patients (26 %) and did not find any association between RPP levels and postoperative fever [40]. In contrast with them, Zhong et al. demonstrated that mean intrapelvic pressure greater than 20 mmHg and accumulated time of RPP greater than 30 mmHg may cause enough backflow to contribute to bacteremia and postoperative fever [41].

Low RPP during surgery is achieved using an open low-pressure access system such as operating through an Amplatz sheath (operating instrument 4 Ch sizes smaller than the access sheath). Inflow of irrigant should be at gravity and never pressurized. We also recommend the use of forced diuresis (furosemide 20 mg at the beginning of irrigation and every 60 min of surgery and irrigation time) to further reduce the pyelorenal reflux potentially causing fluid overload and bacteremia. Other factors that have been related to postoperative fever and risk of

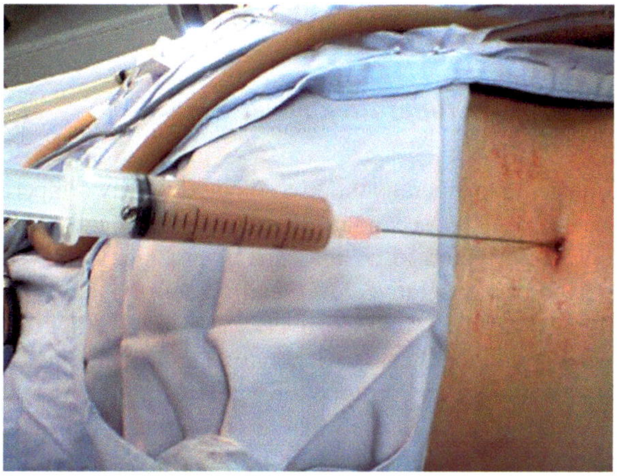

Fig. 21.2 Purulent urine may be obtained during renal access

bacteremia are long operative time, large stone burden, and high amounts of irrigating fluid.

In the presence of an obstruction at the ureteropelvic junction or intrarenal segments, purulent urine may be obtained during renal access despite previous negative cultures of the voided urine (Fig. 21.2). In such instances treatment has to be postponed, the urine cultured and the renal collecting system drained under antibiotic coverage, until eradication of the infection is documented.

According to Ramsey et al. in a recent evidence-based review [42], the effects on the resolution of infected hydronephrosis are similar if a ureteral stent or a nephrostomy tube is used. Nevertheless, Mokhmalji et al., in a prospective randomized study, reported prolonged fever and catheter placement time in the group of patients treated with ureteral stent and suggest that percutaneous nephrostomy is superior to ureteral stents for diversion of hydronephrosis [43].

Small case series have been reported, exploring the possibility of continuing the surgery even if purulent urine is incidentally encountered. Aron et al. in a group of 19 patients reported no difference regarding the incidence of postoperative fever or sepsis between patients with one-stage versus staged surgery with collecting system drainage and 3–7 days of intravenous antibiotic coverage before a second procedure [44]. Hosseini et al. divided 45 patients into two groups: in group 1 ($n = 29$) stones were removed during the first session, and in group 2 ($n = 16$) a nephrostomy tube remained in place, while stone removal was accomplished 3–5 days later when results of urine and nephrostomy fluid cultures were negative [45]. They reported no intraoperative or postoperative complications, other than transient fever in 10.3 and 12.5 % in groups 1 and 2, respectively.

In spite of these recent reports, there is neither sufficient evidence nor well-designed clinical trials to recommend other conduct than performing a staged procedure with drainage and broad-spectrum antibiotic therapy until infection has resolved.

21.6 Treatment of Complications

21.6.1 Postoperative Fever

Transient postoperative mild to moderate body temperature elevation is frequently seen, is usually secondary to the release of inflammatory mediators, and is not always attributed to an infectious cause [4]. In several studies, discordant rates between postoperative fever and bacteriuria have been reported, ranging from 10–35 % to 0–19 %, respectively [5, 23, 28, 32, 46, 47]. Ziaee and coworkers [48], using three simultaneous laboratory tests including postoperative urine cultures, blood cultures, and postoperative polymerase chain reaction, did not show any difference in bacteriuria between febrile and non-febrile patients. Also, Rao and associates [5] demonstrated a lack of this correlation in their study in which 74 % of patients with PNL had fever postoperatively and only 41 % endotoxemia. These discordances may support the hypothesis that the presence of fever might be the result of inflammatory mediators in response to surgical manipulation rather than infectious in origin. On the other hand, a possible explanation is the inhibitory effect of perioperative antibiotics on bacterial growth.

Thus, in patients with absence of bacteriuria or without struvite stone disease, who are given antibiotics preoperatively and maintained postoperatively, temperature rise usually resolves, does not have clinical significance, and does not necessitate immediate bacteriologic evaluation in those who are hemodynamically stable. Treatment of this group of patients consists of continued antibiotic coverage—i.e., intravenous antibiotics during the hospital stay and oral antibiotics for 5 days after discharge. In these patients, the nephrostomy tube is left to drain 24 h after disappearance of any temperature rise (Fig. 21.1). The risk of a more severe infection and systemic bacteremia is low, provided that appropriate preventive measures are taken.

21.6.2 Persistent Postoperative Fever

Noncontinuous, less than 38 °C persistent postoperative fever in patients without hemodynamic instability should be managed with continuous perioperative oral antibiotics for 5 days (or longer if residual infected stone remains inside the collecting system) and maintaining open nephrostomy tube until the urine is clear. If percutaneous renal drainage is necessary for longer periods (second session planned, status post-ureteropelvic junction repair), urine culture should be revaluated and antibiotic therapy modified or restarted 3 days before any further manipulation, such as antegrade pyelography, repeated treatment sessions, or even clamping of the PNL tube. Prolonged percutaneous renal drainage almost invariably leads to bacteriuria; however, the risk of major infectious complications can be kept to a minimum if these precautions are observed.

21.6.3 Postoperative Sepsis: Early Identification and Initial Treatment

Early recognition and management of sepsis optimizes outcome. Therefore, patients in whom this problem is suspected after genitourinary surgery should be prioritized and receive timely care.

To diagnose sepsis and severe sepsis/septic shock as early as possible, it is necessary to have clear definitions of infection, organ dysfunction, and global tissue hypoxia and to recognize the clinical and laboratory findings that are indicative of these conditions. Sepsis is defined as the presence of SIRS caused by a documented or suspected infection. SIRS is defined as the presence of two or more of the following: (1) temperature greater than 38 °C or less than 36 °C, (2) heart rate greater than 90 beats/min, (3) respiratory rate greater than 20 breaths/min (or $PaCO_2$ <32 Torr), and (4) white blood cell count greater than 12,000/mm^3 or greater than 10 % immature band forms. Severe sepsis is defined as the presence of sepsis and one or more organ dysfunctions. Organ dysfunction can be defined as acute lung injury; coagulation abnormalities; thrombocytopenia; altered mental status; renal, liver, or cardiac failure; or hypoperfusion with lactic acidosis. Septic shock is defined as the presence of sepsis and refractory hypotension, i.e., systolic blood pressure less than 90 mmHg and unresponsive to a crystalloid fluid challenge of 500 ml.

As mentioned above, clinical and laboratory recognition of septic problems is mandatory. Procalcitonin is a propeptide of calcitonin, but lacks hormonal activity. During generalized infections with systemic manifestations, its level may rise considerably. In contrast, during severe viral infections or inflammatory reactions of noninfectious origin, procalcitonin levels show no or only a moderate increase. Its exact site of production during inflammatory response is still unknown. The documentation of high levels of early biochemical markers, such as procalcitonin and protein C, in the initial postoperative period may help identify a severe inflammatory response to surgical stress from bacteremia, SIRS, or sepsis/septic shock and prompt the institution of adequate and opportune therapeutic measures [49].

Appropriate therapy is a continuum of infection management ranging from drainage (maintaining indwelling catheter or opening the nephrostomy tube) and broad-spectrum antibiotics to aggressive fluid resuscitation and invasive monitoring with medical management in the intensive care setting, until the causative agent is found and eradicated.

Continuous monitoring of vital signs, pulse oximetry, urine output, and initial laboratory testing to assess the severity of global tissue hypoxia and organ dysfunction, including assessment for lactic acidosis, renal and hepatic dysfunction, acute lung injury, and coagulation abnormalities, should be instituted as soon as possible in patients in whom severe sepsis/septic shock is suspected to facilitate the earliest recognition of this condition.

The usual bacteria cultured from urinary sources are aerobic Gram-negative bacilli and enterococci. Appropriate cultures (including blood and urine) should be obtained before the adjustment of antibiotics. At this point, it is important to reanalyze urine cultures that were obtained preoperatively or during surgery and, based on their results, redirect antibiotic therapy. If results are not available, empiric broad-spectrum antibiotics should be initiated as soon as possible. Suggested primary regimens include the usage of ampicillin/gentamicin, or piperacillin–tazobactam, or carbapenems (doripenem, imipenem, or meropenem). The duration of treatment is determined by the patient's clinical response. It is imperative to modify the antibiotic regimen to a culture directed one when possible. If severe sepsis/septic shock is recognized, besides empiric antibiotic therapy, prompt treatment in the intensive care unit should include repletion of intravascular volume with large amounts of crystalloid intravenous fluids. Pressors are administered as needed to maintain blood pressure, central venous pressures are monitored, and fluids are administered to maintain a pressure of 8–12 cm H_2O. Bicarbonate and low-dose steroids may be used and good blood glucose control maintained. Tight blood glucose control by administration of insulin doses up to 50 U/h is associated with a reduction in mortality. Recombinant activated protein C (drotrecogin alfa) is a new drug that has been approved for therapy of severe sepsis. Multidisciplinary treatment is essential to obtain good results [12, 50, 51].

21.7 Conclusions

Infectious complications represent a potentially life-threatening scenario that has the possibility to be prevented or at least minimized in most of cases; thus it is crucial to identify risk factors. All potential candidates to PNL must be evaluated with a meticulous and strict preoperative work-up. The appropriate time to perform surgery according to the potential infectious sources should be established. A correct preoperative prophylaxis based on provided guidelines and adjusted according to the results of urine cultures or to local or even hospital microbiologic patterns should be provided. As mentioned, there are basic principles and key points that will help us to perform a secure surgery, limiting intraoperative risk. Once an infectious complication is suspected, it is imperative to act accurately with a multidisciplinary approach, to avoid the progression of the natural history of sepsis and to provide better opportunities to obtain a complete recovery.

References

1. Skolarikos A, Alivizatos G, de la Rosette JJ (2005) Percutaneous nephrolithotomy and its legacy. Eur Urol 47:22–28
2. Michel MS, Trojan L, Rassweiler JJ (2007) Complications in percutaneous nephrolithotomy. Eur Urol 51:899–906
3. Skolarikos A, de la Rosette J (2008) Prevention and treatment of complications following percutaneous nephrolithotomy. Curr Opin Urol 18:229–234
4. O'Keefe NK, Mortimer AJ, Sambrook PA, Rao PN (1993) Severe sepsis following percutaneous or endoscopic procedures for urinary tract stones. Br J Urol 72:277–283

5. Rao PN, Dube DA, Weightman NC et al (1991) Prediction of septicemia following endourological manipulation for stones in the upper urinary tract. J Urol 146:955–960
6. Gutierrez J, Smith A, Geaylete P et al (2012) On behalf of the CROES PCNL Study Group Urinary tract infections and post-operative fever in percutaneous nephrolithotomy. World J Urol. doi:10.1007/s00345-012-0836-y
7. Draga RO, Kok ET, Sorel MR et al (2009) Percutaneous nephrolithotomy: factors associated with fever after the first postoperative day and systemic inflammatory response syndrome. J Endourol 23:921–927
8. Bichler KH, Elipper E, Naber K et al (2002) Urinary infection stones. Int J Antimicrob Agents 19:488–498
9. Neal DE Jr (2008) Complicated urinary tract infections. Urol Clin North Am 35:13–22
10. Beutler B (2004) Inferences, questions and possibilities in toll like receptor signaling. Nature 430:257–263
11. Wagenlehner FM, Weidner W, Naber KG (2007) Optimal management of urosepsis from the urological perspective. Int J Antimicrob Agents 30:390–397
12. Nguyen B, Rivers E, Abrahamian F et al (2006) Severe sepsis and septic shock: review of the literature and emergency department management guidelines. Ann Emerg Med 48:28–54
13. Hofmann W (1990) Urosepsis and uroseptic shock. Z Urol Nephrol 83:317–324
14. Foz A (1976) Sepsis of urological origin: microbiological aspects. Antibiot Chemother 21:69–72
15. DasGupta R, Sullivan R, French G, O'Brien TS (2009) Evidence based prescription of antibiotics in urology: a 5-year review of microbiology. BJU Int 104:760–764
16. Thiruchelvam N, Yeoh SL, Keoghan SR (2006) MRSA in urology: a UK hospital experience. Eur Urol 49:896–899
17. DasGupta R, French G, Glass JM (2008) Multi-resistant *Pseudomonas aeruginosa* outbreak in an endourology unit. Eur Urol 53:1009
18. Kashanian J, Hakimian P, Blute M Jr et al (2008) Nitrofurantoin: the return of an old friend in the wake of growing resistance. BJU Int 102:1634–1637
19. Matlaga B, Kim S, Lingeman J (2005) Improving outcomes in percutaneous nephrolithotomy: access. EAU Update Series 3:37–43
20. Book M, Lehmann LE, Schewe JC, Weber S (2005) Urosepsis. current therapy and diagnosis. Urologe A 44:413–422
21. Bootsma AM, Laguna Pes MP, Geerlings SE, Goossens A (2008) Antibiotic prophylaxis in urologic procedures: a systematic review. Eur Urol 54:1270–1286
22. Bratzler DW, Houck PM (2005) Surgical infection prevention guideline writers. Workgroup: antimicrobial prophylaxis for surgery: an advisory statement from the National Surgical Infection Prevention Project. Am J Surg 189:395–404
23. Charton M, Vallancien G, Veillon B, Brisset JM (1986) Urinary tract infection in percutaneous surgery for renal calculi. J Urol 135:15–17
24. Darenkov AF, Derevianko II, Martov AG et al (1994) The prevention of infectious-inflammatory complications in the postoperative period in percutaneous surgical interventions in patients with urolithiasis. Urol Nephrol 2:24–26
25. Mariappan P, Smith G, Moussa SA, Tolley DA (2006) One week of ciprofloxacin before percutaneous nephrolithotomy significantly reduces upper tract infection and urosepsis: a prospective controlled study. BJU Int 98:1075–1079
26. Mariappan P, Smith G, Bariol SV et al (2005) Stone and pelvic urine culture and sensitivity are better than bladder urine as predictors of urosepsis following percutaneous nephrolithotomy: a prospective clinical study. J Urol 173:1610–1614
27. Seyrek M, Binbay M, Yuruk E et al (2012) Perioperative prophylaxis for percutaneous nephrolithotomy: randomized study concerning the drug and dosage. J Endourol 26:1431–1436
28. Dogan HS, Sahin A, Cetinkaya Y et al (2002) Antibiotic prophylaxis in percutaneous nephrolithotomy: prospective study in 81 patients. J Endourol 16:649–653
29. Kumar S, Bag S, Ganesamoni R et al (2012) Risk factors for urosepsis following percutaneous nephrolithotomy: role of 1 week of nitrofurantoin in reducing the risk of urosepsis. Urol Res 40:79–86

30. Wolf JS Jr, Bennett CJ, Dmochowski RR, Urologic Surgery Antimicrobial Prophylaxis Best Practice Policy Panel et al (2008) Best practice policy statement on urologic surgery antimicrobial prophylaxis. J Urol 179:1379–1390
31. Grabe M, Bishop MC, Bjerklund-Johansen TE et al (2009) European Association of Urology. Guidelines on urological infections. European Guidelines Office Publications. Available at www.uroweb.org/guidelines
32. Margel D, Ehrlich Y, Brown N et al (2006) Clinical implication of routine stone culture in percutaneous nephrolithotomy – a prospective study. Urology 67:26–29
33. Dogan HS, Guliyev F, Ceinkaya YS et al (2007) Importance of microbiological evaluation in management of infectious complications following percutaneous nephrolithotomy. Int Urol Nephrol 39:737–742
34. Lojanapiwat B (2011) Role of preoperative and intraoperative factors in mediating infection complication following percutaneous nephrolithotomy. Urol Int 86:448–452
35. McAleer IM, Kaplan GW, Bradley JS et al (2003) Endotoxin content in the renal calculi. J Urol 169:1813–1814
36. Prabakharan S, Teichman J, Spore SS et al (1999) Proteus mirabilis viability after lithotripsy of struvite calculi. J Urol 162:1666–1669
37. Quintero MS, Alvarez UM, Wacher C et al (2008) Interaction of shock waves with infected kidney stones: is there a bactericidal effect? J Endourol 22:1629–1638
38. Gómez-Núñez JG, Alvarez UM, Fernández F et al (2009) Interaction of intracorporeal lithotripters with *Proteus mirabilis* inoculated inside artificial calcium and struvite stones. J Endourol 23:519–522
39. Gutiérrez J, Alvarez UM, Mues E et al (2008) Inactivation of bacteria inoculated inside urinary stones-phantoms using intracorporeal lithotripters. Urol Res 36:67–72
40. Troxel SA, Low RK (2002) Renal intrapelvic pressure during percutaneous nephrolithotomy and its correlation with the development of postoperative fever. J Urol 168:1348–1351
41. Zhong W, Zeng G, Wu K et al (2008) Does a smaller tract in percutaneous nephrolithotomy contribute to high renal pelvic pressure and postoperative fever? J Endourol 22:2147–2151
42. Ramsay S, Robertson A, Ablett MJ et al (2010) Evidence-based drainage of infected hydronephrosis secondary to ureteric calculi. J Endourol 24:185–189
43. Mokhmalji H, Braun M, Martinez-Portillo FJ et al (2001) Percutaneous nephrostomy versus ureteral stents for diversion of hydronephrosis caused by stones: A prospective, randomized clinical trial. J Urol 165:1088–1092
44. Aron M, Goel R, Gupta NP, Seth A (2005) Incidental detection of purulent fluid in kidney at percutaneous nephrolithotomy for branched renal calculi. J Endourol 19:136–139
45. Hosseini MM, Basiri A, Moghadamm SM (2007) Percutaneous nephrolithotomy of patients with staghorn stone and incidental purulent fluid suggestive of infection. J Endourol 21:1429–1432
46. Cadeddu JA, Chen R, Bishoff J et al (1998) Clinical significance of fever after percutaneous nephrolithotomy. Urology 52:48–50
47. Ziaee SA, Kazemi B, Moghaddam SM et al (2008) A study of febrile versus afebrile patients after percutaneous nephrolithotomy regarding bacterial etiologic factors through blood and urine cultures and 16S rRNA detection in serum. J Endourol 22:2717–2721
48. Uzzan B, Cohen R, Nicolas P et al (2006) Procalcitonin as a diagnostic test for sepsis in critically ill adults and after surgery or trauma: a systematic review and meta-analysis. Crit Care Med 34:1996–2003
49. Negrete-Pulido O, Gutiérrez-Aceves J (2009) Management of infectious complications in percutaneous nephrolithotomy. J Endourol 23:1–6
50. Sihler KC, Nathens AB (2006) Management of severe sepsis in the surgical patient. Surg Clin North Am 86:1457–1481
51. Gilbert DN, Moellering R, Eliopoulos GM, Sande MA (eds) (2008) The Sanford guide to antimicrobial therapy, 38th edn. Sanford Guide, Sperryville

Chapter 22
Prone Versus Supine PNL: Results and Published Series

András Hoznek, Julie Rode, Cecilia Maria Cracco, and Cesare Marco Scoffone

Abstract There is still much controversy in the literature concerning the optimal approach for PNL. Although prone PNL remains predominant on a global level, with a superior acquired experience and more training opportunities when compared to supine position, supine PNL is increasingly used and it is now quite consensual that it allows an easier management from the anaesthesiological point of view and may reduce patient morbidity. The available randomized studies demonstrate that in centers which already standardized the supine technique, this procedure may be more ergonomic and quicker and equally efficient in terms of stone clearance and morbidity.

22.1 Introduction

Percutaneous nephrolithotomy (PNL) in prone position has been considered until recently as the gold standard for the treatment of large (more than two centimeters) and/or complex renal stones. However, during the last few years, a new approach in a modified lithotomy and supine position has been proposed, with the purpose of simplifying patient positioning and improving the efficacy of the procedure (see also chapter 9).

The first large clinical series of PNL was reported by Valdivia Uría [1]. His technique was further improved by Ibarluzea [2], opening the era of Endoscopic

A. Hoznek, MD (✉) • J. Rode
Department of Urology, CHU Henri Mondor, 51. Av. du Ml. de Lattre de Tassigny, 94010 Créteil Cedex, France
e-mail: andras.hoznek@gmail.com; rode.julie@orange.fr

C.M. Cracco, MD, PhD • C.M. Scoffone, MD
Department of Urology, Cottolengo Hospital, Via Cottolengo 9, 10152 Torino, Italy
e-mail: cecilia.cracco@libero.it; scoof@libero.it

C.M. Scoffone et al. (eds.), *Supine Percutaneous Nephrolithotomy and ECIRS*, DOI 10.1007/978-2-8178-0459 0_22, © Springer-Verlag France 2014

Combined IntraRenal Surgery (ECIRS). This approach is becoming increasingly popular worldwide, with widely documented advantages: easier anaesthesiological management, one-step patient positioning, and simultaneous antegrade and retrograde access to the urinary tract [2–8]. However, while it is clear that prone position is no longer the exclusive way to perform PNL, many urologists remain reluctant to consider supine positions as a valid alternative in their daily practice [9, 10].

22.2 Heterogeneity of Reporting Outcomes of PNL

In order to establish advantages and inconvenience of both supine and prone position and to decide which method is more efficient and possibly safer, comparative studies are necessary. Unfortunately, the results currently reported by different centers are far from being standardized, and never refer to intra- and postoperative anaesthesiological complications.

First of all, in different series, the complexity of the cases may be very dissimilar. Only recently Thomas and colleagues have recommended a novel scoring system [11]. Guy's stone score takes into account the complexity of the stone burden as well as the patient's anatomy, in order to predict preoperatively the likelihood of a stone-free outcome. This grading system is important because there are currently no predictive models in the urologic clinical practice for this purpose. It comprises four grades (Table 22.1).

The goal of PNL is to obtain a stone-free status with minimal morbidity and optimal cost effectiveness. Therefore, when evaluating the results of the surgery, it is necessary to assess several outcomes, which until now have been mainly stone-free status, operative time, morbidity, costs, and quality of life. However, there is a substantial variability in the reporting of such outcomes among the different studies [12, 13].

Table 22.1 Guy's stone score

Grade I	Solitary stone in mid/lower pole
	Or solitary stone in the pelvis with simple anatomy
Grade II	Solitary stone in upper pole
	Or multiple stones in a patient with simple anatomy
	Or solitary stone in a patient with abnormal anatomy
Grade III	Multiple stones in a patient with abnormal anatomy
	Or stones in a calyceal diverticulum
	Or partial staghorn calculus
Grade IV	Staghorn calculus
	Or any stone in a patient with spina bifida or spinal injury

22.2.1 The Stone-Free Rate

22.2.1.1 The Cut-Off?

Regarding the stone-free status, some authors are faithful to the strict criterion of no fragments visualized on imaging, while others employ a more permissive definition tolerating small, passable, residual stone fragments (CIRF = clinically insignificant residual fragments). In these latter studies, the residual fragment size varies from 2 to 10 mm [12]. Furthermore, nearly one-third of papers evaluating surgical management of urinary calculi do not define stone-free status at all [12].

22.2.1.2 How?

A further difficulty arises from the different sensitivity and specificity of the methods employed for the assessment of residual fragments. These include intraoperative flexible nephroscopy [14], postoperative plain film of the abdomen (KUB), ultrasound (US), and computed tomography (CT). The reliability of these different methods is variable; therefore, the stone-free rate can be overestimated when using a poorly sensitive method. For example, KUB has been found to overestimate stone-free status by 35 % [14]. Although unenhanced computer tomography is the gold standard because it has the best sensitivity and specificity, it is not systematically used because of its cost and high radiation exposure.

22.2.1.3 When?

The timing at which stone-free status should be explored after PNL is also debatable. Many studies report the stone-free rate at 3 months, believing that during this period, most small fragments will pass. Others argue that in the case of PNL, all patients should undergo an immediate postoperative CT scan, before the nephrostomy is removed. This would allow selecting patients in whom a percutaneous second look would be beneficial.

22.2.2 The Operative Time

Operative time is also an ill-defined outcome variable. Many studies report it as the time between the first attempt to puncture the kidney and the suturing of the nephrostomy tube. However, this type of evaluation does not take into account the operative room occupation, which includes also patient positioning, endoscopic access to the bladder, and retrograde pyelography.

Table 22.2 Clavien classification of complications

Grade 1	All events that, if left untreated, would have a spontaneous resolution or need a simple bedside intervention
Grade 2	Complications requiring specific medications, including antibiotics and blood transfusions
Grade 3	Complications necessitating surgical, endoscopic, or radiologic intervention: 3a without general anesthesia 3b under general anesthesia
Grade 4	Neighboring organ injury and organ failures
Grade 5	Death

22.2.3 *The Morbidity*

Concerning complications, the modified Clavien classification seems to be worldwide accepted and increasingly used [15]. Although this classification demonstrates a high validity, it has been found somehow limited by its low inter-rater reliability for minor complications [16]. According to this classification system, perioperative complications are stratified into five grades (Table 22.2).

Standardization of all these criteria would be essential for a more accurate comparison of treatment modalities and outcomes. Unfortunately, at present, there is no consensus on how to report the results of PNL. Therefore, comparison of different series is able to provide only a limited level of evidence. Prospective randomized studies are also available, but only in limited number. Additionally, urologic papers never report clearly on other parameters such as intra- and postoperative anaesthesiological problems.

22.3 Comprehensive Review of Case Series

Two review articles identified a "trend in favour of better outcomes in the prone position over the supine position" [9] and recommend supine position only in "carefully selected patients" [10].

De la Rosette and collaborators conducted a Medline search for articles published during the 10-year period since the first report of supine PNL. Based on the hypothesis that supine position is more fit for physically compromised patients and complex calculi, this study focused on obese patients with a high proportion of staghorn calculi. The authors collected and analyzed 13 manuscripts, nine with supine [1, 3–5, 7, 8, 17–19] and four with prone position [20–23]. They concluded that outcomes in nonobese patients and with small-sized stones seem to favor the supine approach. To assess the outcomes in obese patients and with staghorn calculi, the authors calculated the weighted means for each position separately. This comparison showed a slightly better success rate (84.7 % vs. 81.2 %) and a significantly shorter operative time (79.1 min vs. 94.1 min) in prone position versus supine position respectively. However, a more recent study comparing prone and supine PNL in patients with a body mass index (BMI) >30 kg/m^2 did not confirm any difference in stone-free rates, rather demonstrating an advantage of the supine position in terms of significantly shorter operative time and hospital stay [24].

22.4 The Global Study of the Clinical Research Office of Endourologic Society (CROES)

The largest available observational prospective database was collected in the global study on PNL organized by the Clinical Research Office of Endourologic Society (CROES). Investigators of 96 centers worldwide contributed to the database. Each center was invited to include all consecutive patients during a 1-year period. Five thousand seven hundred and seventy-five patients were eligible for the study.

22.4.1 Patient Positioning

Four thousand six hundred and thirty-seven patients (80.3 %) had their PNL in prone position, whereas 1,138 patients were operated supine (19.7 %). The distribution of supine versus prone position exhibited major regional differences worldwide. While in Europe and South America, respectively, 23.5 % and 98.5 % of the patients were operated supine, patients in North America, Asia, and Australia were almost exclusively treated in prone position (98.5, 98.1, and 100 % of patients, respectively).

22.4.2 ASA Score

Concerning patient demographics, interestingly, an ASA score of 1 was more common among patients in the prone position (54.7 % vs. 46.8 %), whereas an ASA score of 2 was less frequent when compared to supine position (33.4 % vs. 42.1 %).

22.4.3 Renal Access and Tract Dilation

In the prone group, access through the upper pole and access above the 12th rib were more often employed (11.4 % vs. 4.0 % and 17.6 % vs. 5.5 %). Multiple punctures were also more frequent in the prone than in the supine group (9 % vs. 4.1 %). This may be explained by the possibility of a simultaneous ureteroscopy in supine position, offering retrograde access to the ureteropelvic junction or the upper calyces, making an upper pole puncture unnecessary. However, the report did not mention how many patients in the supine group had simultaneous retrograde ureterorenoscopy.

There was also a significant difference in the tract dilation method with the balloon, more frequently used in the supine positioned patients (43.8 % vs. 40.3 % $p = 0.04$).

22.4.4 Operative Time

The mean operative time was significantly shorter in the prone group with 82.7 min versus 90.1 min in the supine ($p < 0.001$). This is somehow unexpected, because one of the supposed advantages of supine position is the elimination of the necessity of patient repositioning after retrograde ureteric catheter insertion, which should shorten operative room occupation. A possible explanation is the dissimilar definition of "operative time" by different investigators. Analyzing the different publications deriving from the CROES database, the operative time is determined based on the sum of the different phases of surgery by some investigators [25], but others recorded the operative time as the time from the first puncture to the completion of the stone removal [26]. If some investigators in the global study used the second definition, this would mean that patient positioning (which should be shorter in supine) was not always taken into consideration during statistical analysis.

22.4.5 Stone-Free Rate

The stone-free rate at 1 month after the procedure was significantly higher in the prone group (77.0 % vs. 70.2 %). However, it remains possible that different factors other than the difference in patient positioning may have at least partly contributed to the better results in the prone group. In this latter group, a more radical treatment strategy could be observed, with more stones managed through multiple punctures. Furthermore, the role of a difference in the acquired experience with either approach cannot be excluded. For example, in high-volume centers performing both supine and prone PNL, the average number of patients treated in the prone position was 74, whereas only an average of 15 patients were treated supine during the 1-year period in the same centers. This suggests that more experience has been accumulated with prone position, which was therefore better standardized. The relative novelty and infrequent use of the supine position suggest that some centers were in their discovery or learning curve.

To eliminate this possible learning curve effect, a further analysis was performed on a subgroup of patients comparing stone-free rates in centers using only supine versus only prone position for PNL. Again, reported stone-free rates were statistically superior in the prone group when compared to supine, i.e., 76.9 % versus 63.3 %. But within this patient population, there was also a significant difference in the assessment modalities of the stone-free status. For example, in the supine group, 20.4 % of patients had a CT scan at 1 month opposed to only 12.7 % in the prone group. The proportion of missing data was only 3.9 % in the supine group but was 11.1 % in the prone group. This suggests that the stone-free rate may have been overestimated in the prone group and that data in this group might be less reliable.

22.4.6 Complications

On the other hand, there was a trend to a higher complication rate in the prone group. Transfusions were more often required (6.1 % vs. 4.3 %; $p=0.026$), and a slightly greater proportion of patients had complications classified as grade Clavien 2 or more (10.0 % vs. 7.2 %; $p=0.064$). One possible explanation for the increased rate of transfusions in prone patients is that this group underwent significantly more multiple punctures than supine patients.

22.5 Prospective Randomized Studies

There were only two randomized prospective studies comparing the outcomes of prone versus supine PNL [3, 27].

Falahatkar compared 40 supine versus 40 prone PNL [27]. The two groups had similar body habitus and stone volume. However, postoperative evaluation was done exclusively with KUB with a relatively tolerant definition of stone-free status, which included also the presence of fragments smaller than 5 mm. But their results can be considered as valid, because the same evaluation method and criteria were used for both groups. Stone-free rate was 80 and 77.5 % in prone and supine position, respectively. The only significant difference was the operative time, favoring the supine approach. Mean operative time in the supine group was 74.7 ± 25.1 min compared to 106.87 ± 17.5 min in the prone group, with a statistically significant difference ($p<0.0001$). It is important to underline that operative time was defined as the procedure beginning with cystoscopy and ureteral catheterization and finishing with final wound closure at the nephrostomy tract site.

De Sio conducted a prospective randomized study with 39 patients operated in supine position and 36 patients in prone position [3]. No significant differences were observed between the two groups in terms of stone-free rate, blood loss, and hospital stay. The only significant difference established was the mean operative time, which was 43 min in the supine group and 68 min in the prone group ($p<0.001$). However, the main limitation of this study is the exclusion of stones in more than one calyx, complete staghorn stones, and BMI >30 kg/m^2.

22.6 Conclusions

There is still much controversy in the literature concerning the optimal approach for PNL. While the CROES study should probably dampen the enthusiasm of pro-supine endourologists, the available randomized studies did not find any difference in the stone-free rate, but operative time was significantly shorter.

Which is the bottom line? Prone position remains predominant on a global level; the acquired experience is still superior when compared to supine position. The CROES global study suggests that urologists worldwide still perform more and feel more comfortable with the classical prone PNL. This is at least partly explained by more training opportunities with prone position. However, prone position is no more the exclusive way to perform a PNL, and supine position is increasingly used. It is now quite consensual that the latter allows an easier management from the anaesthesiological point of view and may reduce patient morbidity. The available randomized studies demonstrate that in centers which already standardized the supine technique, this procedure may be more ergonomic and quicker and equally efficient in terms of stone clearance and morbidity.

References

1. Valdivia Uría JG, Valle Gerhold J, Lopez Lopez JA et al (1998) Technique and complications of percutaneous nephroscopy: experience with 557 patients in the supine position. J Urol 160:1975–1978
2. Ibarluzea G, Scoffone CM, Cracco CM et al (2007) Supine Valdivia and modified lithotomy position for simultaneous anterograde and retrograde endourological access. BJU Int 100:233–236
3. De Sio M, Autorino R, Quarto G et al (2008) Modified supine versus prone position in percutaneous nephrolithotomy for renal stones treatable with a single percutaneous access: a prospective randomized trial. Eur Urol 54:196–202
4. Manohar T, Jain P, Desai M (2007) Supine percutaneous nephrolithotomy: effective approach to high-risk and morbidly obese patients. J Endourol 21:44–49
5. Ng MT, Sun WH, Cheng CW, Chan ES (2004) Supine position is safe and effective for percutaneous nephrolithotomy. J Endourol 18:469–474
6. Scoffone CM, Cracco CM, Cossu M et al (2008) Endoscopic combined intrarenal surgery in Galdakao-modified supine Valdivia position: a new standard for percutaneous nephrolithotomy? Eur Urol 54(6):1393–1403
7. Shoma AM, Eraky I, El-Kenawy MR, El-Kappany HA (2002) Percutaneous nephrolithotomy in the supine position: technical aspects and functional outcome compared with the prone technique. Urology 60:388–392
8. Steele D, Marshall V (2007) Percutaneous nephrolithotomy in the supine position: a neglected approach? J Endourol 21:1433–1437
9. de la Rosette JJ, Tsakiris P, Ferrandino MN et al (2008) Beyond prone position in percutaneous nephrolithotomy: a comprehensive review. Eur Urol 54:1262–1269
10. Basiri A, Mohammadi Sichani M (2009) Supine percutaneous nephrolithotomy, is it really effective? A systematic review of literature. Urol J 6:73–77
11. Thomas K, Smith NC, Hegarty N, Glass JM (2011) The Guy's stone score – grading the complexity of percutaneous nephrolithotomy procedures. Urology 78:277–281

12. Hyams ES, Bruhn A, Lipkin M, Shah O (2010) Heterogeneity in the reporting of disease characteristics and treatment outcomes in studies evaluating treatments for nephrolithiasis. J Endourol 24:1411–1414
13. Deters LA, Jumper CM, Steinberg PL, Pais VM (2011) Evaluating the definition of "stone free status" in contemporary urologic literature. Clin Nephrol 76:354–357
14. Denstedt JD, Clayman RV, Picus DD (1991) Comparison of endoscopic and radiological residual fragment rate following percutaneous nephrolithotripsy. J Urol 145:703–705
15. Tefekli A, Ali Karadag M, Tepeler K et al (2008) Classification of percutaneous nephrolithotomy complications using the modified Clavien grading system: looking for a standard. Eur Urol 53:184–190
16. de la Rosette JJ, Opondo D, Daels FP et al (2012) Categorisation of complications and validation of the Clavien score for percutaneous nephrolithotomy. Eur Urol 62:246–255
17. Neto EA, Mitre AI, Gomes CM et al (2007) Percutaneous nephrolithotripsy with the patient in a modified supine position. J Urol 178:165–168
18. Zhou X, Gao X, Wen J, Xiao C (2008) Clinical value of minimally invasive percutaneous nephrolithotomy in the supine position under the guidance of real-time ultrasound: report of 92 cases. Urol Res 36:111–114
19. Rana AM, Bhojwani JP, Junejo NN, Das Bhagia S (2008) Tubeless PCNL with patient in supine position: procedure for all seasons? – with comprehensive technique. Urology 71:581–585
20. Sergeyev I, Koi PT, Jacobs SL et al (2007) Outcome of percutaneous surgery stratified according to body mass index and kidney stone size. Surg Laparosc Endosc Percutan Tech 17:179–183
21. Koo BC, Burtt G, Burgess NA (2004) Percutaneous stone surgery in the obese: outcome stratified according to body mass index. BJU Int 93:1296–1299
22. El-Assmy AM, Shokeir AA, El-Nahas AR et al (2007) Outcome of percutaneous nephrolithotomy: effect of body mass index. Eur Urol 52:199–204
23. Pearle MS, Nakada SY, Womack JS, Kryger JV (1998) Outcomes of contemporary percutaneous nephrostolithotomy in morbidly obese patients. J Urol 160:669–673
24. Mazzucchi E, Vicenitni FC, Marchini GS et al (2012) Percutaneous nephrolithotomy in obese patients: comparison between the prone and total supine position. J Endourol 26:1437–1442
25. Valdivia JG, Scarpa RM, Duvdevani M et al (2011) Supine versus prone position during percutaneous nephrolithotomy: a report from the clinical research office of the endourological society percutaneous nephrolithotomy global study. J Endourol 25:1619–1625
26. Yamaguchi A, Skolarikos A, Buchholz NP et al (2011) Operating times and bleeding complications in percutaneous nephrolithotomy: a comparison of tract dilation methods in 5,537 patients in the Clinical Research Office of the Endourological Society Percutaneous Nephrolithotomy Global Study. J Endourol 25:933–939
27. Falahatkar S, Maghaddam AA, Salehi M et al (2008) Complete supine percutaneous nephrolithotripsy comparison with the prone standard technique. J Endourol 22:2513–2517

Further Reading

Kumar P, Bach C, Kachrilas S et al (2012) Supine percutaneous nephrolithotomy (PCNL): "in vogue" but in which position? BJU Int 110:E1018–E1021

Duty B, Okhunov Z, Smith A, Okeke Z (2011) The debate over percutaneous nephrolithotomy positioning: a comprehensive review. J Urol 186:20–25

Lardon R, Lacroix B, Lorin S, Mottet N (2012) Prone and supine position for percutaneous nephrolithotomy: is it necessary to change the operative technique? Prog Urol 22:154–158

Wu P, Wang L, Wang K (2011) Supine versus prone position in percutaneous nephrolithotomy for kidney calculi: a meta-analysis. Int Urol Nephrol 43:67–77

Chapter 23
Micro-ECIRS: A Revolutionary New Tool in the Current Endourologic Armamentarium

Cesare Marco Scoffone and Cecilia Maria Cracco

Abstract The present chapter deals with an innovative application of ECIRS, integrated with the recently introduced Microperc technique. Micro-ECIRS is intended as technical refinement of the Microperc technique, solving a variety of recognized limitations of this approach. The idea of combining retrograde flexible ureteroscopy (with or without ureteral access sheath) with Microperc allows Endovision puncture and tract dilation of the chosen calyx, optimal vision due to retrograde illumination and irrigation, maintenance of low intrarenal pressures, sand elimination and fragments extraction. Micro-ECIRS indications are defined, although further large-scale studies are warranted.

23.1 Microperc: An Innovation in the Landscape of Percutaneous Surgery Based on a Brilliant Rationale

The progressive miniaturization of the percutaneous procedure for the treatment of kidney stones started years ago with the proposal of the midi- and mini-PNL [1, 2] and of the MIP (minimally invasive percutaneous nephrolithotomy) [3]. Micropercutaneous nephrolithotomy (Microperc) technique, together with UMP (Ultra-Mini-Perc), is the last born of such family of mini-invasive percutaneous approaches (Fig. 23.1).

Since most of the complications (29–83 % in the literature) of percutaneous surgery are related to renal access and tract dilation, especially bleeding up to 45 % [4],

---

C.M. Scoffone, MD (✉) • C.M. Cracco, MD, PhD
Department of Urology, Cottolengo Hospital, Via Cottolengo 9, 10152 Torino, Italy
e-mail: scoof@libero.it; cecilia.cracco@libero.it

C.M. Scoffone et al. (eds.), *Supine Percutaneous Nephrolithotomy and ECIRS*,
DOI 10.1007/978-2-8178-0459-0_23, © Springer-Verlag France 2014

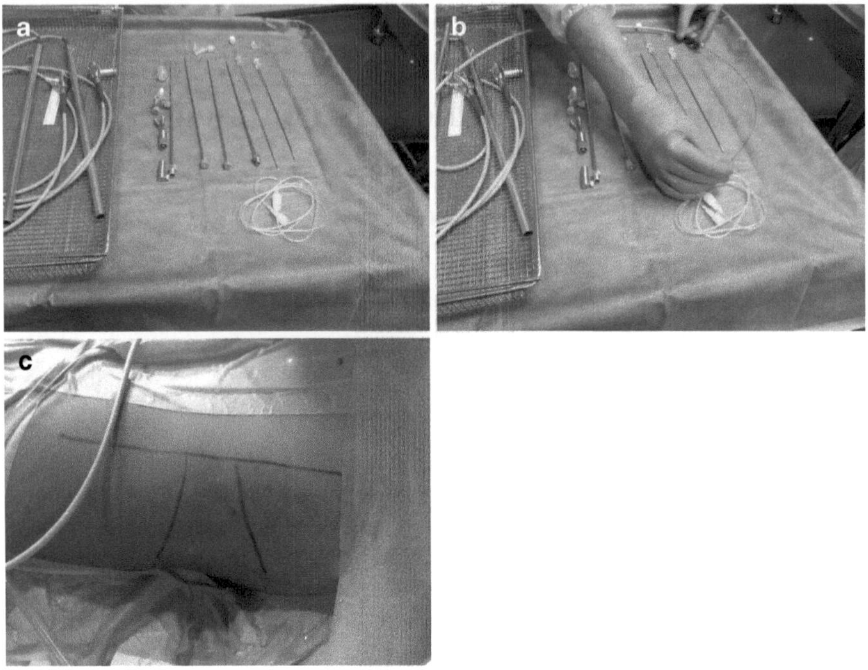

Fig. 23.1 Microperc set with the all-seeing needle (**a**) and flexible micro-optics (**b**) with the final vision of the percutaneous access after the needle removal (**c**)

the reduced size and the one-step creation of the tract without dilation are likely to be a step forward for the safety of the patient. Besides reducing invasiveness and associated morbidity of PNL, Microperc also overcomes the main limitations of the other currently available therapeutic approaches to renal stone disease, i.e. the unpredictable results of ESWL and the recurring costs and the risk of infectious complications of RIRS [5].

The first 15 Micropercs were published in 2011, using a 4.85F (1.6 mm) three-part all-seeing needle, inspired to the laparoscopic Veress needle. This modified and irrigated needle (Fig. 23.1a) has a working sheath, in which a micro-optical system 0.9 mm in diameter with a 120° angle of view and a 10,000 pixels resolution as well as a 200 μm holmium:yttrium-aluminium-garnet laser fibre can be inserted. The optical fibre is highly flexible (Fig. 23.1b) and connected via a zoom ocular and a light adapter to a standard endoscopic camera system, with a Xenon light source of at least 100 W [6]. The all-seeing needle (PolyDiagnost, Pfaffenhofen, Germany) is aided by a surgeon-controlled pressurized irrigation system for vision improvement and stone debris removal, and exploits a variety of disposable devices, like the three-way connector (for optics, laser fibre and irrigation system attached to the outer tip of the shaft) or the multi-jointed mounting arm for the optics. The absence of an Amplatz sheath is one of the possible disadvantages of Microperc [7]; thus, a 6.6F Amplatz sheath has been proposed [8].

23.2 Microperc and the Limitation of the Reduced Quality and Field of Vision

The necessity to employ a thin optics containing few fibres implies the generation of less light, thus a reduced illumination with a reduced image resolution of the working field. Additionally, the rigid optics has a limited field of vision, with no possibility to follow a mobile stone or escaped fragments during lithotripsy and no possibility to check all the calyces for residual fragments at the end of the procedure.

23.3 Microperc and the Limitation of the "Break and Leave" Principle

Microperc is based on the principle of "break and leave", similarly to some RIRS and all ESWL. The lack of stone extraction after lithotripsy might be considered as a limitation factor, may cause renal colics postoperatively and also produce lower clearance rates [9]. Some urologists also succeeded in retrieving stone fragments for analysis using a basket catheter through the 8F microsheath [10].

23.4 Microperc and the Limitation of the High Renal Pelvic Pressures

If lithotripsy is carried out using a 200 μm laser fibre with adequate energy and frequency settings until complete disintegration of the stone, the issue of high renal pelvic pressures (RPP) for a prolonged time interval becomes relevant. From this point of view, Microperc suffers of the limitations of RIRS, working with a mean RPP of 33 mmHg and developing peaks as high as 170–328 mmHg [11].

Normal RPP is 5–15 mmHg, a 30–40 mmHg RPP for more than 10 min causes intrarenal reflux (pyelovenous, pyelolymphatic/pyelotubular, pyelointerstitial) with potential harmful consequences and forniceal damage takes place with 80–100 mmHg RPP [12]. Cadaveric studies revealed that with a 12/14F ureteral access sheath, even with high irrigation pressures, RPP remains within acceptable values [13]. On patients these data were also confirmed [14].

RPP generally remains low during PNL, if no mistakes like Amplatz malpositioning or anatomical problems like narrow infundibula occur [15]. During Microperc the irrigation system creates 50 mmHg RPP with a flow rate of 16 ml/min, and 100 mmHg RPP with 23 ml/min using saline when the optics is within the needle [6]. The question is whether this situation poses Microperc at increased risk of complications, especially in children [16].

23.5 Solving All Microperc Limitations: Micro-ECIRS

To our knowledge here, we report the first technical description of micro-ECIRS, a feasible and safe modification of the well-known one-step Microperc technique [17]. The idea of combining retrograde flexible ureteroscopy (with or without ureteral access sheath) with Microperc, with the patient in the Galdakao-modified supine Valdivia position (Fig. 23.2), is a proposal intended to solve most limitations of Microperc, also providing further advantages:

- The morphology of the collecting system can be preliminarily examined, integrating the preoperative data from CT scans.
- Stone features (mainly position, size, hardness) can be ascertained at the beginning of the procedure for an optimal strategic planning.
- The best calyx to puncture can be chosen in real time, also examining its dynamic features with irrigation.
- Access to the renal collecting system is achieved under fluoroscopic and Endovision control (Fig. 23.3) after preliminary ultrasound for controlling adjacent viscera and for identifying the correct inclination of the needle for the single access, avoiding as much as possible bleeding and multiple puncturing attempts.
- Migration of the stone into the ureter during initial irrigation or subsequent fragmentation is hindered.
- Vision during lithotripsy is improved because of the retrograde illumination of the operating field (Fig. 23.4).
- Vision during lithotripsy is also improved by the retrograde irrigation via the flexible ureteroscope.
- Whether better vision reduces operating time remains to be determined [10].
- Intrarenal pressures are concomitantly maintained low in presence of the ureteral access sheath, thus reducing resorption and uroseptic risk.

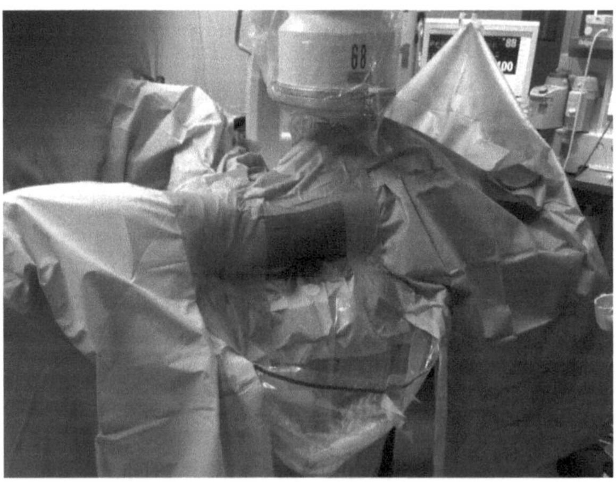

Fig. 23.2 Patient in the Galdakao-modified supine Valdivia position ready for micro-ECIRS

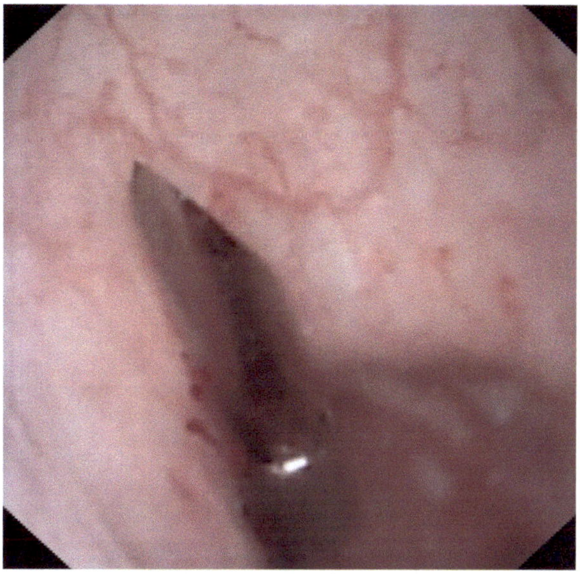

Fig. 23.3 Endovision application of the all-seeing needle

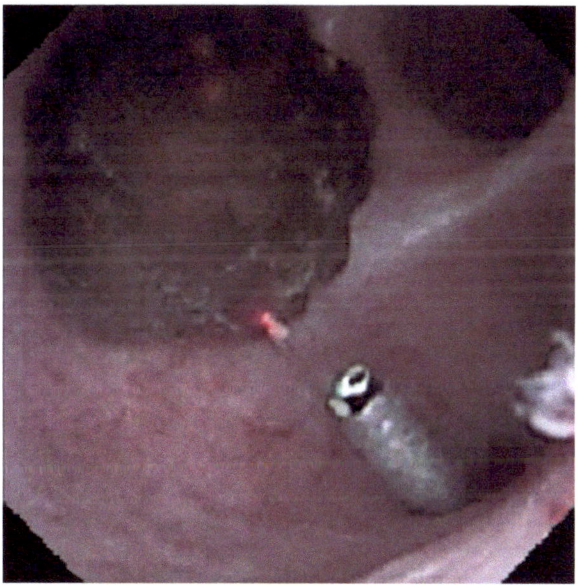

Fig. 23.4 The all-seeing needle with micro-optics and laser fibre inserted (retrograde flexible vision)

- Thanks to the ureteral access sheath, sand from lithotripsy can be washed out retrogradely (Fig. 23.5).
- At the end of the procedure, major stone fragments can be extracted using a retrogradely inserted basket (Fig. 23.6) and the needle extracted under Endovision control (Fig. 23.7).

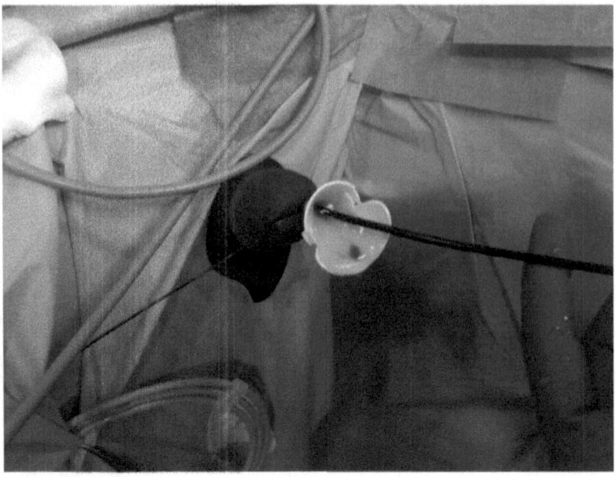

Fig. 23.5 Sand washed down the ureteral access sheath during fragmentation

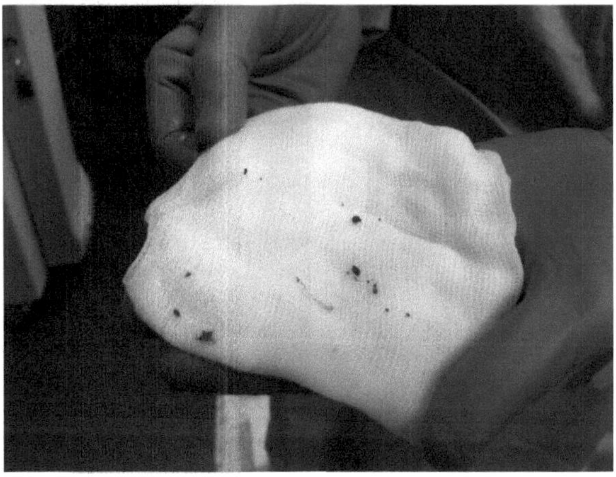

Fig. 23.6 Stone fragments extracted retrogradely using a basket

- At the end of the procedure all calyces can also be explored, in order to exclude migrated or residual stone fragments.
- Both Microperc and micro-ECIRS offer the possibility to avoid prolonged laser lithotripsies in lower calyces/infundibula, maintaining the flexible ureteroscope in constant deflection with the laser fibre inside, thus reducing the risk of rupture of those delicate instruments and reducing costs. In fact, the cost of the disposable Microperc device is very reduced, in comparison to the expenses for a broken flexible analogic or digital ureteroscope, thus more cost-effective (life expectancy of a flexible ureteroscope = 5–14 cases) [17].

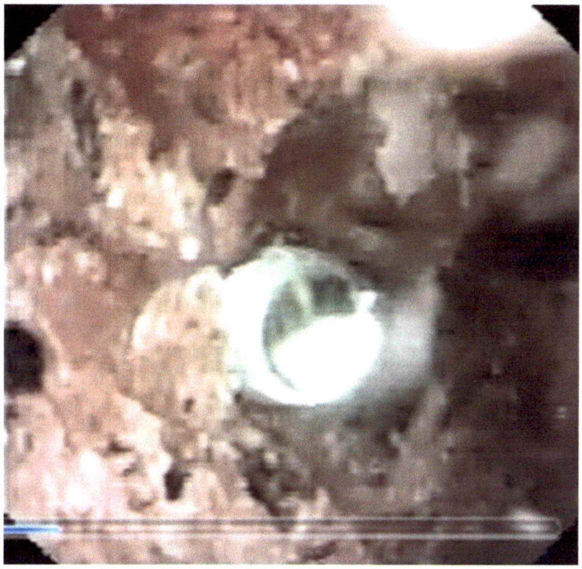

Fig. 23.7 Endovision extraction of the needle at the end of the procedure

23.6 Defining the Selected Indications for Micro-ECIRS

- First-line treatment modality for medium-sized stones, between 1 and 2 cm in diameter, thus also suitable to RIRS, but with unfavourable features such as hard stones and/or stones impacted within a narrow infundibulum or a lower calyx with a narrow and long infundibulum.
- Paediatric patients [17–19].
- Stones in calyceal diverticula.
- Second accesses during a standard PNL, in order to reach calyces parallel to the main percutaneous tract.

23.7 Conclusions

Micro-ECIRS intended as technical refinement of the Microperc technique can be proposed as endpoint percutaneous nephrolithotomy technologies for the next future. Of course efficacy and safety studies are warranted, as well as an evaluation of the cost-effectiveness of such approaches, comparing it to that of RIRS. Comparison of Microperc and micro-ECIRS should also be carried out considering stone-free rates, need of conversion to mini- or midi-PNL and complication rates (especially bleeding and urosepsis).

References

1. Jackman SV, Docimo SG, Cadeddu JA et al (1998) The “mini-perc” technique: a less invasive alternative to percutaneous nephrolithotomy. World J Urol 16:371–374
2. Knoll T, Wezel F, Michel MS et al (2010) Do patients benefit from miniaturized tubeless percutaneous nephrolithotomy? A comparative prospective study. J Endourol 24:1075–1079
3. Abdelhafez MF, Amend B, Bedke J et al (2013) Minimally invasive percutaneous nephrolithotomy: a comparative study of the management of small and large renal stones. Urology 81:241–245
4. Seitz C, Desai M, Haecker A et al (2012) Incidence, prevention and management of complications following percutaneous nephrolitholapaxy. Eur Urol 61:146–158
5. Desai M, Mishra S (2012) “Microperc” micropercutaneous nephrolithotomy: evidence to practice. Curr Opin Urol 22:134–138
6. Bader MJ, Gratzke C, Seitz M et al (2011) The “all-seeing needle”: initial results of an optical puncture system confirming access in percutaneous nephrolithotomy. Eur Urol 59:1054–1059
7. Desai M (2013) Editorial comment on END-2012-0737-TE.R2. J Endourol 27:839
8. Penbegul N, Bodakci MN, Hatipoglu NK et al (2013) Microsheath for microperc: 14 gauge angiocath. J Endourol 27:835–839
9. Tepeler A, Armagan A, Sancaktutar AA et al (2013) The role of microperc in the treatment of symptomatic lower pole renal calculi. J Endourol 27:13–18
10. Armagan A, Tepeler A, Silay MS et al (2013) Micropercutaneous nephrolithotomy in the treatment of moderate-size renal calculi. J Endourol 27:177–181
11. Jung H, Norby B, Frimodt-Moller PC, Osther PJ (2008) Endoluminal isoproterenol irrigation decreases renal pelvic pressure during flexible ureterorenoscopy: a clinical randomized, controlled study. Eur Urol 54:1404–1413
12. Negrete-Pulido O, Gutierrez-Aceves J (2009) Management of infectious complications in percutaneous nephrolithotomy. J Endourol 23:1757–1762
13. Rehman J, Monga M, Landman J et al (2003) Characterization of intrapelvic pressure during ureteropyeloscopy with ureteral access sheaths. Urology 61:713–718
14. Auge BK, Pietrow PK, Lallas CD et al (2004) Ureteral access sheath provides protection against elevated renal pressures during routine flexible ureteroscopic stone manipulation. J Endourol 18:33–36
15. Troxel SA, Low RK (2002) Renal intrapelvic pressure during percutaneous nephrolithotomy and its correlation with the development of postoperative fever. J Urol 168:1348–1351
16. Piskin MM, Guven S, Kilinc M et al (2012) Preliminary, favourable experience with microperc in kidney and bladder stones. J Endourol 26:1443–1447
17. Desai MR, Sharma R, Mishra S et al (2011) Single step percutaneous nephrolithotomy (microperc): the initial clinical report. J Urol 186:140–145
18. Resorlu B, Unsal A, Tepeler A et al (2012) Comparison of retrograde intrarenal surgery and mini-percutaneous nephrolithotomy in children with moderate-size kidney stones: results of a multi-institutional study. Urology 80:519–523
19. Kaynar M, Suemer A, Salvarci A et al (2013) Micropercutaneous nephrolithotomy (microperc) in a two-year-old with the “all-seeing needle”. Urol Int 91:239–241

Chapter 24
Conclusions and Future Perspectives of PNL

András Hoznek, Cecilia Maria Cracco, and Cesare Marco Scoffone

During the last decade, endourology underwent a profound and substantial transformation.

Extracorporeal shockwave lithotripsy lost its predominant role in the management of most stones because of the relative unpredictability of its results.

Few years ago flexible instruments were considered a luxury, but now they are an integral part of the endourologic daily routine. More specifically, flexible ureteroscopy is increasingly used for the treatment of kidney stones even bigger than two centimeters, which represented traditional indications to percutaneous treatment in a near past. The use of new-generation, smaller flexible ureteroscopes considerably reduces the morbidity related to the ureteral access to the upper urinary tract. Additionally, digital ureteroscopes offer an amazing visual quality.

The success of flexible ureterorenoscopy is mainly due to its reputation of having the lowest morbidity with the highest efficacy, while PNL is considered as a procedure with a long learning curve and significant complication rates.

However, concomitantly many improvements affected PNL as well. The modification of patient positioning from prone to supine is part of this evolution. This innovation resulted in a more time-efficient procedure and also opened the era of Endoscopic Combined IntraRenal Surgery (ECIRS). Although most urologists were trained for prone position and still feel more comfortable with the classical method, this positioning has nowadays lost its hegemonic role worldwide. Progressively, a growing number of urologist switched to supine, while many others practice both and choose the technique according to the case or personal preference.

A. Hoznek, MD (✉)
Department of Urology, CHU Henri Mondor, 51. Av. du Ml. de Lattre de Tassigny, 94010 Créteil Cedex, France
e-mail: andras.hoznek@gmail.com

C.M. Cracco, MD, PhD • C.M. Scoffone, MD
Department of Urology, Cottolengo Hospital, Via Cottolengo 9, 10152 Torino, Italy
e-mail: cecilia.cracco@libero.it; scoof@libero.it

C.M. Scoffone et al. (eds.), *Supine Percutaneous Nephrolithotomy and ECIRS*,
DOI 10.1007/978-2-8178-0459-0_24, © Springer-Verlag France 2014

Definitely, supine PNL is here to stay, and this technique represents a major contribution to modern endourology.

But patient positioning is only one aspect of PNL. ECIRS proposal triggered very lively discussions about each PNL step, reconsidered in this new position. Thus, even for those who are not convinced about this alternative positioning and its relevant anesthesiological advantages, it has been a good chance to think over, maximally standardize, and even improve all the steps of the percutaneous procedure, carefully analyzing the clinical results in terms of safety and efficacy. For ECIRS supporters this is a success in any case because the keywords of this procedure are "mental intraoperative versatility" and "meticulous technical standardization."

Presently, as to renal access creation (the crucial step of PNL), we have a better understanding of how to optimize it and of the related renal trauma. Until few years ago renal puncture was highly dependent upon urologist's experience and "feeling," while now the big difference consists in the fact that we can plan in advance the needle's path and then reproduce our planning, knowing exactly the target of our puncture. This allows to make this step reproducible and easy to teach/easy to learn. ECIRS further contributed to the optimization of the renal puncture introducing the possibility of the retrograde flexible ureteropic assistance.

There is now increasing evidence that morbidity (blood loss, postoperative discomfort, and urine leakage) is proportional to the access size. As in most fields of endourology, miniaturization attracts more and more attention of the urologic community concerning PNL as well. We now know that mini-PNL does not only consist in the use of smaller-size instruments and accessories but also facilitates the elimination of fragments due to the vacuum-cleaner effect. In many urologic departments in Europe, standard PNL has been abandoned and only mini-PNL is performed. The role of Ultra-Mini-Perc and Microperc has still to be determined. Any of these mini-invasive approaches can be easily employed during ECIRS.

Another promising innovation is the tubeless technique. Diminishing the period of time during which the kidney and/or ureter is drained has the potential to improve patient comfort postoperatively and reduce hospital stay. The remaining task is to determine objectively which kind of patients may concretely benefit from this technique without any risk in terms of bleeding, urinary extravasation, or obstruction. Again, mini-PNL has the potential of increasing the proportion of the patients which could be included in a tubeless protocol.

Lastly, the next step will be the modernization of our puncture technique. Outcomes of PNL highly depend on the precision, refinement, and accuracy of this step. Image guidance, augmented reality, fusion of different imaging modalities, motion tracking systems, and robotics are rapidly evolving and strongly coming to the attention of the urologic community.

Optimal patient positioning; computer-assisted, image-guided, or robotic puncture; Endoscopic Combined IntraRenal Surgery; miniaturization; and standardized exit strategies will synergistically contribute to give birth to the percutaneous technique of tomorrow.

MIX
Papier aus verantwortungsvollen Quellen
Paper from responsible sources
FSC® C105338

If you have any concerns about our products,
you can contact us on
ProductSafety@springernature.com

In case Publisher is established outside the EU,
the EU authorized representative is:
Springer Nature Customer Service Center GmbH
Europaplatz 3, 69115 Heidelberg, Germany

Printed by Libri Plureos GmbH
in Hamburg, Germany